Evoked Potential Audiometry

Evoked Potential Audiometry

Fundamentals and Applications

Robert Goldstein
Professor Emeritus, University of Wisconsin-Madison

William M. Aldrich
Private Consultant
Orange, California

Allyn and Bacon
Boston • London • Toronto • Sydney • Tokyo • Singapore

Executive Editor: Stephen D. Dragin
Editorial Assistant: Elizabeth McGuire
Editorial-Production Administrator: Joe Sweeney
Editorial-Production Service: Walsh & Associates, Inc.
Composition Buyer: Linda Cox
Manufacturing Buyer: Dave Repetto
Cover Administrator: Jennifer Hart

Internet: www.abacon.com

Library of Congress Cataloging-in-Publication Data

Goldstein, Robert, 1924–
    Evoked potential audiometry : fundamentals and applications /
Robert Goldstein and William M. Aldrich.
       p.   cm.
    Includes bibliographical references and index.
    ISBN 0-13-299603-0
    1. Auditory evoked response.   2. Audiometry, Evoked response.
3. Speech disorders.   I. Aldrich, William M., 1941– . II. Title.
    [DNLM: 1. Evoked Potentials, Auditory—physiology.   2. Audiometry,
Evoked Response—methods.   WV 270 G625e 1998]
RF294.5.E87G64   1998
617.8′07547—dc21
DNLM/DLC
  for Library of Congress
                                             98-23831
                                               CIP

Printed in the United States of America

10 9 8 7 6 5 4 3 2 1   02 01 00 99 98

Contents

Preface

Authors naturally want many readers for their books. However, authors who try to cater simultaneously to the fullest spectrum of readers usually end up with books that are too disorganized and diffuse to satisfy any of their intended readers. We have targeted two primary groups of readers. The first group is graduate students in audiology and speech/language pathology who are familiar with fundamentals of audiologic evaluation accomplished by behavioral-response, acoustic-immittance, and otoacoustic-emission procedures. Persons in the second main target group are practicing audiologists and other clinicians who wish to revive or expand their knowledge of evoked potential audiometry (EPA).

We have not ignored potential readers outside the two main target groups. University instructors who teach beginning students in audiology and speech/language pathology will find material in the book that can be adapted easily for introductory courses for less advanced students. Our book assumes little prior knowledge of auditory electrophysiology. The book also contains some material for students and clinicians at the other end of the experience spectrum who want to extend themselves beyond the fundamentals of EPA.

Use of averaged auditory averaged evoked potentials (AEPs) in clinical service or for research is not restricted to audiologists. Speech/language pathologists and researchers in normal hearing, language, and speech already have contributed to the understanding of auditory AEPs and their use in EPA. Similarly, clinicians and researchers in other fields (e.g., neurologists, psychologists) use auditory AEPs as well as AEPs in other modalities in their work. We believe that these people and others outside the targeted groups will find material of interest and value in our book.

The book is not a treatise. Nevertheless, its scope is wide enough to acquaint graduate students with most of the technicalities and procedures that confront them in their first job and to provide them with sufficient bases for on-the-job learning. However, the book does include some approaches to EPA that are not commonly used but should, and probably will, be used more frequently in the future.

Basic or *fundamental* does not mean *short* or *brief*. It takes more words to impart understanding about basics to novices than it does to explain advanced concepts and procedures to experienced professionals. Some students and professionals may be insulted by how far we back up in laying the technical foundations for EPA. We risk the unintentional slur on their background because in our teaching experience we encountered too many students with weak technical background despite evidence from their academic transcripts that they did take appropriate background courses. We know, too, that practicing clinicians do not have enough time to review the fundamentals that they once knew. Our backing up will aid them in restoring their previous background knowledge.

Completely logical sequencing of topics acceptable to everyone is impossible. What is presented in early chapters cannot be fully understood without knowledge of what is in later chapters. Everything has to come first. Given this impossibility, we summarized in the first chapter what will be covered in the remaining chapters. This overview will give readers some idea of the relevance of the subsequent, more technical chapters. In addition, we backtracked in several chapters to repeat some of the same material in different contexts.

Three sequencing issues were particularly difficult to resolve. (1) Should major clinical applications of various components of averaged evoked potentials (AEPs) follow immediately after the initial description of each of the components or should applications be discussed separately after the AEP components had been described? We took the latter approach with the belief that major clinical applications would be understood better if the reader could see how any or all of the components might be used in a particular application. Some insight is given during the description of the individual components about how the component being described can be used clinically. (2) AEP components are defined in this book along time dimensions: early, middle, and late. Wouldn't it be logical, therefore, to describe cochlear potentials (cochlear microphonic, summating potential, and action potential) first? We chose to place the peripheral potentials later because the emphasis of the book is on brain potentials; the potentials discussed in Chapter 13 (Electrocochleography) come from the ear. Much of the material in Chapters 5 through 8 can serve as background for electrocochleography; less of what is discussed in Chapter 13 can be extrapolated to Chapters 5 through 8. Also, the major application of electrocochleography is in otologic diagnosis; therefore, placing it next to the chapter on otoneurologic diagnosis (Chapter 12) seemed appropriate. (3) The material in Chapter 16, the last chapter, provides a basis for understanding AEPs and their clinical applications. Why, then, is it not the first chapter after the summary overview? Our teaching experience convinces us that the material in the chapter cannot be understood well or appreciated without fuller understanding of how AEPs are elicited, recorded, and applied. More experienced readers may benefit by reading Chapter 16 first and then going back to Chapter 2. Less experienced readers can, and probably should, reread Chapters 2 through 15 after reading Chapter 16.

Books on EPA, and on other topics as well, often begin with a full historic account. Unfortunately, novices in EPA do not have enough vocabulary in this area to absorb the details of the history at the beginning of a book. In addition, some readers have difficulty appreciating the impact of history on procedures about which they know little. We opted against a separate history chapter. Instead, in most chapters, we present a brief historic background to the chapter's topic.

Applications of auditory averaged evoked potentials (AEP) are broad, and the breadth of their applications is increasing. Auditory AEPs are used in such things as intraoperative monitoring and assessment of psychiatric disorders. Visual and somatosensory AEPs also have broad clinical applications. This introductory book only touches on these broader applications. Nevertheless, the principles underlying the basic clinical applications of auditory AEPs that are stressed can be extrapolated to other applications and to other modalities. We know, too, that writings become obsolete before the ink is dry on the page. Nevertheless, we believe that most of the generalities and concepts that we present will last beyond technical advance or technical obsolescence.

As we wrote, we wrestled with two closely related presentation problems that were resolved with difficulty and apprehension: (1) documentation (or lack of it) versus readability, and (2) popular procedures and concepts versus more valid procedures and unproven but promising directions for the future. Critical, experienced readers want published references for authors' claims. Novice readers, on the other hand, are distracted by lines of authors and dates that break the flow of what they are reading. We opted for less rather than more. We did not reference everything that is generally accepted. In most instances we gave just a sampling of helpful references. Often, we chose some of the oldest applicable references, mainly to give a historic basis for the topic. Omissions from the samples in no way denigrates the relevance or importance of the omitted references. We resolved the second issue by putting less stress on what is popular and more stress on what we believe to be more valid and of greater future value.

Purchasers of any book should know that they buy the packager along with the package. Similarly, writers should realize that they sell themselves along with their product. This awesome realization had an immense sobering effect as we wrote. Despite the trepidation it induced, we decided that when it was essential we would inject ideas (*biases* may be more accurate) derived from our years of varied, extensive experience in the classroom, library, research laboratory and, especially, the clinic. In other words, we weighted our own preferences more heavily when our views differed from more conventional views on the same clinical question.

We describe the preferences just mentioned but cannot provide illustrative examples to buttress all of the preferences and recommendations. EPA, like other clinical procedures, evolves and changes. Readers can find chronicles of changes, and of proposed changes, in the periodic literature. Book authors, on the other hand, generally look back as they attempt to consolidate views of the field. Authors must pick some cut-off point in time to begin. Otherwise, books would never be written. This time constraint, unfortunately, prevents us from providing graphic substantiation of everything that we recommend to clinicians. We would, if we could, redo some illustrations to be certain that recommendations and figures agreed with no exception. At some point, however, we are forced to say in certain instances, "Do as we say, not as we did."

Prior to 1935, several different composers had written well-liked variations on Paganini's 24th violin caprice. When Rachmaninoff's *Rhapsody on a Theme of Paganini* was premiered in 1935, music lovers and critics said, "Oh, no. Not another one!" Nevertheless, without hurting the acceptance of previous versions, the Rachmaninoff *Rhapsody* became a standard concert piece. Others have written good books on evoked potential audiometry. In fact, we used those books as resources for some of our material. Why do we presume to offer another version? We believe that our version differs sufficiently from others to be considered usable by many without diminishing the value of other versions. We trust that readers will agree.

Many colleagues contributed in various ways to development of this book, more than we can acknowledge in our limited space. We would be remiss, however, if we did not single out Kathryn A. Barrett, PhD, and her students at the University of North Carolina-Greensboro, for providing us many original traces of averaged evoked potentials that we could not generate ourselves. Her material appears in Figures 1-3, 1-6, 3-6, 5-1, 5-2, 5-4, 6-1, 6-5, 8-1, 8-2, 8-3, and 12-1.

We also thank the reviewers of the manuscript for this book for their time and valuable input: Craig A. Champlin, The University of Texas at Austin; and T. Newell Decker, University of Nebraska–Lincoln.

Part *I*

Overview

1

Overview of Evoked-Potential Audiometry (EPA)

Electrophysiologic Audiometry

Audiometry implies measurement of hearing. However, no form of audiometry measures directly what the patient hears. In some audiometric procedures, the clinician presents an acoustic signal, looks for some reaction to that signal, and then *infers* what the patient hears. The reaction can be an involuntary overt change (e.g., the Moro reflex in a neonate), a voluntary overt response (e.g., raising a finger), a biophysical reaction (e.g., contraction of the stapedius muscle resulting in a change of acoustic impedance at the tympanic membrane), an acoustic signal coming from the ear (e.g., transient otoacoustic emission), or a change in some electric property of the body (e.g., electric resistance of the skin). Clinicians come closer to knowing what patients hear when they ask patients to repeat words delivered through earphones or loudspeakers.

Historically, the emphasis in audiometry has been on voluntary behavioral responses. For most purposes and for most patients, voluntary behavioral response audiometry is the least expensive and most definitive of all procedures. What purpose is served, then, by audiometry that uses an electrophysiologic index, that is, **electrophysiologic audiometry**?

A major justification for electrophysiologic audiometry is that we can obtain reasonable measures of threshold hearing level for some patients only through electrophysiologic procedures. Neonates provide the prime example. Other patients for whom electrophysiologic audiometry may be the procedure of choice are children and adults who are severely mentally handicapped, patients with psychiatric disorders whose voluntary behavioral responses are too erratic to be used with confidence, and patients involved in litigation whose lack of cooperation negates the results of more conventional audiometry. Even when other forms of audiometry can be carried out with compliant patients, test results on some of them may not be reliable enough for the clinician to draw valid conclusions about their threshold hearing levels. Electrophysiologic threshold audiometry, when used as a supplement to behavioral response threshold audiometry, can help the clinician quantify hearing threshold levels with more confidence. Another justification for electrophysiologic audiometry is that it can provide diagnostic information beyond what may be derived from the threshold audiogram determined behaviorally or electrophysiologically. Some forms of electrophysiologic audiometry may help to confirm (or reject) diagnoses derived from other procedures.

EPA Instrumentation, Signal Averaging, and Averaged Evoked Potentials (AEPs)

The core of any instrument that measures electrophysiologic response to sound is a voltmeter that registers potential differences or voltages between any two points on the body where electrodes are attached. If sound presented is above the patient's threshold, changes can occur in the potential differences or voltages. Often, however, the changes are too small or weak to activate the voltmeter. Therefore, an amplifier is used to magnify the potential differences so that the voltmeter will register them.

The spectrum of the voltage changes or response to sound is complex, and not all of the electricity registered by the voltmeter helps to define the response of interest. Unwanted electricity from head and neck muscles and from the stimulating and recording instruments often are registered as well. This extraneous electricity acts like noise, interfering with the clarity of the electricity associated with the response. Therefore, filters are inserted in the circuit to reject as much of the extraneous noise as possible while retaining those spectral components that contribute most to defining the response. The measuring instrument also includes a mechanism for storing the voltages of interest and for providing a hard copy or printout of the voltage changes as a function of time.

Clinicians have used a variety of electrophysiologic indices in audiometry. The most popular indices have been changes of heart rate detected in the **electrocardiogram** (Beadle & Crowell, 1962; Miller, Morse, & Dorman, 1977; Morrongiello & Clifton, 1984), changes of electric resistance or of electric potential of the skin detected in the **electrodermogram** (Goldstein, 1956; Hardy & Pauls, 1952; Ruhm & Carhart, 1958), and changes in the ongoing brain activity detected in the **electroencephalogram** or EEG (Davis, Davis, Loomis, Harvey, & Hobart, 1939; Derbyshire & Farley, 1959; Eisenberg, 1966; Goldstein, Kendall, & Arick, 1963; Marcus, Gibbs, & Gibbs, 1949). The most successful index has been some change in the EEG and it is this index that is the basis for **evoked potential audiometry** or EPA.

EEG changes constantly and is influenced greatly by the state of alertness or of sleep. Ongoing EEG patterns and their changes, however, are not random. For example, the person who is alert but relaxed quietly with eyes closed can have an EEG dominated by voltage changes occurring about 10 per second, the so-called **alpha rhythm** (see strips A and B in Figure 1-1). The same person asleep may have larger voltage fluctuations occurring at about 3 per second. If sound is presented to a patient during any stage of wakefulness or sleep, a change can occur in the ongoing EEG. If distinct changes occur, as in strips B, C, and D of Figure 1-1, the clinician may conclude that the sound was above the patient's threshold. Successively weaker sounds are presented until no apparent change, synchronized with the sound, takes place in the EEG. The audiologist then concludes that the patient's threshold has been reached. Thus, threshold can be measured without having to ask the patient to signal whether the test sounds have been heard.

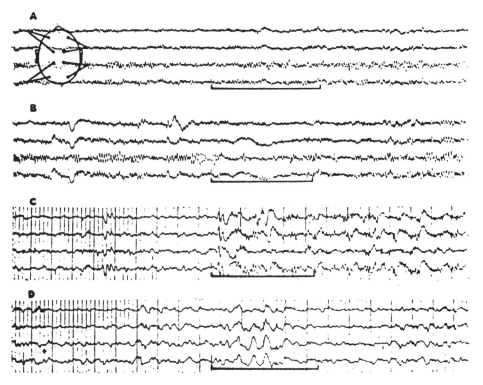

FIGURE 1-1. Sample 4-channel electroencephalograms (EEGs) from a 10-year-old hearing-impaired boy during evoked potential audiometry in which changes in the raw EEG were used as response indices. Line under each strip indicated the 5-second duration of the test tone. (A and B) patient awake; (C and D) patient asleep. Distinct electroencephalic responses in B, C, and D.

[Reprinted with permission from Withrow & Goldstein, "An electrophysiologic procedure for determination of threshold in children." *Laryngoscope*, *68*, 1676–1699,1958.]

The procedure just described has been used successfully in audiometry. However, several limitations curtail its use. One major shortcoming is that the changes in the ongoing EEG in response to sound often are too small to be detected against the larger, spontaneously changing activity, which, for audiometric purposes, is considered noise. A second shortcoming is that the largest changes elicited by sound apparently are generated by neural mechanisms that habituate quickly (Marsh, McCarthy, Sheatz, & Galambos, 1961; Pampiglione, 1952). Thus, a sound that evokes a clear change in the raw EEG may evoke a smaller change the second time it is presented or, perhaps, no discernible change at all. Characteristic undramatic responses are shown in the three segments of Figure 1-2. Habituation requires that long intervals be interspersed between successive test signals making the test procedure uncomfortably long for both clinician and patient (Davis, Mast, Yoshie, & Zerlin, 1966). Although some smaller changes in voltage do not habituate, usually they are too small to be distinguished from the larger, spontaneous voltage changes in the ongoing background EEG.

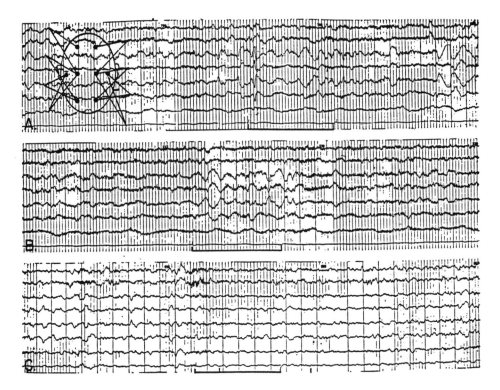

FIGURE 1-2. Examples of common electroencephalic responses recorded from three different hearing-impaired children. (A) K-complex; (B) increase in slow-wave activity and then return to previous ongoing pattern; (C) reduction in slow-wave activity. These records illustrate definite but undramatic responses. Sometimes the responses are more obvious, as in Figure 1-1; more often, however, they are less discernible. Seven channels were recorded instead of the four in Figure 1-1. Sensitivity of the channel producing the last line purposely was reduced to allow greater visibility of the artifact showing onset and offset of the 5-second test tone.

[Reprinted by permission of the American Speech-Language-Hearing Association from Goldstein, Kendall, & Arick, "Electroencephalic audiometry in young children." *Journal of Speech and Hearing Research*, *28*, 331–354, 1963.]

If one takes EEG traces following repetitions of identical test signals (Figure 1-3A) and superimposes them (Figure 1-3B), and if the signal is above the patient's threshold, the traces can reveal commonalities among them that are not apparent when the traces are viewed separately. The audiologist may interpret the commonalities as a response. By contrast, superimposed traces usually show no apparent commonalities (as in Figure 1-3F) if the signal is below the patient's threshold.

Commonalities between the traces, or lack of commonalities, can be found another way. A baseline can be drawn through the middle of the individual traces. Then, positive or negative amplitudes are measured at successive small intervals after the onset of the signal.

Many traces are obtained under identical test conditions, and the values at the same intervals or time points for each trace are added algebraically. Those deflections that are random with respect to signal onset time, theoretically, should add to zero. The sums become closer to zero, or to a straight line when plotted, as the number of superimposed samples or traces

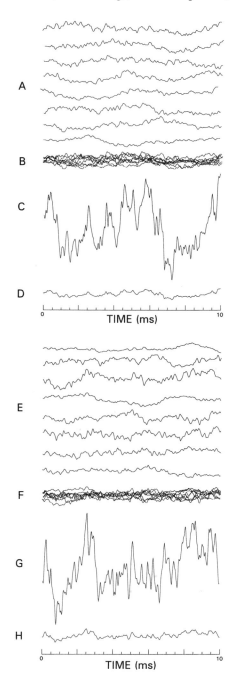

FIGURE 1-3. **(A) Eight EEG traces obtained under identical signal conditions. Onset of a brief acoustic signal above the patient's threshold is at the beginning of the traces. (B) Overlap or superimposition of the eight traces in A. Commonalities between the eight traces are more apparent in the superimposition than when the traces are viewed apart as in A. (C) Algebraic sum of positive and negative voltages in the eight traces in A and B. This is a *summed evoked potential*. (D) Average of the eight traces in A and B. This is an *averaged evoked potential (AEP)*. The configuration of the AEP is identical to that of the summed evoked potential in C, but is only one-eighth its amplitude. (E-H). Same recording conditions as in A–D. However, the acoustic signal was below the subject's threshold. This is equivalent to a silent-control condition. Theoretically, the silent-control AEP could be a straight line. In practice, however, straight lines (i.e., summed values at all addresses = 0) rarely occur, especially when the number of samples (N) per AEP is as few as eight. Even with as few as eight samples, the configuration of the signal-related traces (C and D) resembles typical traces obtained with larger samples (see Figure 1-4). The deflections in the silent-control waveforms (G and H) are almost as large. However, the configuration of G and H does not resemble that of C and D.**

increases. Those small deflections that are signal-related are not random but have the same polarity (negative or positive) in each trace. The sum of the amplitudes of these deflections is significantly more positive or more negative than zero. When the sums are plotted as a function of time, they define a response by a sequence of positive and negative deflections (Figure 1-3C). If the signals are below the patient's threshold and no signal-related deflections occur, then the resulting trace comes closer to being a flat line (Figure 1-3G).

Traces C and G in Figure 1-3 are **summed evoked potentials**. If one divides the sums by the number of signals used to obtain them, then the resulting traces (Figures 1-3D and 1-3H) are **averaged evoked potentials** or **AEPs**.

The manual procedure just described for response extraction is valid and can be used clinically (Davis & Derbyshire, 1972; McRandle, Smith, & Goldstein, 1974). However, it is too cumbersome, tedious and time-consuming to have achieved widespread clinical use. Fortunately, the advent of digital computers and the **averaged response computer** has made the averaging process practical. Instead of using hard copy EEG traces, the computer digitizes the electric activity from the brain, stores the positive and negative voltages at successive time points, and does the averaging electronically. The resulting time-amplitude waveforms are displayed on an oscilloscope and can be printed for permanent records. This is how the traces in Figure 1-4 were generated.

When neurologists use the EEG for neurologic diagnostic purposes, they record voltage changes between multiple pairs of electrodes placed on different areas of the scalp. Then they examine many minutes or hours of the ongoing EEG. In most applications of EPA, however, activity is recorded with only one or two pairs of electrodes. A common pairing is between the vertex or top of the head and either the mastoid or the earlobe. In EPA, the analysis window or epoch seldom is longer than one-half second or 500 **milliseconds (ms)**. For the most common form of EPA, the analysis window is only 10 ms, as in Figure 1-4.

AEPs are characterized by a complex sequence of large and small positive and negative deflections called waves or peaks. The pattern or configuration of the waves or peaks depends on equipment variables (e.g., size of the analysis window, width of the filter passband), signal variables (e.g., spectrum of the signal, presentation rate), subject variables (e.g., age, gender, normal versus pathologic), subject state (e.g., attentive or in reverie, awake or asleep), and circumstances under which the AEP is elicited. The specific clinical purpose of the EPA dictates the selection of those variables that can be controlled.

Clinical Applications of AEPs

Signal-Related AEPs

Figure 1-5 illustrates two ways in which the time-amplitude configuration of AEPs can be used as a response index for threshold audiometry. First, the clinician observes the similarity between AEP traces obtained at the same signal level. Two or three AEPs obtained under identical conditions should resemble each other. Similarities in the AEPs are best seen when the traces are superimposed. Traces that are replicable at a given signal level argue that the eliciting signals were suprathreshold. Signal levels are lowered until the superimposed traces no longer are replicable. The clinician then infers that threshold has been reached.

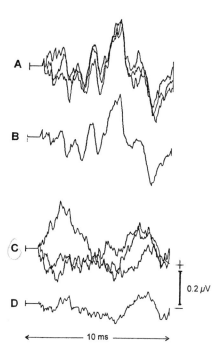

How can data be recorded if sound is inaudible?

FIGURE 1-4 (A) Three superimposed averaged evoked potentials (AEPs) from a normal-hearing subject in response to clicks at 60 dB nHL; number of samples (N) per AEP = 800. (B) Composite AEP of the three traces in A (sum of the three traces divided by 3). (C) Three superimposed AEPs from the same subject for clicks at –10 dB nHL, which were inaudible. (D) Composite AEP of the three traces in C. Conditions for all traces: click rate = 11.1/s; filter passband = 100-3000 Hz.

[Process]

A second thing that the clinician observes are changes in the latency and amplitude of the positive and negative peaks of the AEP as a function of signal level. **Latency** of the peaks (that is, time from signal onset to the peak) is expected to increase and peak **amplitude** can be expected to decrease as the eliciting signals become weaker. The changes in latency and amplitude can be observed with successively weaker signal levels until the peaks are small and bear no apparent relation to the peaks in AEPs elicited by stronger signals. The clinician then concludes that threshold has been reached. Certain time-amplitude configurations, that is, waveforms, are common across most patients. Sometimes, however,

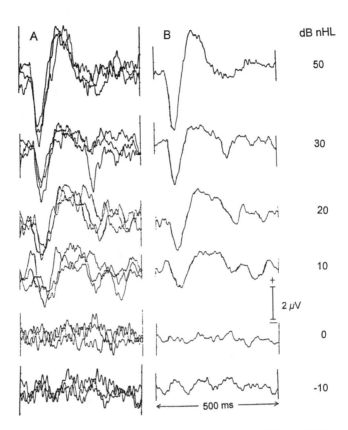

FIGURE 1-5 AEPs from normal-hearing adult to 1000 Hz tone bursts (10 ms rise/fall time; 10 ms plateau) presented at 1 per second. Recording filter passband: 1–70 Hz. (A) Three replications of 90 samples each. (B) Composite AEPs (average of the three replications). Tone bursts were audible to subject at 10 dB nHL but not at 0 dB nHL.

a patient's waveform is not typical for the recording and test circumstances. Nevertheless, the peaks that do occur for that patient will show the same systematic increase in latency and decrease in amplitude with decreasing signals levels.

An audiogram obtained through EPA, just as an audiogram obtained from voluntary behavioral response audiometry, yields an important bit of information. It tells the clinician something about the integrity of the patient's peripheral auditory mechanism. If the audiogram is not normal, that is, if there is some manifestation of hypacusis, the audiologist is safe in assuming that something (or several things) from the external auditory meatus to the entry of the auditory nerve in the brainstem is not functioning normally. Further, if EPA thresholds are obtained by bone conduction as well as by air conduction, similarities or differences in the two thresholds can tell the audiologist whether the patient's loss is conductive, sensorineural, or mixed.

The components of AEPs discussed so far depend largely on the nature of the eliciting signals and, thus, are called **signal-related potentials** or **SRPs**. Their latencies and amplitudes vary predictably with the level of the eliciting signals. When they are elicited by tones or other narrow-spectrum signals, the AEP peaks will be larger and later for low-frequency signals than for high-frequency signals (McFarland, Vivion, & Goldstein, 1977; Sininger, Abdala, & Cone-Wesson, 1997). As a rule, the earlier the component—that is, the shorter the latency—the more replicable it is, and the less susceptible it is to changes in subject state such as going from alertness to drowsiness to sleep. Replicability of early SRPs makes them more reliable than later SRPs as indices for threshold audiometry.

Those peaks that occur within the first 10 ms after the onset of a click usually are called **auditory brainstem responses (ABR), brainstem evoked potentials (BSEP)**, or similar names with corresponding initials. The popularity of the ABR has led to a confusing practice of genericizing all AEPs as "brainstem responses" and all instruments used to obtain AEPs as "brainstem machines."

Early SRPs also are used as indices of the integrity of the **central auditory nervous system** or **CANS**, and even of the auditory nerve (VIIIth cranial nerve) that delivers auditory messages to the brain. AEP waveforms, especially in response to distinctly suprathreshold clicks as in Figure 1-4, have a definable sequence of positive and negative deflections or peaks with certain expected peak latencies, interpeak intervals, and relative peak amplitudes (Bauch, Olsen, & Pool, 1996; Elberling & Parbo, 1987; Weber, 1992). Significant deviations from expected AEP configuration prove useful in determining or confirming lesions of the VIIIth nerve and of various parts of the brain (e.g., vestibular neurilemmoma, brainstem tumor, multiple sclerosis). These same early SRPs can be monitored during surgery (e.g., removal of a vestibular neurilemmoma) to provide the surgeon information about the integrity of the structure being incised or otherwise manipulated (Aravabhumi, Izzo, & Bakst, 1987; Fisher, Raudzens, & Nunemacher, 1995).

Event-Related Potentials

Event-related potentials (ERPs) are another category of AEPs that can be used clinically. In contrast to SRPs, ERPs are not related to the absolute physical characteristics of the eliciting signals, such as sound pressure level or frequency, but to the circumstances under which the eliciting or target signals are presented. The most common way of eliciting ERPs is through an **oddball paradigm** or procedure (Picton, 1992; Polich, 1990). In this paradigm, one signal (e.g., 1000 Hz tone-burst) is presented in a regular sequence (e.g., 1 per second). Infrequently (e.g., one out of five) and randomly, a different signal (e.g., 2000 Hz tone-burst) is presented in the sequence instead of the 1000 Hz tone burst. The 1000 Hz tone burst (80% probability of occurrence) is referred to as the **frequent, standard** or **expected** signal; the 2000 Hz tone burst (20% probability) is called the **unexpected, deviant, infrequent, rare,** or **oddball** signal.

In the oddball paradigm, the electroencephalic activity following each frequent signal is stored in one memory bank of the evoked-potential system, and the activity following each oddball signal is stored in a separate memory bank. Both the frequent and the oddball AEPs will contain SRP components differing slightly from each other because they were elicited by tone bursts of different frequencies. The oddball AEP also will contain components not found in the frequent AEP; these components are ERPs.

A commonly discussed ERP is a large positive deflection with its peak at or just beyond 300 ms (see Figure 1-6). It is usually called **P300**. Its latency and amplitude depend on several factors including the probability of occurrence of the oddball signal and the magnitude of the physical difference between the frequent and oddball signals (Donchin &

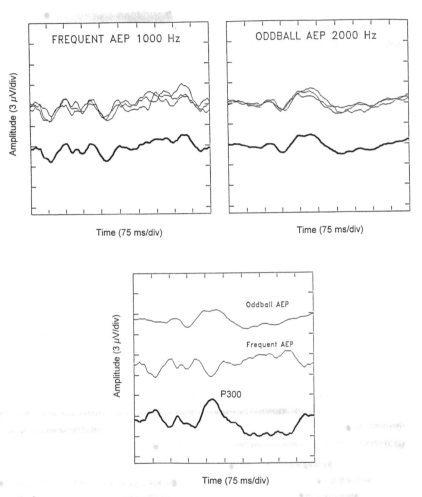

FIGURE 1-6   AEPs from a 23-year-old normal-hearing woman. Frequent AEP: 1000 Hz tone burst at 85 dB nHL, probability 81%. Superimposed traces: 73 sweeps each. Heavy trace below, composite AEP (sum of the three individual traces divided by 3). Oddball AEP: 2000 Hz tone bursts at 85 dB nHL, probability 19%. Superimposed traces: 17 sweeps each. Heavy trace below, composite AEP (sum of three individual traces divided by 3). Subject kept mental count of number of oddball signals during each trial. P300 trace obtained by subtracting composite frequent AEP from composite oddball AEP. Although P300 is the most prominent deflection in the heavy trace, other differences between oddball and frequent AEPs also are evident.

McCarthy, 1979; Polich & Kok, 1995). The P300 also depends on the subject's state during its elicitation. It is most distinct if the subject is asked to count the number of oddball signals during a test trial or to attend to the oddball signal in some other manner (Adams & Benson, 1973; Davis, 1964).

So much attention has been given to the P300 that this designation has been genericized, that is, it is often applied to any component of the ERP and to any procedure used to elicit ERPs. However, under the test circumstances just described, the ERP obtained consists of several negative and positive deflections before and after the prominent P300. Earlier components of the ERP are less dependent than the later ones on subject participation, attention, or state.

ERPs may be used to assess the way in which the brain can differentiate between similar signals differing only slightly along one dimension (e.g., frequency, sound pressure level) (Alho, Sams, Paavilainen, & Näätänen, 1986; Chertoff, Goldstein, & Mease, 1988). With oddball speech signals differing from the frequent speech signals along phonemic, semantic or syntactic dimensions, even language functions and dysfunctions can be assessed (Bentin, McCarthy, & Wood, 1985; Martin, Sigal, Kurtzberg, & Stapells, 1997; Rubin, Newhoff, Peach, & Shapiro, 1996). ERPs also are used to help evaluate site, nature, and extent of brain lesions (Baran, Long, Musiek, & Ommaya, 1988; Coburn, Campbell, Kuhn, & Moreno, 1996; Kraus, McGee, Ferre, Hoeppner, Carrell, Sharma, & Nicol, 1993).

Basic Technique

Electric Activity in the Brain and Auditory System and Principles of Signal Averaging

The goal of Part II is to expand on the biologic substrate of auditory averaged evoked potentials and on the instruments used to elicit and record them. Further elaboration will be given in subsequent chapters in conjunction with the descriptions of AEPs and their clinical applications.

Electricity associated with auditory function takes place at the cellular level. Audiologists and other clinicians, however, cannot invade the patient's ear or brain with intracellular electrodes to record the auditory related electricity. Even if intracellular recordings were technically feasible, they might not provide enough clinical information about how the patient hears. Auditory averaged evoked potentials (AEPs) recorded extracranially also have their clinical limitations. Nevertheless, they can be obtained noninvasively and they can yield much practical clinical information valuable for diagnosis and management. The purpose of this chapter is to describe (1) the biologic substrate of auditory AEPs and (2) the signal averaging process used to extract them from other electric activity registered by the recording electrodes.

General Background

Electrodes attached to different parts of the head register differences in electric potential or voltage between those electrodes. The potential differences result from electricity generated in the ear and the brain. However, neither the ear nor the brain generates the electricity as a conglomerate organ. Rather, constituent components of the ear and of the brain generate electricity at the cellular level. The principal generators in the ear are hair cells of the organ of Corti and fibers of the auditory nerve. Potential changes in the ear induced by sound are multicomponent and complex.

The complexity within the brain is incalculably greater than that of the ear. The brain has a greater variety of cell forms and synaptic connections than the ear. Pre- and post-synaptic potentials overlap in time and space with all-or-none axonic discharges. Potentials are influenced by caudal-rostral interactions and by interactions between both sides of the brain. Potentials generated by cells associated primarily with audition blend with potentials generated by cells serving other sensory and motor modalities. In addition, potentials arise from interactions between sensory modalities and from sensory-motor interactions. Interactions between the autonomic and voluntary nervous components add to the complexity.

Complexities within the brain are even greater than implied by the examples just cited. These examples alone, however, justify caution in interpreting the physiologic significance of the peaks of AEPs recorded from extracranial electrodes. Any deflection in an AEP trace is the sum of all the positive and negative potentials in the brain registered between the two extracranial electrodes at one given instant. Similar caution is given to attempts to predict the configuration of an AEP from the potentials generated at the cellular level within the brain.

Despite the limitations imposed by neural complexities, much can be learned from AEPs about the underlying functions of the ear and the brain. Further, some predictions can be made about extracranial AEPs from knowledge of ear and brain integrity. Clinical attributes of AEPs will be expounded in later chapters. The goal now is to provide insight into the auditory-related electricity in the brain, how we record it, and how we extract that activity through the process of signal averaging.

Recording Auditory-Related Electric Activity from the Brain

Various diagrams can be found in the literature of what many call the central auditory nervous system or CANS (Ades & Brookhart, 1950; Møller, 1994). Figure 2-1 is our rendition of what traditionally is called the CANS. It resembles the drawings of others in most respects. We elaborate further on this traditional or classical CANS in Chapter 16. When suprathreshold sounds are presented to a patient, the stimulated auditory or VIIIth cranial nerve delivers its all-or-none messages to the CANS. In turn, the electric status of the CANS changes. Measuring these changes or responses directly from the neural structures of the brain is impractical. Therefore, audiologists and others attempt to measure the electric activity with **far-field** electrodes, that is, with electrodes attached to the scalp, far from the neural generators.

Two related conditions make far-field recordings difficult to interpret. These conditions can be appreciated by reference to Figure 2-2, a photograph of an actual cross-section through the brain. First, electrodes on the vertex and on the mastoid or earlobe, a common electrode montage, pick up activity not only from the heavy lined pathways and their interconnecting nuclei structures shown in Figure 2-1 but from billions of other neurons as well. Second, the heavy-lined structures shown in Figure 2-1 are not the only ones that react to sound, although they may be the only brain structures that respond exclusively to sound. Many other structures distributed throughout the brain also respond to sound, even though they may respond as well to signals from other modalities. The combination of these two

Cochlea
↓
Ventral Coch. Nuc.
Dorsal Coch. Nuc.
+ Trapezoid Body
↓
SOC
↓
LL (Nerve Tract)
↓ (also has nucleus)
Inf. Colliculus
↓
MGB
↓
Aud. Radiations /
Aud. Cortex

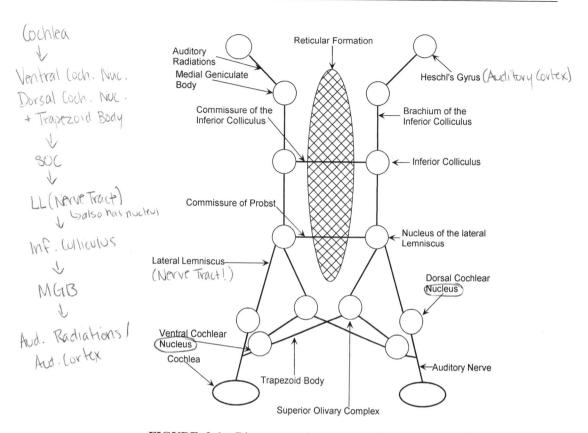

FIGURE 2-1   Diagrammatic representation of what traditionally is called the central auditory nervous system or CANS. The reticular formation is not considered a distinct part of the CANS but is attributed important roles in audition in the traditional or classical view of the CANS. See text of this chapter and of Chapter 16 for further discussion of structures depicted in this figure.

conditions leads to a response-related electricity distributed in time and space, accompanied by unrelated or extraneous electric activity (considered noise in the recordings) from other structures of the brain. These two conditions will be revisited after a more general discussion of recording the brain's electric activity with extracranial electrodes.

Billions of neurons of the brain produce electricity and electric fields at all times. The nature and extent of that **electroencephalic activity** vary with the nature, size, location, and state of the individual neurons. Extracranial electrodes do not register activity of isolated neurons but of all the neurons. The conglomerate activity is complex, ranging from direct current to alternating current of various frequencies. In addition, other electrophysiologic activity, such as muscle potentials and skin potentials, often contaminates recordings of electroencephalic activity.

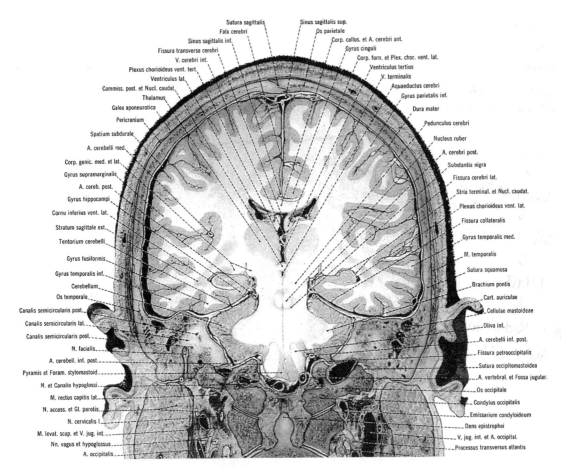

FIGURE 2-2   Coronal section through a head. The primary auditory projection system (PAPS) as diagrammed in Figure 2-1 is only a small part of the total brain. Electricity recorded between an electrode on the vertex and one on the mastoid (or the earlobe) comes not only from the PAPS but from billions of other brain cells, most of which ordinarily are not considered part of the central auditory nervous system (CANS). All of the brain's electricity, which is small to begin with, is even smaller at the recording sites because of attenuation by cerebrospinal fluid, meninges, skull, and scalp. Names of the structures indicated by the dashed lines are not relevant to the message of this figure.

[Copyright 1985 by Otto Kampmeier. Used with permission of the University of Illinois Press.]

Differences in electroencephalic activity between any two extracranial electrodes on the scalp are registered by a voltmeter as a difference in potential or voltage. However, the voltmeter may not be sensitive enough to register any deflections (Figure 2-3A). The electroencephalic activity, which is small to begin with, is attenuated by the meninges, skull, and scalp. The difference in potential between the voltmeter leads now is in the range of **microvolts (μV)**, that is, millionths of a volt. This is too weak to cause any visible deflection of the needle. It is necessary, therefore, to insert an **amplifier** in the circuit (Figure 2-3B).

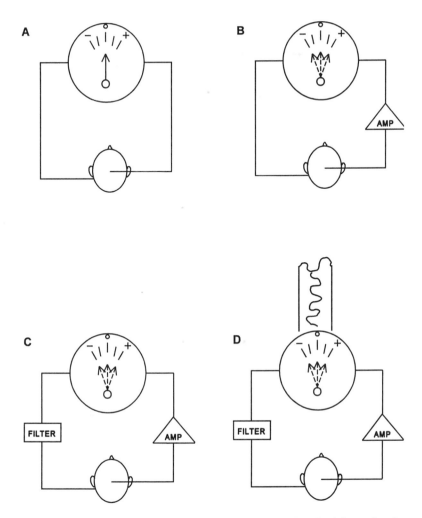

FIGURE 2-3 **(A) Voltmeter attached to human head with one lead or electrode on the vertex of the head and the other on one mastoid. The brain always produces both direct current (DC) and alternating current (AC) electricity. The voltmeter registers no electricity, however, because the voltage is too weak to cause the needle to deflect. (B) An amplifier is inserted into the circuit to make the initially weak voltage strong enough to cause the needle to deflect. (C) A filter is inserted in the circuit to help eliminate extraneous electric activity that might ordinarily cause unwanted and confusing deflections in the needle. (D) Ink flows through the voltmeter's needle and paper is pulled underneath the needle, which is now a pen, to trace a permanent record of the needle's deflections as a function of time. The total circuit in D is essentially a one-channel electroencephalograph (EEG machine) and the paper trace is an electroencephalogram (EEG).**

Not all of the electricity registered by the voltmeter contributes to the definition of the response to sound. Extraneous electricity acts like noise and interferes with the identification of the electric changes that constitute the response. Therefore, **filters** are inserted in the circuit to reject as much noise as possible while retaining the spectral components that contribute most to defining the response (Figure 2-3C).

The clinician cannot remember the sequence of voltage changes that help to distinguish response-related voltage changes from ongoing changes that are not associated with the test signal. However, if ink flowed through the tip of the needle making it a pen and if paper were pulled at a steady rate underneath the needle (Figure 2-3D), a permanent record would be made of the movement of the needle, that is, of all the voltage changes at the extracranial electrodes.

The instrument depicted in Figure 2-3D is an **electroencephalograph**, and the paper trace is an electroencephalogram or EEG. Electroencephalographers usually record from 16 to 32 sets of electrodes when they examine the EEG for neurologic diagnosis. Their large awesome instruments with arrays of complicated looking controls are, in reality, a collection of 16 to 32 voltmeters that enable electroencephalographers to record voltage changes simultaneously from 16 to 32 different portions of the head.

EEG changes constantly and is influenced greatly by the state of alertness or of sleep. Ongoing patterns and their changes, however, are not random. For example, the person who is alert but relaxing quietly with eyes closed can have an EEG dominated by voltage changes occurring at about 10 per second, the so-called alpha rhythm (Davis, 1936; Yardanova & Kolev, 1996). The same person asleep may have larger voltage changes occurring at about 3 per second (Davis et al.,1939). If sound is presented to a patient during any stage of wakefulness or sleep, a change can occur in the ongoing, spontaneously changing EEG (Davis et al.,1939; Oken and Salinsky, 1992). If a change does occur, the clinician may conclude that the sound was above the patient's threshold. Weaker sounds can then be presented until no apparent change, synchronized with the sound, takes place in the EEG (Derbyshire, Fraser, McDermott, & Bridge, 1956; Marcus, 1951). The clinician concludes that the patient's threshold has been reached. Thus, threshold may be measured without having to ask the patient to signal whether the test sounds have been heard.

Some kinds of changes that can be seen in the EEG in response to sound are illustrated in Figure 1-1, Chapter 1. The traces were obtained from a 10-year-old boy with a hearing loss (Withrow & Goldstein, 1958). EEG was recorded simultaneously from four different sites as shown diagrammatically in Figure 1-1A. Prominent alpha rhythm from the occipital region of the head indicates that the boy was awake. The dark line underneath the traces indicates the duration (five seconds) of the tone that was presented. Little happened in the EEG during those five seconds that differed appreciably from the EEG pattern preceding the tone, except, perhaps, for the slow waves occurring about midway through the tone. This change may have been an electrodermal response from the scalp. In Figure 1-1B, however, during which the child still was awake, there was a dramatic change in the EEG shortly after the onset of the tone. Alpha rhythm diminished, large slow waves were introduced, and the EEG did not return to its pre-stimulus state until several seconds after the tone ceased.

In Figure 1-1C, the ongoing EEG indicates that the child was asleep. Again, the sound, depicted by the line under the traces, caused a change in the EEG. It differs considerably from the change in strip B, but is as dramatic. The combination of abrupt, large, low-frequency waves on which faster activity is superimposed is the **K-complex**, first described by Davis and colleagues at Harvard (Davis et al.,1939). In this strip, the EEG change induced by the sound continued even after the cessation of the sound. According to the EEG pattern in Figure 1-1D, the child was in a different state of sleep than he was during the acquisition of strip C. Consequently, the change induced by the sound—large slow waves— also was different. Nevertheless, the change in strip D is a clear response to the test signal.

If suprathreshold signals always evoked EEG changes as clear as those in Figure 1-1, threshold audiometry with changes in the ongoing EEG as the response index could be used routinely on difficult-to-test patients. Unfortunately, changes in the EEG evoked by the sound, that is, **electroencephalic responses,** usually are not so clear. EEG changes that do take place are not singular events. They are made up of activity from several different systems or sets of generators within the brain. Those generators responsible for the largest changes apparently habituate quickly, especially for rapid repetitions of the same signal (Marsh et al., 1961; Pampiglione, 1952). Therefore, long intervals must elapse between successive signals for each signal to elicit clinically useful, large changes. Normal habituation is healthy. It keeps the brain from reacting precipitously to each repetition of a similar sound that has little meaning for the listener. However, it is perplexing for the clinician who now either must look for subtler changes in the EEG as an indicator of response or prolong the intervals between successive test signals so much that the test procedure becomes prohibitively long.

Figure 1-2 depicts electroencephalic responses from three different patients (Goldstein et al., 1963). The EEG was recorded from seven different sets of electrodes; the eighth channel was used to mark the onset and offset of the 5-second test signal. Small but noticeable changes occurred in each set of tracings. They are more typical of changes that clinicians are likely to encounter than are the dramatic changes shown in Figure 1-1. Sometimes, changes are even less distinct and, at times, the clinician can discern no signal-related change in the EEG in response to suprathreshold signals.

We know that if the test signal is suprathreshold, electric changes will occur within the brain, especially in those portions of the brain (Figure 2-1) specifically dedicated to auditory function. If we remove the scalp, lay back a flap of bone covering the temporal lobe, pry open the Sylvian fissure, and place electrodes on Heschl's gyrus, those electrodes will register electric activity in response to the test signal. Why, then, is this electric activity not visible in the activity registered by the extracranial electrodes? First, that activity even at Heschl's gyrus is small. Second, Heschl's gyrus and other structures of the primary auditory projection system are buried deep within the brain. Electricity arising from them is attenuated by other brain tissue, meninges, skull, and scalp. Third, the small auditory-related voltages registered by the extracranial electrodes are superimposed on the larger ongoing EEG, and are not readily distinguished from the larger, constantly changing EEG.

Principles of Signal Averaging

As mentioned earlier, the large generalized responses to sound shown in Figures 1-1 and 1-2 habituate quickly, require long inter-stimulus intervals to recover, and vary considerably in their form. In contrast, the primary auditory projection system and closely associated neural structures of the CANS produce smaller, earlier activity with little habituation. The neurons can fire after short inter-stimulus intervals and produce patterns of electric activity that vary little with successive firings. Properties of the auditory-specific activity make it possible to extract their activity from the larger ongoing EEG in which they are indistinguishably buried. Figures 2-4 through 2-7 illustrate how that extraction can be accomplished.

The first line in Figure 2-4 shows an artificially constructed EEG trace recorded between an electrode on the vertex of the head and one on the mastoid process. A brief suprathreshold sound, for example, a click, is presented to the patient at the time marked by the heavy vertical line. The tester allows several seconds to elapse, begins recording the EEG again (Trace 2) and at the time marked by the arrow presents another click. After several more seconds, the EEG recording resumes (Trace 3) and another click is presented. The process is repeated two more times. The five traces in Figure 2-4 are not simultaneous recordings from five different locations on the scalp but are successive recordings from one set of electrodes. In none of the five traces is there an obvious electroencephalic response

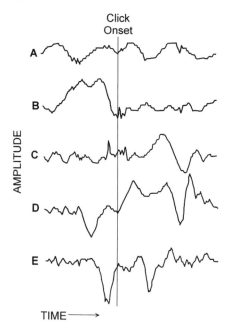

FIGURE 2-4   Hand-drawn traces made to resemble electroencephalic activity recorded between one electrode on the vertex another on the mastoid. Both the time and amplitude axes represent relative, not absolute, values. All five traces come from the same set of electrodes with enough time between successive clicks for full recovery of the response, which, though not obvious, is embedded in the post-signal portion of each trace.

to the click; the EEG following the click does not differ distinguishably from the pre-stimulus EEG. Furthermore, the five traces seem to have little in common with each other except their apparent randomness. Nevertheless, a small stimulus-related change was drawn into the post-stimulus portion of each trace. How can that small change be extracted from the larger ongoing EEG?

Figure 2-5 shows the first step in the extraction process. A baseline is drawn through the middle of each trace. Everything above the baseline is considered a positive voltage and everything below the baseline is considered negative. The next step (Figure 2-6) is to draw vertical lines through the traces. The lines are separated by fixed time intervals. Those intervals will be small (e.g., 1 millisecond [ms]) if only a short post-stimulus period is to be analyzed, or large (e.g., 25 ms) if the clinician wishes to examine much more of the post-stimulus activity. Then, voltages are measured in each trace at each of the time lines and added algebraically. The final step in the extraction process is plotting the algebraic sums as a function of time (Figure 2-7). Had all the post-stimulus activity been completely random with respect to the click onset, the sum of the traces would have been small, like the pre-stimulus portions of the traces and, with sufficiently large numbers of samples, would

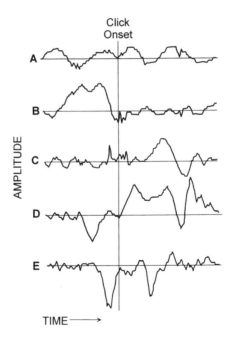

FIGURE 2-5 Same hand-drawn traces as in Figure 2-4 with an arbitrary baseline drawn through each of them. Deflections above the baseline represent positive voltages or potentials and deflections below the baseline are negative.

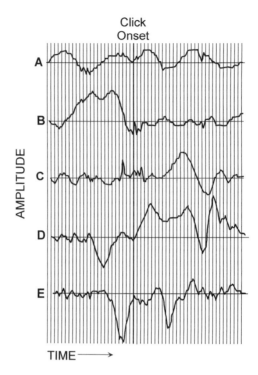

Click
Onset

A

B

AMPLITUDE

C

D

E

TIME ⟶

**FIGURE 2-6   Same hand-drawn traces
as in Figure 2-5 with the traces intersected by equally spaced vertical time lines or
addresses.**

approximate zero or a straight line. At each time point, sometimes the deflections would be
positive and other times negative; sometimes the deflections would have been large and at
other times small, and all of the algebraic values would approximate zero. However, if one
looks along the time lines at those points in the post-stimulus portion of the summed trace
that show the largest positive or negative deflections, one notes that the ongoing EEG
waves in the individual traces are made more positive (or less negative) or more negative (or
less positive) at those particular time points. That is the way in which the individual traces
were artificially constructed. They were constructed in that way to resemble what happens
in actual recordings.

The electric changes evoked by the click are not absolutely identical after each click.
Nevertheless, they are more alike than different. Certain positive and negative changes
apparently are **time-locked** to the onset of each click. When many real EEG samples,
obtained under identical circumstances, are summed algebraically, summed traces with
distinctive forms result, as in Figure 1-3.

As stated, the trace on the bottom of Figure 2-7 is a summed response. If one wishes
to know the contribution of each individual response to that sum, one divides the sum by the
number of samples added, in this case five. The resulting trace will be identical in form or

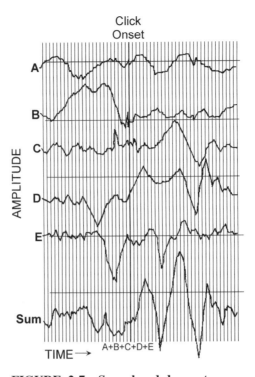

Click
Onset

FIGURE 2-7 **Same hand-drawn traces as in Figure 2-6. Bottom trace is actual addition or sum of the five positive or negative voltages at each time line or address. Pre-signal summed voltages are smaller and less well-defined than post-signal summed voltages.**

configuration to the summed response but the positive and negative deflections will be one-fifth the size (see Figure 2-8). Most of the older literature and some contemporary literature refer to the smaller trace as an averaged evoked response or AER. In this case, "evoked" is redundant because nothing can be considered a response unless it is evoked. The choice in this book is to call the resulting trace an averaged evoked potential or AEP.

In audiometry, the AEP, instead of distinctive changes in the raw or ongoing EEG, is used as the response index. In threshold audiometry, the clinician observes changes in the AEP pattern or configuration with successively weaker sets of test signals. When the signals are so weak that they no longer elicit an identifiable configuration, the judgment is that the signals are at or below the patient's threshold sensitivity.

The form of the trace on the bottom of Figure 2-7, although an actual addition of traces 1 through 5, is contrived. Actual waveform configurations depend on many factors including the size (in ms) of the post-stimulus recording window or epoch, bandwidth of the recording filters, acoustic properties of the test signals, and age of the patient. Also, usually

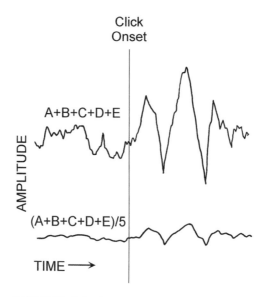

FIGURE 2-8   **Upper trace is the same
summed voltage or potential as the bottom
trace of Figure 2-7. The lower trace in this
figure is the summed potential divided by
5, the number of traces from which the
upper trace was derived. This lower trace
is the** *averaged evoked potential* **(***AEP***). Its
configuration is the same as that of the
summed potential but its amplitude is only
one-fifth that of the summed potential.**

more than five samples are acquired per AEP. As few as 16 and as many as 15,000 samples have been used. The number of samples will be dictated largely by the signal(response)-to-noise ratio.

The manual method of signal averaging just described is too laborious and time-consuming to be used routinely clinically. Signal averaging is done today by means of digital computers. Most signal averagers or averaged response computers have a fixed number of **stations** or **addresses** placed at equal intervals throughout the **analysis window** or **recording epoch**. An electric signal that is concurrent with the onset of the electric signal delivered to the test earphone **triggers** a **sweep** of the signal averager. The electroencephalic activity following the onset of each test signal is examined sequentially at each address in the analysis window. If there are 100 addresses and if the analysis window is 100 ms, the electroencephalic activity will be sampled every 1 ms. If the analysis window is 500 ms, electroencephalic activity will be sampled every 5 ms; if the analysis window is only 10 ms, electroencephalic activity will be sampled every 0.1 ms.

At each address, the **analog** electroencephalic activity is **digitized**, and the signed (plus or minus) digital value is stored at that address. This is an **analog-to-digital (A-to-D) conversion**. With the next sweep, the electroencephalic activity evoked in the analysis window again is digitized and the new value is added algebraically to the first value at each address. The process continues until a preset number of sweeps has been completed or until the tester is satisfied with the signal-to-noise ratio. (As a reminder, signal here refers to the potential change evoked by the acoustic test sound and the noise is the electric activity unrelated to the acoustic signal presentations.) At the completion of the process, the digital values are converted to analog values. This is the **digital-to-analog (D-to-A) conversion**. The analog values are displayed as a continuous trace on an oscilloscope.

The fidelity with which the analog voltages are converted to digital values and then back to analog voltages depends on the digital resolution. Figure 2-9 displays an analog trace digitized with differing degrees of **amplitude resolution** or precision. In the first example, the amplitude resolution is so coarse or wide that the evoked potential component of interest falls completely within the first set of lines and is not reproduced at all. In the second example, the digitization is narrow or fine enough to reproduce the larger, slower wave but not the smaller, faster wave. In the third example, the digitization is fine enough to reproduce both components faithfully. Because the smaller deflections usually have a high-frequency spectrum, coarse resolution can lead to inadvertent high-frequency (low-pass) filtering.

Fidelity of A-to-D and D-to-A conversions also depends on **temporal resolution**. Figure 2-10 displays a trace superimposed on time grids of differing resolution. In the three examples shown, the slow or low-frequency waves are reproduced with reasonable fidelity. However, with coarse resolution, the high-frequency waves can fall between the set time lines and not be digitized and reproduced. Therefore, coarse temporal resolution also can lead to inadvertent high-frequency (low-pass) filtering.

The AEPs shown in Figures 2-9 and 2-10, and elsewhere in the book, are not simple sinusoids, although a few frequencies may dominate the spectrum of the complex AEPs. For a specific frequency component in the original evoked activity to be reproduced in the A-to-D and D-to-A conversions, the temporal resolution of the signal averager must be fine enough to intersect at least two points on the cycle for that frequency (Hyde, 1994). For example, if it is important to reproduce a 1000 Hz component, one must first calculate the period of that frequency. The period (T) is the reciprocal of the frequency or $T = 1/f = 1/1000$ cycles/s $= 0.001$ s or 1 ms. Because at least two points on the cycle are to be reproduced, the separation between successive addresses must be no greater than 0.0005 s or 0.5 ms. If still higher frequencies are to be reproduced, then the temporal separation between successive addresses must be even shorter.

If one has the instrumental capacity to provide as many addresses as needed, then one repeats the above calculation for the highest frequency expected to be reproduced in a given analysis period and provides the number of addresses accordingly. Most affordable commercial signal averagers, however, do not have infinite flexibility. The clinician, therefore, is limited to a finite number of addresses that must be distributed evenly throughout the analysis window of choice. The user then must calculate the highest frequency that the signal averager can reproduce. By way of example, a given signal averager has 500 addresses, and the clinician wishes to examine 100 ms of post-stimulus activity. 100 ms/500 addresses = 0.2 ms or 0.0002 s per address. At least two points per cycle must be intersected before any one frequency can be reproduced. The highest frequency that can be reproduced must have a period no shorter than 2×0.0002 s or 0.0004 s. Frequency is the reciprocal of period or $f = 1/T$; therefore, $f = 1/0.0004$ s or 2500/s or 2500 Hz. This highest frequency that can be reproduced is called the **Nyquist frequency**. If a 500 ms epoch is to be analyzed, the period of the

ANALOG TO DIGITAL CONVERSION

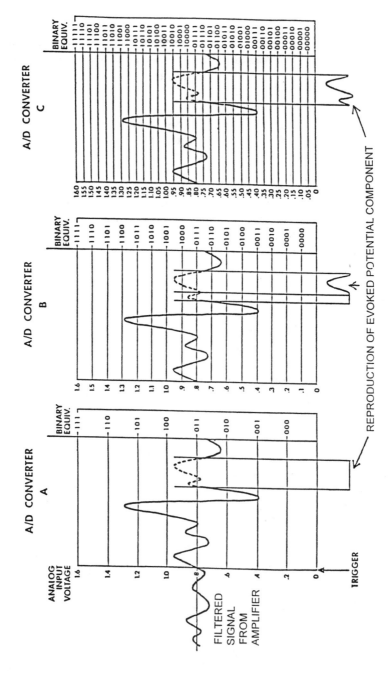

FIGURE 2-9 Effect of amplitude resolution on analog-to-digital conversion of electroencephalic activity. If amplitude digitization is not fine enough, the potentials of interest will not be reproduced accurately.

[Reprinted with permission of Grass Instruments Division, Astro-Med, Inc.]

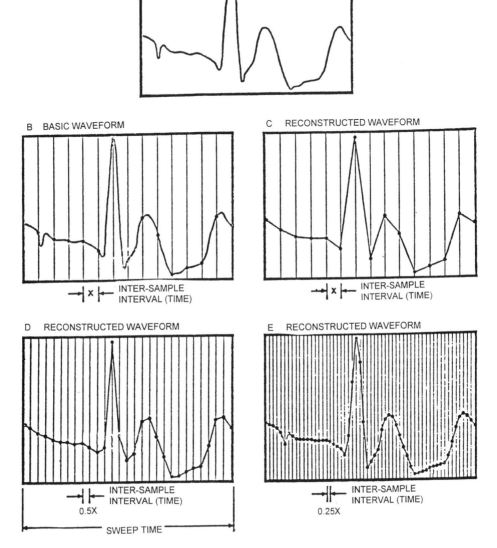

FIGURE 2-10   Effect of temporal resolution on analog-to-digital conversion of electroencephalic activity. If temporal sampling is not fine enough, all of the potentials of interest will not be reproduced accurately.

[Reprinted with permission of Grass Instruments Division, Astro-Med, Inc.]

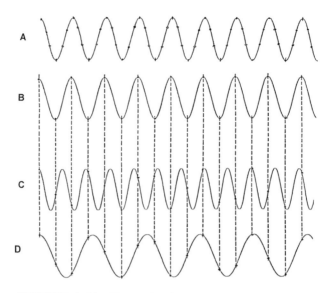

FIGURE 2-11   Example of how aliasing occurs. (A) With 6 points per cycle or period, the original frequency is accurately reproduced. (B) Even with only 2 points per cycle (as indicated by the intersection with the vertical hatched lines) the original frequency can be reproduced. (C) When the same time resolution is used for a higher frequency, fewer than 2 points per cycle results. (D) Digital-to-analog reproduction of the frequency in C leads to a wave with distinctly lower frequency than the original frequency.

Nyquist frequency for the same signal averager would be (500 ms/500 addresses) × 2 = 2 ms or 0.002 s. The Nyquist frequency would then be 1/0.002 s or 500/s or 500 Hz. For a 20 ms analysis time, the period of the Nyquist frequency would be (20 ms/500 addresses) × 2 = 0.08 ms or 0.00008 s; the Nyquist frequency would be 1/0.00008 s or 12,500 Hz.

A phenomenon called **aliasing** occurs if temporal resolution is not adequate (Hyde, 1994a). An example is shown in Figure 2-11. The large dots superimposed on the traces show the addresses at which the A-to-D amplitude conversion takes place. In trace A, more than two dots occur per cycle of the sine wave; this resolution is more than sufficient to reproduce the sine wave. In trace B, exactly two dots occur per cycle; this is still sufficient resolution for faithful frequency reproduction. If, however, the resolution in trace B were to be used for the higher frequency sine wave shown in trace C, fewer than two points would intersect each cycle. The resulting reproduction would be a lower frequency than the original frequency. In other words, the D-to-A conversion would show a frequency not present in the original signal. The error, which is sometimes described as folding back, is called aliasing. To insure that aliasing will not take place, the operator should calculate the Nyquist frequency and then set the low-pass end (high-frequency cut-off) of the recording bandpass filter at or lower than the Nyquist frequency.

Chapter 3

Response Acquisition System

Most instruments used for evoked potential audiometry (EPA) are designed for general purpose electrodiagnosis. They can obtain a variety of electrophysiologic data besides auditory averaged evoked potentials (AEPs): averaged visual and somatosensory evoked potentials, electroretinograms, electronystagmograms, electromyograms, and measures of nerve conduction. The general purpose instruments evolved from special purpose recorders, each configured for a specific task. They are basically sophisticated voltmeters with digital oscilloscopes.

[Other tests]

Multipurpose commercial instruments can be configured by setting their operating parameters to optimize observations of a particular bioelectric event. Specific parameters vary according to the goal of the procedure. Parameters include, but are not limited to, preamplifier gain, filter passband, and signal selection. In this chapter, we discuss instruments only as they are used to elicit and record auditory AEPs. Further, we limit the discussion to parameter generalities. Misulis (1989) provides a broader, useful reference tutorial on basic electronics for clinical neurophysiology.

All instruments have the same functional components. They are characterized by the block diagram in Figure 3-1. Most instruments have multichannel capability. For simplicity only one channel is depicted. If the instrument is multichannel, each channel has its own preamplifier and filter, which, ordinarily, are analog devices. Analog-to-digital (A/D) conversion must be available to each channel but often several channels share one converter.

The chapter concentrates on the purpose of and operator-adjustable settings for each component, starting with the recording electrodes and ending with the printout or other visualization of AEPs. We direct attention to how these components and their controls affect the recorded responses. When studying a particular AEP, the clinician has to recognize the effects and account for them.

[handwritten: A/D → switches to binary code]

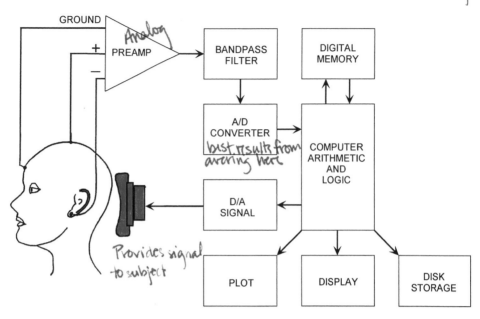

[handwritten annotations: Analog; best results from averaging here; Provides signal to subject]

FIGURE 3-1   Functional components of an evoked potential instrument.

[handwritten: AEP can only be seen by signal processing, can't be seen by naked eye]

Instrument Components

Electrodes

An **electrode** is the surface contact or interface between the patient's skin and the instrument. The most commonly used electrode is a metal contact surface and a wire with a connecting pin at the other end. The pin plugs into the input of the **preamplifier**. Different kinds of metal can be used for the contact surface. Gold, silver, and tin are most common. The metal does not contact the skin directly. An electrolyte preparation in the form of a gel or a paste, which promotes conductivity, is sandwiched between.

At least two electrodes are required to make a complete circuit with the preamplifier. The preamplifier responds to the potential difference between the two electrodes (Figure 3-2). An additional electrode connected to a convenient place on the body serves as a **ground**. The ground electrode functions as a as a common reference point, not as an instrument- or patient-to-earth connection. Each of the two electrodes is referred separately to this third or ground electrode. Thus, single-channel measurement requires three connections to the patient. When additional channels are used, each preamplifier must be connected to two electrodes but only one ground is required for all of the preamplifiers.

Amplifiers

Amplifiers magnify the tiny voltages at the head to make them large enough to register on the voltmeter, which in this case is the signal averager of the evoked potential equipment. Two factors dictate the amount of **amplification** or **gain**: (1) magnitude of the voltages at

Stimulus artifact:

Braiding: all wires will radiate (better) in the electro- magnetic field. Acts as a shield

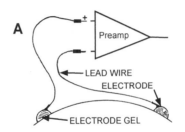

A

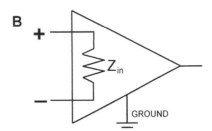

B

FIGURE 3-2 (A) Electrode connections from the head to the preamplifier (Preamp); (B) Pre- amplifier, showing input imped- ance (Z_{in}) and ground.

Good @ minimizing passing of electrical conduction (artifact)

the recording electrodes on the head, and (2) voltage needed to fill the full range of the analog-to-digital (A/D) converter. Gains reported in experimental and clinical studies range between 10,000 and 2,000,000.

Amplification usually is accomplished in two stages. Preamplification ordinarily is done by an amplifier located close to the patient. Further amplification takes place in the main evoked-potential system that may be in the same room with the patient or outside a sound-attenuating electrically shielded test booth. If all amplification were remote from the patient, the long electric leads into the evoked-potential system could be susceptible to elec- trostatic or electromagnetic noise anywhere along their lengthy passage. The need for large amplification of the tiny electroencephalic signals would lead to correspondingly large amplification of the unwanted noise as well. However, with some gain already provided by the preamplifier close to the patient, the subsequent amplification can be less. Therefore, the additional noise picked up after the preamplifier will be less and the resulting signal-to- noise ratio will be better. Careful shielding of all cable leads with secure connection of the shield to a single or common earth ground reduces noise interference from stray electric fields along their course.

Electrode leads from the patient to the preamplifier should be short. However, a com- promise usually is made between the electric desirability of short leads and the freedom that has to be given to patients to move their head without constantly exerting tension on both ends of the electrodes.

The preamplifier (or simply preamp) is the first component of the instrument proper. Usually, it is housed separately from the main chassis. It is connected to the chassis by a cable that includes control lines and power supply. The preamp most often used is a **differential amplifier** designed to accept two inputs and to produce an output proportional to their difference. The operator has access to the gain control and input pin jacks.

Manufacturers mark the two inputs to each preamp in various ways. The most popular designation is "active" and "reference." These labels may be proper in a few instances. One electrode (active) may be close to the generator in the head and the other (reference) so remote that it is essentially neutral. However, in recording AEPs of most clinical value to audiologists, both electrodes are active. They are remote enough to be considered far-field and they are placed on the head in such a way to be on opposite sides (or as nearly opposite as is feasible) of the dipole(s) generating the electricity of interest.

Another common designation of preamp inputs is "+" (plus) and "–" (minus). The + and – signs are not absolutes, that is, the place on the head to which the + electrode is attached is not always electrically positive with respect to the place on the head where the – electrode is attached. Different polarities indicate only that the electrodes may be on opposite sides of the generator(s) in the head producing the potential differences relevant to the particular application of EPA. At one moment during the analysis epoch one electrode may be more positive than the other. Several milliseconds later, polarities may reverse. As will be explained later, one input is **inverted** (usually the one labeled either "reference" or "–") and the other remains **noninverted**.

Preamps have three functions: amplification, source loading, and noise rejection.

Amplification

Bioelectric potentials range from tens of millivolts to less than a microvolt. Electronic instrument circuits usually operate in the range of several volts. Consequently, bioelectric potentials must be increased or amplified before they can be measured by the electronic instrument. The clinician must know how much the bioelectric potentials are amplified in order to measure the voltage and, therefore, must be able to control the amplification.

Gain is used to specify the amount of amplification. It is defined as the ratio of output voltage to input voltage.

$$\text{Gain} = V_{out}/V_{in}$$

For example, an input of 1 millivolt (0.001 volt) subjected to a gain of 1000 becomes an output of 1 volt. Gain is dimensionless because volts divided by volts is 1, in essence canceling the dimensional units.

In practice, gain often is not explicitly specified. Instead, the term "sensitivity" is used, defined in terms of a vertical unit of measurement on the oscilloscopic display. It is the increment of voltage that corresponds to one vertical division on the display graticule.

$$\text{Sensitivity} = \text{Voltage Unit/Vertical Scale Division}$$

Thus, it has a dimension of volts/division or, in most applications, microvolts/division.

Sensitivity information is applied in one of two reciprocal ways. When gain is fixed and sensitivity is known, measuring the amplitude (in voltage units) of a waveform in question is possible. Conversely, if the approximate amplitude of an expected waveform is known, selecting the appropriate display sensitivity for the instrument is possible.

Source Loading

When a measuring instrument is connected across a voltage source, it acts as an electric load, similar to placing a light bulb across a battery. For measurement to be made, some current must be allowed to flow from the voltage source through the instrument. Typical sources of bioelectricity are weak and cannot be loaded to any extent without altering the voltage that is to be measured. Therefore, bioelectric preamps are designed to have a large **input impedance** (Z_{in} in Figure 3-2); 10 megohms or more is typical. This allows measurement from a weak source such as the scalp with minimal source distortion.

Noise Rejection

A fundamental problem of auditory AEPs is that small signals of interest are obscured by the simultaneous presence of a much larger electric noise. Signal averaging alone may not be sufficient to unmask the AEP. Good practice dictates using all available techniques to limit noise before the averaging stage of processing.

Of particular concern is a class of interference called **common-mode noise**, which is any noise in the measurement environment that appears as equal voltage and phase at both inputs of the differential amplifier. An example of common-mode noise is environmental 60 Hz electric interference. However, one input is inverted. The inversion causes the preamp to subtract the noise from itself, thus canceling the noise (Figure 3-3). At the same time, the target signal, which has opposite phase relations in both portions of the amplifier, is enhanced as it is added to itself. The common-mode rejection just described works best when the impedances between each of the active electrodes and the ground electrode are nearly equal.

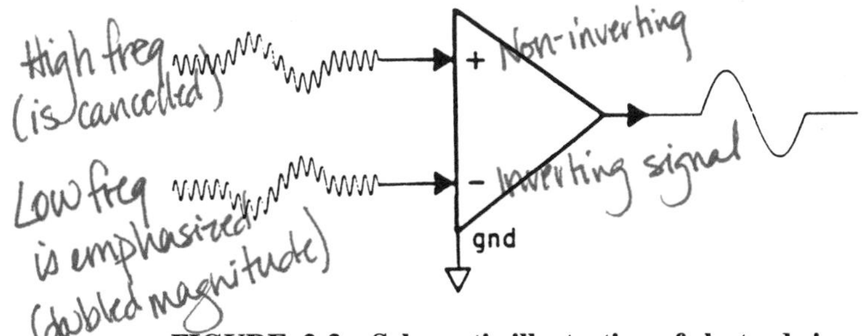

FIGURE 3-3   Schematic illustration of electrode input inversion and common-mode rejection. Upper left trace (+ input) is from the vertex electrode (non-inverting) and lower left trace (– input) is from the mastoid electrode. The high-frequency ripple (noise) has the same phase and amplitude at both electrodes but the low-frequency signal (response) has opposite phases at the same electrodes. When the electroencephalic activity represented by the lower trace is inverted in the preamplifier and added to the activity from the upper trace, the noise adds to zero (i.e., is canceled) while the signal portion is doubled in amplitude.

[© American Speech-Language-Hearing Association. Reprinted by permission.]

The degree to which a differential amplifier rejects common-mode noise is given by its **common-mode rejection ratio (CMRR)**. It is actually the preamp's gain for common-mode signals or noise. Typical CMRRs in contemporary equipment are -90 to -100 dB. The negative sign verifies that the output is smaller than the input. Noise rejection performance of preamps is the second opportunity, after using a careful electrode attachment technique, to limit noise in a measurement that is characteristically noisy.

Filters

In each channel of the measuring instrument, the preamplifier is followed by an analog filter. The evoked potential signal of interest and the background noise each has its own spectrum. Most often, the noise bandwidth exceeds that of the signal of interest. Because the signal and the noise occur simultaneously, their spectra are superimposed. Therefore, both signal and noise contribute many of the same frequencies in the resulting spectrum. An operator may set the filter passband to reject or reduce noise above and below the anticipated spectral range of the response signal. This filtering improves the signal-to-noise ratio by reducing the noise. Filtering, however, cannot remove the noise that shares spectra with the signal. Therefore, signal averaging still is necessary to uncover or unmask the AEP even after filtering.

In the future, most, if not all, of the commercial evoked potential systems probably will be equipped only with digital filters. However, most contemporary systems depend primarily on analog filters. Therefore, the stress in this section is on analog filters. Details about the actual structure of either analog or digital filters are beyond the scope of this book but the general nature and performance of filters are discussed. Cook and Miller (1992) and Marsh (1988) provide helpful tutorials on digital filtering of AEPs.

Filters may be either **low-** or **high-pass** or they may be **bandpass** (Figure 3-4). In reported clinical applications of EPA, only bandpass filters have been used. The particular clinical application determines the filter passband. In common clinical applications of early potentials or the ABR, for example, the high-pass end (often labeled "low-cut" by instrument manufacturers) of the passband may be 100 Hz and the low-pass end (often labeled "high-cut") may be 3000 Hz. Other passbands are more favorable for other AEP indices and their applications.

The **frequency response** of the filter is displayed in a graph that shows the relation between the input signal components and those at the output. Filter parameters of major concern to the operator are the cutoff frequencies, slope of the rejection skirt and evenness or linearity of the output/input function between the cutoff frequencies. Differences in the electronic configuration of filters also affect the nature of the energy that passes through the filter (Hyde, 1994a).

Ideally, the filter output at each frequency should be equally proportional to the input. Said differently, the graphic function between the cutoff frequencies should be a horizontal straight line, a plateau. Filters in most contemporary commercial evoked-potential systems do have linear or nearly linear plateaus. For a given input voltage, the output usually differs by no more than 1 to 2 dB at any frequency. Nevertheless, filter frequency response characteristics should be measured before clinical work with a new unit begins, and periodically thereafter.

Cutoff frequencies for filter passbands are those low and high frequencies at which the

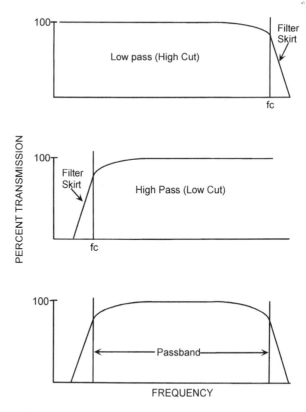

FIGURE 3-4   Schematic representation of low-pass (high-cut), high-pass (low-cut), and bandpass filters. The frequency at which transmission is 3 dB down from 100% is designated by fc.

output for a given input is 3 dB lower (half power) than the output in the linear plateau. Operators must set the high- and low-pass frequencies according to the requirements of the target AEP. Ideally, clinicians should be able to set their filters at any frequency. This requires filters with continuous adjustment. Filter settings on most commercial systems are not continuous. Instead, certain discrete cutoffs are designed into a given instrument. If a test protocol specifies filter settings that are not available, settings that are as close as possible should be used.

Attenuation for frequencies outside the filter passband can be configured many different ways. Usually, attenuation is linear when output is plotted with relative dB on the ordinate and frequency on the logarithmic abscissa. Slope generally is specified as dB per octave. Filter cutoff slopes or skirts vary in steepness from as shallow as 3 dB/octave to as steep as 96 dB/octave. Commercial units often have linear filter skirts of 12 dB/octave. Steep slopes have the obvious advantage of excluding more energy outside the filter passband than can be excluded by shallow slopes. The downside of steepness is increased distortion, especially for the frequencies close to the cutoff frequencies. **Phase shift** is one troublesome distortion. **Phase lags** and **phase leads** can lead to *apparent* latency shifts

(Figure 3-5). The word apparent is stressed because neural activity that generates a peak of interest is not affected by the filtering. It is the time of appearance of the peak in the AEP trace that can be advanced or delayed.

A second form of filter distortion is the attenuation of some spectral energy that helps to define the peak. Filtering out unwanted noise also may lead to reduction of valuable or contributory spectral energy. Through a combination of phase and amplitude distortion, analog filtering can eliminate some peaks entirely.

Consequences of distortion are serious if the clinician or experimenter wishes to use the **time-amplitude configuration** of the AEP to determine exactly when an event occurred in the brain, what its possible source or generator might be, and what the peaks may imply physiologically. On the other hand, distortion may have no negative consequences, and may even be desirable, if only correlative information is being sought from the AEPs. An example of the value of intentional distortion is in threshold EPA. Distortions in the AEP caused by the recording filter may allow the operator to be more certain about response replicability and about the systematic change in AEP peak latencies and amplitudes as a function of signal level. Therefore, correlation between EPA thresholds and probable behavioral response thresholds may be made more confidently.

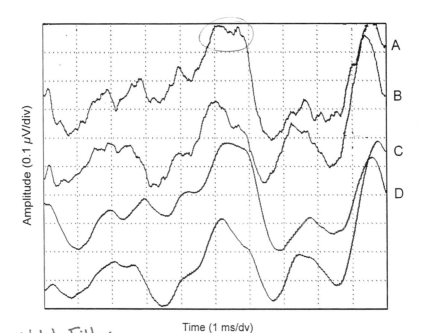

Time (1 ms/dv)

FIGURE 3-5   AEP recorded simultaneously from a single electrode pair (Cz-M1) through four different filter passbands: (A) 100-3000 Hz, the usual filter passband; (B) 1–3000 Hz; (C) 100-1000 Hz; (D) 1–1000 Hz. Differences in peak amplitudes and peak latencies are artifacts of the analog filters. An upward deflection represents positivity of the vertex electrode (Cz) relative to the mastoid electrode (M1).

One of the largest and most troublesome artifacts is 60 Hz from power outlets and from adjacent active equipment being powered by those outlets. In clinical environments that are electrically hostile, a disturbing 60 Hz artifact may bleed through the bandpass filter even though the high-pass end of the filter is 100 Hz or higher. Some evoked-potential systems are equipped with **notch filters**. The notch with its antiresonant point at 60 Hz is narrow (e.g., 6 Hz) and can reduce 60 Hz by as much as 30 dB. The notch filter may reduce the 60 Hz artifact effectively (Marsh, 1991) but it is plagued by two problems. First, it can distort the resulting AEP in a major way through phase shifting. Second, although 60 Hz and neighboring frequencies may not be major spectral components of the ABR, the most commonly used response index, they are major contributors to the definition of other AEP indices used for audiometric and otoneurologic purposes. Effects of filters on specific AEP components will be discussed further in later chapters. At this point, clinicians are advised to use 60 Hz notch filters only in exceptional circumstances, or not at all.

A big risk of large 60 Hz artifact is that the signal repetition rate could lock in on one phase of the 60 Hz. The process of signal averaging will then enhance rather than wash out the 60 Hz artifact. Risk of artifact enhancement increases if the signal repetition rate is 60/s or some even harmonic or subharmonic of 60/s. When early and middle latency auditory AEPs were first studied, using a 10/s signal rate was common. Now it is more customary to use a non-integer rate—for example, 11.1/s—to reduce the likelihood of locking in on the 60 Hz artifact.

When a clinician does threshold EPA, the expectation is that thresholds obtained will be the same as they would have been had an audiologist been able to evaluate the patient by reliable behavioral response audiometry for the same test signals. For this specific purpose, no physiologic interpretations are expected to emerge from the time-amplitude configuration of the AEP. Distortions in the AEP caused by the recording filter when it is used to reduce the obscuring noise may allow the clinician to be more certain about response replicability and about the systematic changes in AEP peak latencies and amplitudes as a function of signal level. Therefore, as pointed out earlier, correlation between EPA thresholds and probable behavioral response thresholds may be made more confidently.

Response filtering with its attendant distortion also occurs in voluntary behavioral response audiometry, especially pure-tone threshold audiometry. The audiologist does not put earphones on a patient without instruction, present sounds from the adjacent control room, and expect the patient to free-associate about the test signals. Instead, the patient is placed in an unnatural listening environment, fitted with earphones, which are not the sources of sounds to which the patient ordinarily listens, asked to listen to sounds that never occur by themselves in nature, and asked to attend carefully to uncustomarily weak sounds. Further, the patient is asked to respond by raising a finger or a hand or by pushing a button, actions rarely taken in daily response to sound. Nevertheless, behavioral response thresholds obtained in this filtered and distorted way yield powerful information about the integrity of the patient's peripheral auditory mechanism and even some insight into the patient's ability to communicate through hearing. Similarly, EPA thresholds reliably obtained from filtered and distorted AEPs yield powerful information about some aspects of the patient's ability to hear.

Digital filters, properly constructed and integrated into the recording system, do not cause the phase shifts that one sees with analog filters (Cook & Miller, 1992). Also, some digital filters are more effective than analog filters in reducing noise for equivalent passbands (Møller, 1988). Unfortunately, however, digital filters are more expensive than analog filters and usually are not standard features of most contemporary commercial evoked potential systems. Nevertheless, many commercial systems have the capacity for post-averaging digital filtering. The AEP, which may be stored on a hard drive or on accessory disk units, can be retrieved from storage and filtered through a passband or several different passbands of the clinician's choice. This post-averaging filtering causes no phase leads or lags, or what appear to be actual latency changes. Furthermore, the post-averaging filtering does not alter the original waveform held in storage. An example of post-averaging filtering is shown in Figure 3-6.

Some systems that do not have either front-end digital filtering or post-averaging capabilities still can do a form of post-averaging digital filtering known as **smoothing**. In 3-point smoothing, for example, the amplitude value at each address in the analysis window is weighted with the amplitude in the address on either side and then averaged. The net result

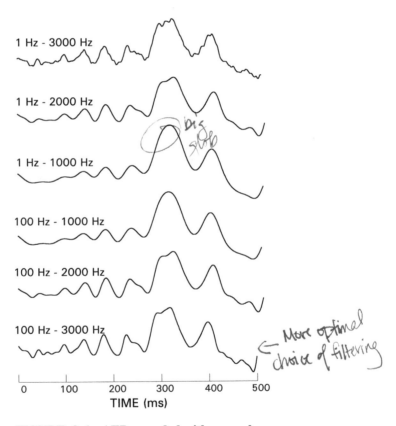

FIGURE 3-6   AEP recorded with an analog filter passband of 1–3000 Hz, and then, post-averaging, was digitally filtered through several selected narrower passbands. Note that that there are no phase shifts.

is a reduction in some of the high-frequency ripple that often is superimposed on the larger, lower-frequency peaks. No phase shifts occur. An example of 3-point smoothing is shown in Figure 3-7. The smoothing, which is, in effect, low-pass filtering, makes the resulting AEP trace less jagged than the original and may make peak identification and measurement easier. The smoothing process can be repeated if the clinician still is not satisfied with the cleanliness of the trace. Information lost through 3-point smoothing cannot be retrieved. Therefore, careful forethought must be given to its use. If many traces are obtained in a test procedure, which usually is the case, then the same number of 3-point smoothings should be applied to each trace. Otherwise, inter-trace comparisons may be hampered.

Because of the uncertainties attendant to filtering, no one kind of filter and no one specific passband can be recommended for all EPA applications. It will become even more apparent in later chapters that the peculiar circumstances of each EPA application dictate the filter conditions. If the clinician has no clear guidelines for filter conditions, less rather than more filtering should be used. When in doubt, use the widest filter passband and the shallowest filter skirts that the noise in the recording will allow.

Artifact Rejection

The need for filtering noise in a recording can be reduced by using an **artifact reject circuit**. These are standard in most evoked potential systems. Each successive digitized trace first goes to a buffer where it is examined for any voltages that exceed some pre-set level. If all voltages are at or below a pre-set level, then the digitized voltages are dumped to the memory unit for averaging with prior and succeeding traces. Conversely, if excessive volt-

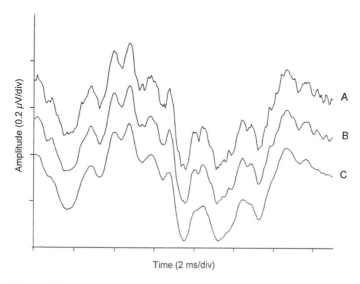

FIGURE 3-7 **(A) AEP obtained with a 100–3000 Hz passband. (B) Same AEP after 3-point smoothing. (C) Same AEP after second 3-point smoothing.**

age is found at any address in the analysis window or epoch, then that sample in the buffer is erased instead of being forwarded to the averaging memory. This process prevents spuriously large potentials that are essentially noise from dominating and distorting an AEP.

Analog-to-Digital Conversion

All signal processing discussed to this point, except artifact rejection, has been performed by analog devices. Electrodes, preamps, and filters all operate on continuously variable voltages. *Continuously variable* implies that there are no time gaps during which the signal does not exist. By contrast, the averaging process that removes the masked evoked potentials from the background noise is performed by a digital computer. This presents two problems. First, no digital computer has enough memory to store all values of a continuous analog voltage. Second, calculations are made with digital numbers instead of with ordinary arithmetic. Converting analog voltage into digital form (A/D conversion) is a two-step process that solves both problems.

The problem of insufficient memory is solved by sampling. The solution is provided by reference to Figures 2-9 and 2-10. Each figure shows a continuous analog voltage that varies with time. The curves show that voltage is defined for every instant of time between 0 and T seconds. It is not necessary, however, to know all of the continuous values to represent the shape of the curve. At the instant the A/D converter is given a start command, samples of the continuously changing voltage are taken at regular intervals. Each sample voltage is converted to digital form before the next sample is taken. Commercial instruments commonly will take 256 (2^8), 512 (2^9), or 1024 (2^{10}) samples over the interval during which the A/D converter observes the incoming voltage. The clinician sets the appropriate observation interval at the time of testing.

Figure 2-10 shows a series of sample points taken at the successive time points. The sampling theorem of Nyquist specifies the minimum sampling frequency. It requires that samples be taken at twice the frequency of the highest spectral component in the analog function. (Examples were given in Chapter 2.) If that is accomplished, the analog waveform can be reconstructed faithfully from the samples. Insufficient sampling frequency results in distortion of the analog waveform through aliasing (see Figure 2-11). The final panels in Figure 2-9 and 2-10 show the result of conversion from a continuously varying waveform to a set of samples. The curve now is defined only at times for which there is a sample. Inside the computer memory, the samples are represented as a list of values and their corresponding times.

The second problem, requiring a digital representation of each sample, is solved by a process called **quantizing**. Inside a digital computer, numbers are represented in binary form, that is, the numeric base is 2. Each place or bit in the binary number is rendered either as a zero (0) or a one (1). The whole binary number is a series of zeros and ones. Its length establishes the number's precision. Common number lengths range from 8 bits to 32 bits. An 8-bit number can assume any of 256 (2^8) values (0 through 255); therefore, it can specify a number to a precision of better than $\frac{1}{2}$%. Sixteen-bit (and larger) numbers obviously have still finer precision.

The first job of the A/D converter is to sample the input at a given instant and to determine which of the finite possible values of the digital number most closely matches it. Then, that value is given to the computer for storage in a predetermined location in memory. Now that both problems have been solved, a digital representation of the original analog waveform is stored in the computer and available for computation.

Precision of digitizers is wasted if the signal to be digitized is small. Therefore, amplification should be great enough to fill the digitizer so that its full range is used. No one amplification can be specified because of the variety of AEPs used clinically and the variety of circumstances under which they are used. However, a useful guideline is to amplify the electrophysiologic activity sufficiently so that responses to about 5% of signals presented during any test run will be rejected by the artifact reject system.

Computer

The term computer can refer to anything from a single microprocessor chip to a massive mainframe system like the one used by the Internal Revenue Service. A general purpose neurodiagnostic instrument can be viewed as a special purpose digital computer. It consists of a microprocessor that serves as the central processor unit (CPU), a number of forms of input/output (I/O), and memory. The memory contains the controlling program, space for storage of waveforms, and room for computations with intermediate results.

The special-purpose computer has several key functions. Most obvious, perhaps, is the averaging needed to reveal an AEP waveform. Just as critical, however, are generation and timing of test signals, control of data collection, organization of data in memory, and communication with the operator. Commercially available instruments vary in the amount of computer literacy needed to operate them. Some units have their program in read only memory (ROM) while others require the program to be loaded from a floppy diskette or internal hard drive.

Manufacturers usually provide in-service training in the use of their evoked potential systems. Nevertheless, clinicians should study the instrument manual provided thoroughly before attempting to operate new equipment. Also, becoming computer literate is useful. Literacy enables the clinician to exploit the full capabilities of the instrument and to recognize its limitations.

Stimulus Generation

The computer generates the electric signal that is then delivered to the earphone or other acoustic transducer. Electric signals may be as simple as a 100 μs rectangular pulse or more complex such as a gated sinusoid with specified rise/fall time and plateau. Stimulus generation usually is done in one of two ways. In one, the CPU supplies a trigger pulse to an external analog circuit that produces the required electric waveform. In the other, the CPU calculates digitally the values that define the waveform and then uses digital-to-analog (D/A) conversion to produce the waveform.

Display

The display is the primary means by which the clinician obtains information from the instrument. The information takes two forms. First, like any computer terminal, the instrument displays alphanumeric characters, those entered by the operator and those generated by the program. This exchange of information allows the operator to control the instrument and the instrument to inform the operator of its status. Second, the instrument uses the display to present the evoked potential data. Many instruments allow the operator to view both the real-time input from the amplifiers and the averaged waveform from the computer memory. Waveform display is in the same format as on any digital oscilloscope. The vertical axis is voltage defined by the operator-set sensitivity (i.e., μV/division). The horizontal axis is time, defined by either total sweep time (i.e., ms) or by the time rate of the sweep trace (i.e., ms/division). It is common for the display to register both character and waveform information simultaneously.

Storage

The clinician collects more than one waveform during EPA. Storage of waveforms with their descriptive information can be done in one of two ways. Each instrument has a volatile memory, as described above. It is called volatile because it loses its information when the instrument is turned off. Not only is this memory temporary, but usually the amount of it that the program assigns to waveform storage is limited. For example, it may hold only four responses including the one being collected. When temporary waveform memory is filled, the waveforms must be plotted out and the memory cleared before continuing with the data collection protocol.

Magnetic disks, either diskettes or hard drive, are another form of storage. They have the advantage of permanent storage capability. Data stored on magnetic media are compact. Thus, large quantities of clinical information occupy little space. Data in magnetic storage can be retrieved into the computer for later inspection or analysis. Further, diskettes can be copied and exchanged between users of the same or compatible instruments.

Plotter

Waveforms obtained from patients have little value if they remain in instrumental storage. The simplest way of externalizing the computer's data is to plot them on paper. The paper can be incorporated into a formal clinical report. Forms taken by plotters and printers are diverse. A printer may be a general purpose add-on device or it may be integrated into the instrument's main chassis. Printout varies from draft quality dot-matrix to publication quality laser print. Some instruments print/plot waveforms with the barest labeling while others allow the audiologist to enter test data and impressions that are incorporated into a finished report. Whatever the print-out mechanism, it is usually the component of the entire evoked potential system most likely to malfunction.

Chapter 4

Test Signals

The focus of this chapter is on signals commonly used to elicit stimulus-related potentials (SRPs). Circumstances under which event-related potentials (ERPs) are elicited are too varied to allow discussion of signals used to elicit ERPs apart from the specific test circumstances.

Customary clinical applications of SRPs are threshold audiometry and otoneurologic diagnosis. Clicks are the most commonly used signals for both purposes, although other signals also are used for threshold audiometry. We shall discuss signals only in relation to threshold audiometry.

The word signal is used here instead of the more popular **stimulus**. Stimulus implies sound strong enough to have activated the cochlea and auditory nerve. A signal, on the other hand, still is a signal even if it is not above a patient's threshold. In threshold audiometry, audiologists commonly present test signals below a patient's threshold, that is, too weak to have been a stimulus.

Thresholds determined by EPA are the same as thresholds determined by behavioral response audiometry when the same signals and the same criteria for threshold are used for both procedures. Furthermore, the clinical interpretation of an audiogram or other threshold measure derived from either procedure is the same. EPA has not displaced behavioral response audiometry as the routine procedure of choice for threshold audiometry. However, thresholds cannot be assessed in some populations (e.g., neonates, adults who are severely retarded) by behavioral response procedures, especially with procedures that require voluntary responses.

The question to be asked by the clinician who does threshold EPA is "What would threshold have been had I been able to determine it reliably by voluntary, behavioral threshold audiometry?" Ideally, then, the clinician should use the same signals for EPA as are used in conventional behavioral response audiometry: tonal signals with a minimum of 20 ms rise/fall time and a minimum plateau of 150 ms (ANSI, 1989). Unfortunately, recording circumstances required to observe SRPs to these conventional signals force clinicians to look at long-latency SRPs whose configuration and general properties are influenced greatly by subject state (e.g., awake or asleep, degree of alertness when awake, medication). Wide swings in subject state, especially in patients for whom threshold EPA is most necessary, lead to serious limitations in the confidence with which the tester can judge whether the test signal elicited a response. Response reliability usually makes clinicians favor SRPs that occur within the first 50 ms after signal onset. This time restriction in turn dictates the use of test signals test signals of shorter duration than those used in conventional behavioral response audiometry.

Types of Test Signals

Clicks

Clicks are the most commonly used short-duration signals. They are generated by delivering rectangular electric waves or pulses (Figure 4-1A) to an earphone or other transducer. The electric pulses cause the transducer to ring and to produce short-duration acoustic signals described as clicks because of how they are perceived audibly. The most commonly used pulse duration is 0.1 ms or 100 μs, although no clinical rationale has been given for this specific duration. The resulting sound often is called a "100 microsecond click"; however, as shown in Figure 4-1A, the measurable duration of the acoustic signal is longer. Click duration ordinarily ranges between 1 and 2 ms depending on the voltage delivered to the transducer and on the physical characteristics of the transducer.

An example of the click spectrum is shown in Figure 4-1B. Spectrum varies with the transducer and closely parallels the frequency response curve of the transducer. For reasons that are not entirely appropriate, the click often is called a "high-frequency click." Nevertheless, because of the resonance characteristics of most earphones, usually there is slightly more energy in the 2000–4000 Hz region than in lower and higher frequency bands.

The polarity of the electric pulse (+ or –) determines whether the initial portion of the acoustic signal will be rarefaction or condensation (see Figure 4-1A). For some patients, the early potentials (EP or ABR) differ significantly for what is called a **rarefaction click** compared to a **condensation click** (Borg & Löfqvist, 1981; Coats & Martin, 1977; Jacobson, Jacobson, Ramadan, & Hyde, 1994). Therefore, the clinician should be certain of the acoustic polarity of the click.

Polarity of the electric pulse is no predictor of the polarity of the acoustic pulse, that is, a positive-going electric pulse is no guarantee of an initial acoustic condensation, and a negative-going electric pulse is no guarantee of an initial acoustic rarefaction. The way in which the electric generator is wired to the transducer is the main determinant. Manufacturers of signal averagers check polarity relations at the factory so that when their instrument reads RARE (a common prompt), the initial acoustic wave is a rarefaction; likewise, COND will lead to an initial condensation wave. If the clinician modifies the manufacturer's wiring or if there is uncertainty about the validity of the instrument panel's prompts, the relation between the prompt and the polarity should be verified acoustically.

For weak signal levels, rarefaction clicks will be nearly mirror images of condensation clicks (see Figure 4-1A). When signal levels are strong, click symmetry may break down. Therefore, the clinician may err in believing that rarefaction and condensation clicks are identical at strong signal levels except for polarity. Levels at which the clicks deviate from symmetry vary with the nature of the transducer and with the abuse to which the transducer may have been subjected.

DC pulse will not always create a condensation; no relationship (depends how it was set up + measured)

Signal could've been created w/ either + or - polarity

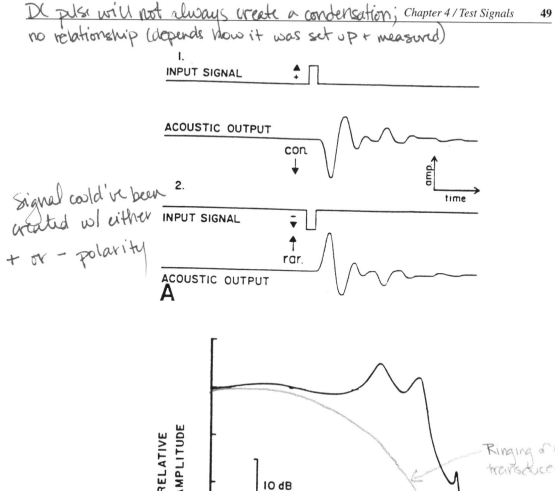

OE + ME response will effect this response

Ringing of the transducer

FIGURE 4-1 **Transduction of a 100 µs DC pulse by an earphone (Telephonics TDH-39). (A1) Condensation (con.); (A2) rarefaction (rar.). Note the opposite phases of the acoustic output for the two input signals and the greater than 100 ms duration of both acoustic outputs. (B) Spectrum of the acoustic click.**

[Modified and reprinted with permission from Durrant, "Fundamentals of sound generation." In E. J. Moore (Ed.), *Bases of Auditory Brain-Stem Evoked Responses*. New York: Grune & Stratton, 1983.]

Clicks are useful signals for obtaining a general estimate of the patient's auditory sensitivity. However, because the click spectrum is so broad, determining a patient's AEP threshold as a function of frequency, such as one does in conventional pure-tone audiometry, is impossible. A procedure (detailed in a later chapter) has been described for extrapolating some frequency-specific information from what is called the **latency-intensity function** of the auditory brainstem response (ABR). Those extrapolations are crude, however, and are clinically limited.

Narrow-Spectrum Signals

As mentioned earlier, it is impractical to use the same long tonal signals for EPA as are used conventionally in voluntary behavioral response audiometry. However, shorter duration signals with relatively narrow spectra and some tonality can be used. EPA thresholds with these signals yield a closer approximation of the pure-tone audiogram than can be extrapolated from AEPs to clicks. One type of narrow-spectrum signal used for threshold EPA is the **tone pip** (Davis, Silverman, & McAuliffe, 1951; Davis & Zerlin, 1966; Zerlin & Naunton, 1974). The tone pip is generated by ringing an electric filter with a brief rectangular electric pulse.

Although not a pure sinusoid, the main activity of the tone pip has the periodicity of the resonant frequency of the filter. Tone pips usually have unequal rise and fall times. Time-magnitude characteristics of the acoustic signal are determined by the electronic filter characteristics, by the characteristics of the transducer, and by the signal level. The tone pip has no plateau; its amplitude begins to diminish after the maximum magnitude is attained. The spectrum of a tone pip has the largest concentration of acoustic energy in one frequency region but there is considerable spread of energy above and below that frequency region. Tone pips are used infrequently now for tonal threshold EPA mainly because of wide spectral spread of acoustic energy. They have been supplanted by **gated tone bursts**. The distinction between tone pips and tone bursts is not always clear in the literature because at times the term "tone pips" is used for either tone pips or tone bursts. The name for short-duration narrow-spectrum signals is inconsequential clinically. However, we maintain the distinction here because of the dissimilar ways by which they are generated.

Gated tone bursts are generated by allowing an ongoing electric signal of a given frequency to be passed through an electronic gate. The gate will determine the nature and rate of the onset, the plateau duration (if any), and the nature and rate of the fall time. Usually, the rise time and the fall time are identical. The gated electric signal is delivered to the transducer whose acoustic output should resemble the electric input. Figure 4-2 shows the time-amplitude configuration and the corresponding spectra of tone bursts with 3 ms rise/fall times and no plateau. The tone bursts are not pure tones, that is, they do not have single-line spectra. Nevertheless, the spectra of these short tone bursts have most of their energy concentrated around the fundamental frequency. The 3 dB down or half-power bandwidth is about 200 Hz. The strongest sidebands are well below the level of the fundamental. When weak levels are used, as in a threshold search, the fundamental clearly dominates the signal. Nevertheless, sidebands still may be of concern for those patients with steeply sloping high-frequency or low-frequency hearing losses.

Figure 4-3 shows the acoustic waveforms and power spectra for 500 Hz tone bursts with different rise/fall times and equivalent durations ($\frac{2}{3}$ rise time + plateau) (Dallos &

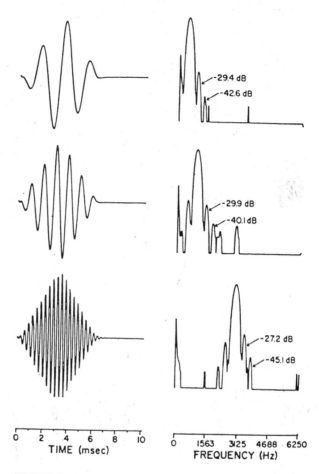

TIME (msec)

FREQUENCY (Hz)

FIGURE 4-2 Acoustic waveform and acoustic spectrum for tone bursts with 3 ms rise/fall time and no plateau. The half-power bandwidth (3 dB down from the power of the fundamental frequency) is about 200 Hz.

[Reprinted by permission from McFarland, Vivion, Wolf, & Goldstein, "Middle components of the AER to tone-pips in normal-hearing and hearing-impaired subjects." *Journal of Speech and Hearing Research, 20*, 781–798. ©American Speech-Language-Hearing Association.]

Olsen, 1964). Half-power bandwidth for a tone burst with 5 ms rise/fall time and no plateau is about 100 Hz. We recommend tone bursts with 5 ms rise/fall time and 1 ms plateau for threshold EPA. With that configuration, the strongest sidebands are nearly 30 dB below the level of the fundamental.

The type of window through which the electric signal for the tone burst is passed affects the spectral spread of the resultant acoustic energy (Gorga, Beauchaine, Kaminski,

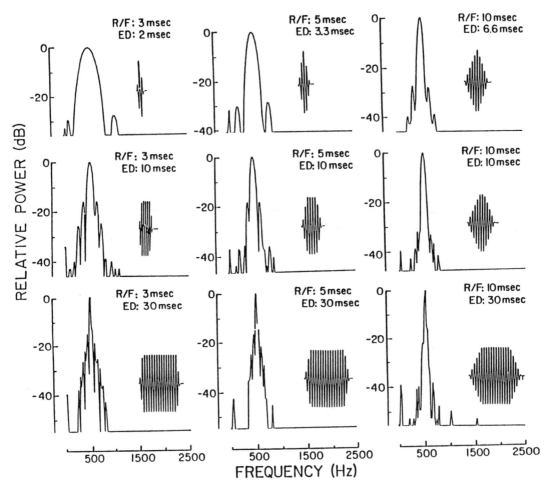

FIGURE 4-3   **Acoustic waveforms and power spectra of 500 Hz tone bursts with various rise/fall times, plateaus, and equivalent durations (ED)(2/3 rise time + plateau). Waveforms and spectra for other frequencies are the same except for fundamental frequency.**

[Reprinted from Vivion, Hirsch, Frye-Osier, & Goldstein, "Effects of stimulus rise-fall time and equivalent duration on middle components of AER." *Scandinavian Audiology*, 9:223–232, by permission of Scandinavian University Press, Oslo, 1980.]

& Bergman, 1992; Gorga & Thornton, 1989; Robier, Fabry, Leek, & Van Summers, 1992). However, unless sidebands are less than 25 dB below the fundamental tone, differences in resulting threshold measures will be small in comparison to the precision of EPA thresholds achievable under most circumstances. When signal levels are reduced close to the level of audibility, as is always the case in threshold audiometry, the fundamental or test frequency dominates the spectrum of the test signal.

Some investigators have used the same temporal configuration across all frequencies (e.g., 5 ms rise/fall time and no plateau)(Kupperman & Mendel, 1974; Thornton, Mendel,

& Anderson, 1977; Vivion, Hirsch, Frye-Osier, & Goldstein, 1980). Other investigators have used rise times with a fixed number of cycles, especially when examining the first 15 to 20 ms of post-stimulus activity (Beattie & Kennedy, 1992; Davis, Hirsh, Turpin, & Peacock, 1985; Gorga & Thornton, 1989). In the latter case, the rise time for a low-frequency signal is longer than the rise time for a high-frequency signal. If, for example, the rise time is to be two complete cycles, the rise time will be 4 ms for a 500 Hz tone burst and only 1 ms for a 2000 Hz tone burst. No convincing evidence argues that one kind of rise time is more valid than another for threshold EPA in practical clinical situations in which wider analysis windows may have to be used and in which precision of threshold estimation is limited. Therefore, we recommend using a fixed rise time just as is done with the longer duration signals used in conventional behavioral response audiometry.

Either tone pips or tone bursts may be used as narrow-spectrum signals for threshold EPA, and the thresholds determined with each may be the same if the spectra are nearly the same. Tone bursts have the advantage of being more manipulable than tone pips in terms of rise/fall time and total duration, and can be adjusted to have considerably narrower spectra than can be achieved with tone pips. Still other kinds of narrow-spectrum signals have been used for threshold EPA (e.g., logon, notched noise) but none has been shown to be more clinically valid or convenient than tone bursts.

Transducers

Air Conduction

Test signals most often are delivered monotically through one of several types of earphones. One type is the standard electromagnetic earphone (e.g., TDH-39 or TDH-49) mounted in supra-aural cushions (e.g., MX41/AR) (see Figure 4-4A). Sometimes the standard phone and cushion are mounted in a sound-attenuating circumaural casing (Figure 4-4B). Testing must be done at times in hostile acoustic environments; the casing provides some attenuation beyond that provided by the standard cushions.

Standard electromagnetic earphones have two disadvantages. First, because they are usually mounted in tension-producing headbands, they become uncomfortable during the test. This is especially true for the dome-mounted earphones. Second, standard earphones are close to those recording electrodes attached to the mastoid or the earlobe. The electromagnetic and electrostatic fields generated by the earphone may induce **signal artifacts** in the recording electrodes. These artifacts can be considerably larger than the electroencephalic activity, especially at strong signal levels, and can interfere seriously with response identification. Interference is especially disturbing if the clinician is trying to observe the **cochlear microphonic (CM), summating potential (SP),** and waves I and II of what is called the auditory brainstem response (ABR). It is important, therefore, that these earphones be carefully shielded and grounded to reduce artifact induction.

One ploy to reduce signal artifact in the recording is to alternate the polarity of each successive click. The rationale for this is that the AEP will differ only little as a function of polarity. Adding and averaging the responses, therefore, should result in an AEP closely resembling the response to either a rarefaction or a condensation click. The artifact, on the

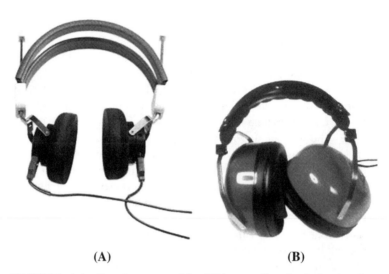

(A)   (B)

FIGURE 4-4   Earphones used for EPA as well as for behavioral
response audiometry. (A) TDH-39 mounted in supra-aural cushions;
(B) same TDH-39 with earphone covered by circumaural sound-
attenuating casing.

[Photos courtesy of Cadwell Laboratories, Inc. Cadwell is a registered trademark of Cadwell Laboratories, Inc.]

other hand, will be exactly out of phase as a function of polarity; therefore, adding and averaging with alternating rarefaction and condensation clicks should lead to a complete can-
cellation of the signal artifact in the resulting AEP.

Two cautions are given about the use of alternating polarity clicks. First, as previously
mentioned, in some patients, AEPs for rarefaction and condensation clicks will be distinctly different. AEPs to alternating clicks can disguise what might be a diagnostically
important abnormality. Some evoked-potential systems allow the electroencephalic activity
following rarefaction clicks to be stored in one memory bank and the activity following the
condensation clicks in a separate bank. If, on viewing the separate AEPs, the audiologist
notes little difference, then the two traces can be added and averaged to help cancel the
early signal artifact. The second caution is that the rarefaction and condensation artifacts
may not be exact mirror images of each other, especially with strong signal levels when the
artifacts may be huge and the polarity symmetry tends to break down.

One way of reducing large signal artifacts is to use a loudspeaker sufficiently remote
from the patient and the recording electrodes. A major disadvantage of loudspeakers is the
difficulty of keeping the non-test ear from being stimulated. Also, because of the large
mass of air to be driven, it may not be possible to present undistorted signals at a sufficiently high level to reach threshold for the seriously impaired patient. The patient whose
sensitivity is not seriously impaired ordinarily can be tested under earphones because the
test signals can be weak enough not to induce interfering artifacts in the recording system.
Loudspeakers, of course, eliminate the problem of trying to constrain a squirmy child or
adult under earphones. The downside of that advantage is that movements of the patient's

head invalidate the calibration of the loudspeaker, which is measured with a stationary instrument.

A transducer (Etymotic ER-3A) that reduces the problems of signal artifact in the recording and the discomfort of ordinary earphones is shown in Figure 4-5A. The output of the transducer is delivered through a 25 cm long plastic tube. The other end of the tube is passed through a pliable ear protector (Etymotic ER3–14) that can be molded snugly and comfortably in the external auditory meatus. Distance of the electroacoustic transducer from the recording electrode limits the amount of electromagnetic artifact that can be induced in the recording electrodes. The length of the tube increases the acoustic transmission time from the transducer to the ear. Therefore, about 0.8 ms has to be subtracted from the peak latency measurements of the AEP if the clinician wishes to report absolute latencies.

Figure 4-5B shows the frequency response of the transducer system illustrated in Figure 4-5A. The curve is acceptably flat throughout most of its range. However, the output drops too sharply beyond 4000 Hz to be used for measuring the threshold of auditory sensitivity above that frequency.

A related type of transducer system was developed primarily for use with newborn babies and young infants. The transducers are mounted in a headband that does place them a little closer to the recording electrodes than with the other system. In this system, however, the plug that is inserted into the external auditory meatus is so constructed that it doubles as one of the recording electrodes. Its mesh-like material is impregnated with an electrode jelly. Because that electrode is in the ear canal, it is closer to the generator of the **whole nerve action potential (WNAP)** than is an electrode either on the earlobe or on the mastoid.

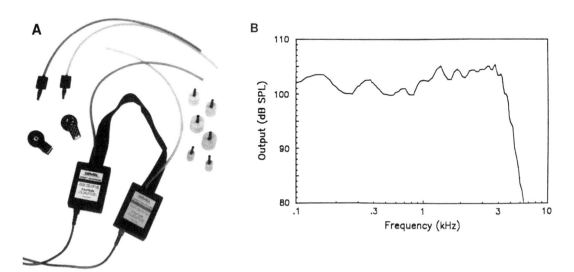

FIGURE 4-5 **(A) Popular form of insert earphone transducer (Etymotic ER-3A) with plastic tubing and other accessories. (B) Frequency-response curve for the earphone.**

[Photo of earphone system courtesy of Cadwell Laboratories, Inc. Cadwell is a registered trademark of Cadwell Laboratories, Inc.]

Bone Conduction

Test signals for EPA can be delivered by bone conduction just as they are in conventional voluntary behavioral response audiometry. Two problems plague bone-conduction EPA. First of these is large signal artifact. More electric energy is required to drive a bone-conduction transducer than an air-conduction transducer for threshold level signals. Correspondingly, electromagnetic radiation is greater. If one recording electrode is near the mastoid placement of the bone-conduction vibrator, the recording, especially the first few milliseconds, can be completely obscured by signal artifact.

A second problem with bone-conduction EPA is that the bone-conduction vibrator output for a 100 μs electric pulse input differs from the click output of a standard earphone for that same input. The bone-conduction vibrator output contains proportionately less high-frequency energy than the output of most air-conduction earphones (Cone-Wesson, 1995; Schwartz, Larson, & DeChicchis, 1985; Yang, Stuart, Stenstrom, & Green, 1987). The spectral difference is particularly important if one tries to compare the air-conduction and bone-conduction EPs (ABRs) from the same patient. On the other hand, tone bursts with more gradual rise/fall times (e.g., 5 ms) than clicks produce outputs that are more nearly comparable across all transducers. The down side of bone-conducted tone bursts is the long signal artifact that is almost impossible to control or to filter without serious distortion to the resulting AEPs. However, if bone-conduction thresholds as a function of frequency is the goal of EPA, then the first 10 to 12 ms of the resulting AEP can be ignored. Judgments of response or no response can be made from the remaining 38 to 40 ms of a 50 ms AEP.

Calibration

No physical calibration standards exist for clicks or for narrow-spectrum signals as they do for longer duration signals used in conventional pure-tone audiometry. Juries of young normal-hearing listeners have to be convened to establish psychophysical thresholds for the short-duration signals to be used in the specific EPA application, and under the conditions (e.g., signal rate) appropriate to that application. The 0 dB Hearing Levels so established have been designated as **HL, nHL** or **HLn**, where **n** stands for normal.

Measuring the physical equivalent of 0 dB HL for purposes of clinic calibration and inter-clinic comparisons is important. Acoustic output at some fixed hearing level, e.g., 70 dB HL, should be measured with a sound level meter having impulse-measuring capability. Calibration also could be in peak-equivalent SPL (peSPL), that is, the peak amplitude of a long-duration tone having the same peak value as the click. The peSPL may be a more appropriate measure than peak SPL for short-duration tone bursts. Acoustic calibration also should include the linearity of the attenuator of the signal-generating system. More details on calibration of signals used in EPA can be found in Gorga and Neely (1994) and in Hall (1992, pp. 263–268).

Part *III*

Auditory Averaged Evoked Potentials (AEPs) and Their Protocols

Signal-Related Potentials: Early Potentials

We define early-latency AEPs or **early potentials (EPs)** as those replicable positive and negative peaks that occur between 0 and 10 ms after the onset of the eliciting signals. Characteristic EPs—as commonly displayed and labeled—are shown in Figure 5-1. Peaks occurring between 0 ms and about 3 ms arise from the cochlea and auditory nerve. Peaks between 3 and 10 ms arise from neural structures in the lower brainstem. The earliest activity will be described more fully in Chapter 13 on electrocochleography. Nevertheless, we include some discussion of this peripheral activity here because it often is used in conjunction with the 3–10 ms activity from the lower brainstem.

There is consensus about the probable *regions* of the ear and of the brainstem from which the principal EP waves arise (Møller, 1994a, 1994b; Musiek & Baran, 1986). Waves I and II come from the distal and proximal portions, respectively, of the auditory or VIIIth cranial nerve. The cochlear nucleus complex of the brainstem gives rise to wave III, the superior olivary nucleus complex to wave IV, and the lateral lemniscus to wave V. The certainty is less about the microstructures in or around the principal generators of the typical waveform depicted in Figure 5-1. It is not clear how much of the AEP is determined by all-or-none discharges of the heavily myelinated neural pathways, by pre- or postsynaptic potentials, by graded changes within nuclear cell bodies and their dendrites, by interactions between sides or levels of the brain, and so on. As mentioned in previous chapters, clarification of these uncertainties is not crucial for gross clinical correlations between EP properties and either estimates of auditory sensitivity or of otoneurologic integrity. However, if the clinical goal is fine or detailed correlation, then more exact elucidation of generating structures and their responding mechanisms may be required.

EPs have been so closely associated with the brainstem that the term "brainstem" has nearly supplanted "early" as a modifier for the potentials. Various anatomic terms, along with their corresponding initials, have been used as descriptors. The most common designations for EPs are *auditory brainstem response (ABR)*, *brainstem evoked response (BSER*

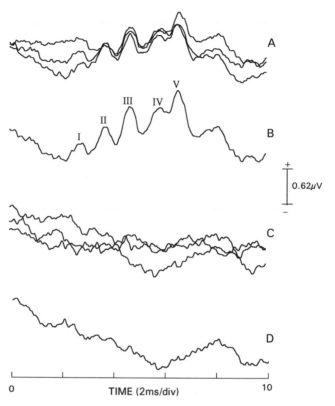

FIGURE 5-1 Early potentials (EPs) from normal-hearing young woman. Filter passband 30–3000 Hz. (A) Clicks at 60 dB nHL; rate = 11.1/s; N per AEP = 800. (B) Composite AEP from the three replications shown in A. Roman numerals designate the five successive peaks commonly observed and measured in threshold audiometry and otoneurologic diagnosis. (C) Clicks at –10 dB nHL, inaudible to subject. (D) Composite AEP from the three replications shown in C.

or *BER)*, and *brainstem auditory evoked response (BAER)*. The popularity of the first term leads some to genericize all averaged evoked potentials (AEPs) as "brainstem" or "ABR," all evoked potential instruments as "brainstem machines," and all forms of evoked potential audiometry as "ABR." We prefer the term **early potentials (EPs)** to designate the first 10 ms of post stimulus-onset activity. It implies no specific generators of the activity or specific physiologic or psychologic function.

Comparison of evoked potentials along the time dimension (early, middle, and late potentials) is simpler than comparisons along the dimensions of anatomy, physiology, or psychology. Also, it avoids questionable comparisons *across* dimensions (e.g., brainstem [anatomic], middle latency [temporal], cortical [anatomic], cognitive [psychologic]).

Historic Background

Several investigators before and around 1970 reported what they considered replicable activity recorded extracranially within the first 10 ms following signal onset. However, the landmark descriptions of EPs appeared independently from two different groups: Sohmer and Feinmesser (1967, 1970), and Jewett and colleagues (Jewett, 1970; Jewett, Romano, & Williston, 1970). Each used different designations for the equivalent peaks. The Roman numeral designations used by Jewett and Williston (1971) have had the wider international acceptance.

EPs quickly became popular as response indices for threshold evoked potential audiometry (EPA). Before then, late potentials (LPs) had been the most popular indices for threshold audiometry and other audiologic measures. EPs were more replicable than LPs for patients of all ages, including premature neonates (Schulman-Galambos & Galambos, 1975). EPs, unlike LPs, could be elicited with little modification from patients who were asleep as well as awake (Jewett & Williston,1971; Picton, Hillyard, Krausz, & Galambos,1974), and they were not seriously affected by most sedatives or related drugs (Mokotoff, Schulman-Galambos, & Galambos, 1977; Starr & Achor, 1975). Their validity as auditory response indices never was questioned seriously. They arose from peripheral and central neural structures that are clearly part of the auditory mechanism. Middle potentials (MPs), which also were proposed as substitutes for LPS, were considered as much myogenic as they were neurogenic, and probably triggered more by vestibular than cochlear stimulation (Bickford, Jacobson, & Cody, 1964; Davis, Engebretson, Lowell, Mast, Satterfield, & Yoshie, 1964).

Otologic and neurologic applications also helped to propel EPs into clinical prominence (Clemis & Mitchell, 1977; Selters & Brackmann, 1977; Starr & Achor, 1975). Certain aberrations in the expected characteristics of EPs were correlated with lesions or dysfunctions of the VIIIth nerve, the lower brainstem, or both. Many diagnosticians bypass EPA for more definitive anatomic diagnostic procedures such as CAT scans, PET scans, and MRI. Nevertheless, using EPs for otoneurologic diagnosis still is valid clinically and less expensive than such things as CAT, PET, and MRI. Applications of EPs for otoneurologic diagnostic purposes are described in Chapter 12.

Before the popularity of EPs, clinicians used LPs to diagnose or to explain the mechanisms underlying such entities as aphasia in children (Beagley, 1970) and various psychoses (Bertolini & Dubini, 1969; Callaway, 1966). Two factors frustrated the use of LPs for these purposes. The more apparent problem was the variability of the LPs under ordinary clinical conditions even for normal subjects against whom the patients' LPs were to be compared. The variability led to too much overlap between normal and patient populations to allow confident diagnosis in individual patients. The less recognized problem was the absence of clear psychophysiologic rationale for relating observed LP aberrations to the character of the patients' disorders.

The replicability or the invariability of the EPs led investigators to try to relate them, instead of LPs, to various clinical entities such as autism (Student & Sohmer, 1978), mental retardation (Squires, Aine, Buchwald, Norman, & Galbraith, 1980), and speech and language disorders ascribable to brain rather than ear dysfunction (Finitzo-Hieber, Freeman, Gerling, Dobson, & Schaefer, 1982; Mason & Mellor, 1984). Some statistically significant differences were reported between the EPs of groups of patients with these disorders and matched groups of normal subjects. However, despite the small measurement variability, the absolute differences were too small to allow EPs to distinguish individual patients in these groups from normal subjects with clinical confidence. Furthermore, the psychophysiologic rationale for relating EPs to high-level disorders was even more tenuous than it was for LPs. This critique of the limitations on relating EPs to high-level dysfunctions does not imply that no relation(s) exist, or that clearer relations will not be discovered. The critique merely cautions against overenthusiastic clinical expectations.

Characteristics of EPs

This chapter covers only general descriptions. A few specific values are given for illustrative purposes.

Recording Parameters

Analysis Window or Recording Epoch

As defined earlier, EPs are those replicable positive and negative peaks that occur between 0 and 10 ms after onset of the eliciting signals. Accordingly, the analysis window should be 10 ms. However, the American EEG Society [now the American Clinical Neurophysiology Society] (1994a) suggests "An analysis time of 10–15 msec from stimulus onset. . . ."

The issue of what window size should be is treated again in chapters on MPs, LPs, and ERPs. Our general advice is that any definition of EPs (or MPs, LPs, or ERPs) established for intra- and interclinic comparisons should not inhibit expansion or contraction of the analysis window. If solution to a specific clinical problem will benefit from alteration of protocol-dictated window size, then window size should be changed. For example, wave V of the neonatal EP occurs later than in adults for a given physical click level. Close to threshold, neonatal wave V occurs beyond 10 ms (Galambos & Wilson, 1994; Stuart, Yang, & Green, 1994). Without extending analysis time to 12–15 ms, wave V, particularly its trailing edge, would not be identified and defects in auditory sensitivity would be overestimated. As another example, hypothermia, a common condition during surgery, can prolong the latencies of the peaks of the EP (Hall, Bull, & Cronau, 1988; MacKenzie, Vingerhoets, Colon, Pinckers, & Notermans, 1995). Therefore, intraoperative monitoring would be hampered and perhaps even invalidated if analysis time were limited to 10 ms, the defined limit for EPs. Analysis time also can be shortened for convenience—for example, to 5 ms during electrocochleography, when the clinician wants to use only the cochlear microphonics, summating potentials, and whole-nerve action potentials as the response indices.

Extending analysis time beyond 10 ms, as in two of the examples just cited, means encroaching on the defined early limit of the middle potentials (MPs). In these cases, the index of interest, wave V, which ordinarily is an EP occurring before 10 ms, now becomes an MP. This intrusion is of no clinical consequence. The EP, MP, and LP time zones are established for descriptive convenience. They do not connote any specific wave, generator, or functional process.

Filters

The most commonly recommended filter passband for recording EPs is 100–3000 Hz. That passband usually suffices when clicks are the eliciting signals and the goal of EPA is a gross estimate of (a) auditory sensitivity or (b) the integrity of the peripheral auditory system and lower brainstem. However, the recommendation to use a 100–3000 Hz passband should serve only as a guideline, not as a rigid straitjacket. The American EEG Society (1994) recommends that a lower high-pass setting of 10–30 Hz be used when possible. It also specifies that the high-pass filter skirt or roll-off not exceed 12 dB/octave; the limit for the low-pass (high cut) roll-off should be no greater than 24 dB/octave.

Experience dictates that a high-pass setting lower than the customary 100 Hz should be used for assessment of auditory sensitivity in neonates and young infants (Davis et al., 1985; Goldstein & Frye-Osier, 1984). A high pass lower than 100 Hz also may be desirable if one wants to go beyond just establishing a region of otic or brainstem abnormality to obtain more information about the underlying pathophysiologic process.

The filter low pass (high cut) can be set below the commonly used 3000 Hz because the bulk of the energy that defines EPs lies below 1000 Hz (Doyle & Hyde, 1981; Hall, 1992, pp. 494–495). Eliminating some high-frequency energy (e.g., above 2000 Hz) eliminates some physiologic and instrumental noise that can interfere with peak identification and measurement. On the other hand, keeping the energy above 2000 Hz sharpens the peaks, giving greater precision to measurements.

In our discussion of filters in Chapter 4, we recommended that whenever possible, use as little filtering as possible. We repeat that recommendation here and again in later chapters. Control noise as much as possible through proper electrode placement, instrumental shielding and grounding, and patient comfort. Disturbing noise that remains can be reduced through post-averaging filtering or post-averaging smoothing. However, we paraphrase the general advice given about the size of the analysis window. Let the clinical question dictate the filter conditions. If a 100–3000 Hz passband suffices, use it. If the answer to the clinical question demands a different passband, adapt accordingly.

Electrode Montage

Largest EPs usually are recorded when an electrode on the vertex (Cz) is referred to an electrode either on the earlobe (A) or the mastoid (M) ipsilateral to the ear stimulated (Parker, 1981; van Olphen, Rodenburg, & Verwey, 1978). The earlobe electrode can be designated A1 or A2, depending on whether it is the left or the right earlobe; or can be designated Ai or Ac, depending on whether it is ipsilateral or contralateral to the stimulated ear (American EEG Society, 1994a). The same designations can be used for the M electrode. With this montage for the recording electrodes, the ground electrode usually is placed somewhere in the middle of the forehead, although it could be placed elsewhere on the head or on another part of the body. Recording can be single-channel, usually from the side of the head ipsilateral to the stimulated ear (e.g., Cz-M1), or two-channel from both the ipsilateral and contralateral sides of the head (e.g., Cz-Ai and Cz-Ac).

Clicks presented to one ear of adult subjects elicit similar EPs from both sides of the head (Figure 5-2). Some differences in the contralateral EP are smaller or absent wave I, clearer separation of wave IV and wave V, and slightly shorter latency for wave III (Durrant, Boston, & Martin, 1990; Rosenhamer & Holmkvist, 1982).

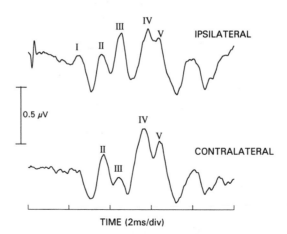

FIGURE 5-2   Ipsilateral and contralateral early potentials (EPs) from a normal-hearing young woman. These are composite AEPs from three replications of 800 samples each. Clicks: 70 dB nHL at 11.1/s. Filter passband: 30–3000 Hz.

Secure attachment of a vertex electrode often is difficult. Many clinicians avoid this difficulty by using only three electrodes, two attached either to the earlobes or to the mastoids and the other to the forehead (FPZ), where attachment is more secure than on the vertex. During recording, the forehead electrode is referred to the ipsilateral earlobe or mastoid electrode. The contralateral earlobe or mastoid electrode serves as ground. Using three instead of four electrodes also reduces electrode application and removal time. The configuration of the EP with this montage is about the same as when the vertex electrode is used. Peak amplitudes, however, usually are a little smaller. Simultaneous ipsilateral and contralateral recordings are not possible with this three-electrode montage.

EP Measures

Peak latency in milliseconds (ms) is the most common EP measure. Latency is measured from the onset of the electric pulse that is delivered to the earphone for click (or other test signal) generation to the positive or negative peak of interest. Absolute latencies and differences in latencies between peaks (**interpeak** or **interwave intervals**) are prime measures in otoneurologic assessment. Absolute latencies and interpeak intervals are of less consequence in threshold EPA. Change in peak latency with change in signal level, however, is an important observation or measure in threshold EPA.

Peak or peak-to-peak amplitude in microvolts (μV) is another measure. The measure can be absolute for a given signal level or can be change in amplitude with change in signal level. Amplitude measures have been played down because of their intra- and intersubject variability (Schwartz, Morris, & Jacobson, 1994). This common view has led to general shunning of amplitude as a clinical measure, even though within-group measures are much less variable (Hoth, 1986; Kjœr, 1979). However, relative amplitude of waves I and V may be of value in otoneurologic assessment. Normally, the V/I amplitude ratio is greater than 1.00, with a ratio less than 0.5 being considered abnormal.

Signal Parameters

Temporal and Spectral Characteristics

The most commonly used signals to elicit EPs are clicks generated by delivering electric rectangular waves of 0.1 ms duration to a transducer. The acoustic output often is called a "100 microsecond click." The output of the transducer, however, as depicted in Figure 4-1, lasts about 1.5 ms. Actual duration varies with the input voltage, nature of the transducer, and mode of coupling of the transducer to the ear. The electric input is a step function that causes the transducer to ring at its own resonant frequencies. Therefore, the spectrum of the click closely resembles the frequency-response curve of the transducer.

Most electromagnetic transducers (such as those of the Telephonics TDH series) have several small but distinct resonant peaks between about 2000 and 6000 Hz. Therefore, when voluntary behavioral response thresholds for clicks are compared with similarly obtained thresholds for pure tones, correlation between click and tone thresholds is slightly higher for high frequencies than for low frequencies. Usually, the correlation is highest for 2000 Hz. This correlation is one of the bases for referring to signals commonly used to elicit EPs as "high-frequency clicks."

Two accidents of conventional recording parameters, 10 ms window and 100–3000 Hz filter passband, also lead to a misconception that high frequencies are the most effective portions of eliciting clicks. First, because of cochlear mechanics, responses to low frequencies have longer latencies than responses to high frequencies. Therefore, much of the low-frequency response lies beyond 10 ms, outside a narrow analysis window. Second, again largely because of cochlear mechanics, responses to low frequencies are distributed over a wider time range than are responses to high frequencies. This temporal distribution leads to a lower frequency concentration in the spectrum of the responses to low frequencies. The typical high-pass end of the filter passband at 100 Hz eliminates much of the low-frequency energy in response to the low-frequency components of the click. This helps to reduce the recognizability of the response to the low-frequency components of the click.

There is clinical support for the contribution of the low-frequency components of the click to typical EPs such as shown in Figure 5-1. Patients with normal or nearly normal low-frequency sensitivity but with distinct high-frequency hypacusis have longer than normal wave V latencies for a given nHL than persons with totally normal sensitivity (Fowler & Mikami, 1992; Gorga, Reiland, & Beauchaine, 1985). By contrast, a patient with low-frequency sensorineural losses but normal high-frequency sensitivity can have normal wave V latencies, but usually at the *short* end of the normal range (Goldstein, Karlovich, Tweed, & Kile, 1983). Further evidence of the contribution of low-frequency energy to EPs comes from studies on the derived band technic and the notched noise technic for eliciting EPs. These latter technics are described briefly in Chapter 10.

Narrow-spectrum signals also have been used in experimental and clinical studies. As pointed out in the previous chapter, sometimes the signals are equated across frequencies by their temporal envelopes, that is, equal rise/fall times and plateaus. In other clinics and laboratories, rise/fall time and plateaus of signals are equated by number of cycles. If all signals are to have the same number of cycles, for example, 1 cycle rise/fall time and 1 cycle plateau, then a 500 Hz tone burst will have a total duration of 6.00 ms and a 4000 Hz tone burst a total duration of 0.75 ms duration.

The principal use of narrow-spectrum signals is in threshold EPA. The obvious advantage of narrow-spectrum signals over clicks is that narrow-spectrum signals can be used to obtain audiograms that more nearly resemble threshold audiograms obtained with conventional long-duration tones in voluntary behavioral response audiometry. High-frequency tone bursts do elicit EPs similar to those elicited by clicks although waves prior to wave V usually are not as distinct as in EPs to clicks (Beattie & Kennedy, 1992; Maurizi, Paludetti, Ottaviani, & Rosignoli, 1984). Overall, the lower the frequency, the less distinct are the early waves. Also, the lower the frequency the less likely is the tone burst even to elicit an identifiable wave V with the usual recording parameters.

Clicks continue to be the main signals used for eliciting EPs for understandable reasons. First, they elicit more distinct EPs than are elicited by narrow spectrum signals of equivalent level. Second, because of their longer onset, compared with that of the click, narrow-spectrum signals usually do not elicit well-defined waves I and II, and sometimes even wave III. This limits use of narrow spectrum signals for otoneurologic assessment. Third, the electric artifact created during generation of the click is brief. If it is necessary to present strong level clicks to a patient with hearing impairment, the artifact, which often is larger than the response itself, will obscure the earliest waves of the EP. However, if waves III and V are unaffected by the artifact, they often can provide enough information for threshold or for otoneurologic assessment. On the other hand, for a signal to be truly narrow spectrum, its duration must be longer than the 1.5 to 2.0 ms of the strong click. This means that at strong signal levels the attendant artifact could even obscure the clarity of wave V.

Signal Rate

The EPs in Figure 5-1 were elicited by clicks presented to the subject at a rate of 11.1/s. Latencies and amplitudes would have been essentially indistinguishable had click rate been slower. Also, as shown in Figure 5-3, virtually no change in latencies and amplitudes occurs even with rates at least as high as 30/s. With further rate increases, especially above 40/s, two changes in the EP are apparent: (a) latency of wave V increases and (b) earlier waves become less identifiable (Fowler & Noffsinger, 1983). Normal differences in wave V latency between the slowest and fastest (about 90/s) rates range between 0.4 and 0.8 ms (Gerling & Finitzo-Hieber, 1983).

Signal Level

EPs behave predictably to changes in signal level. Peak latencies increase and peak amplitudes decrease as signal level decreases. Figure 5-4 shows this signal-related phenomenon for clicks, a 10 ms analysis window, and a 100–3000 Hz filter passband. Changes in wave V latency with changes in signal level often are plotted as a "latency-intensity function" (see Figure 5-5). The quotation marks call attention to the questionable use of "intensity." The abscissa of these graphs never is plotted in units of intensity (watt/cm^2 or watt/m^2), or even in intensity level (dB re 10^{-16} watt/cm^2 or 10^{-12} watt/m^2). Most commonly, the units of **signal magnitude** are Sensation Level (SL), dB nHL, or dB peSPL. The hatched lines in Figure 5-5 represent the range of normal values. Some clinicians use 2.0 standard deviations around the mean values as the range of normal. Others consider values within the range of 2.5 or 3.0 standard deviations as normal.

The latency-magnitude function is not linear. It is steep in the low-magnitude range, that is, near threshold, but the slope is nearly flat in the high-magnitude range because

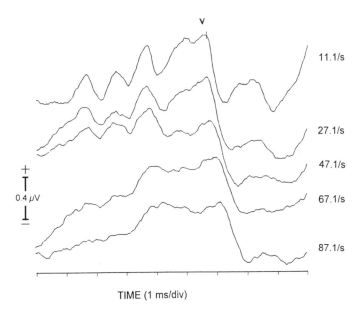

FIGURE 5-3 **Early potentials (EPs) from normal-hearing young woman as a function of click rate. These are composite AEPs from three replications of 800. Level: 70 dB nHL; filter passband: 100–3000 Hz.**

latency decreases little with further magnitude increases above 60 dB nHL. Clinicians compare a patient's latency-magnitude function with the normal curve as an aid to estimating the patient's threshold sensitivity and determining whether the patient's impairment (if any) is conductive or sensorineural. Clinical use of the latency-magnitude function is discussed further in Chapter 10.

Monotic versus Diotic Stimulation

When the identical signal is presented simultaneously to both ears (diotic) of a normal-hearing, normal-brained subject, the EP amplitude is nearly twice as large as with monotic stimulation of either ear. A similar effect is observed with MPs and LPs.

A phenomenon often labeled **binaural interaction component (BIC)** has been postulated because diotic EPs are not exactly twice as large as monotic EPs (Ainslie & Boston, 1980; Dobie & Norton, 1980). The phenomenon usually is quantified by subtracting the diotic EP from a doubling of a monotic EP. A reason given for the difference between the two—that is, the BIC—is that part of the response mechanism for monotic EPs is shared by the input from the separate ears during diotic stimulation.

Some audiologists speculate that certain patients with CANS disorders will not show the BIC because their central nervous systems are unable to integrate the simultaneous input from the two ears (Ivey, 1986; Katz, Chertoff, & Sawusch, 1984). Clinical application of the BIC, however, has been frustrated by the failure of experimentalists to find a consistent BIC in the EPs in subjects with normal ears and brains (Levine, 1981; Wilson, Kelly-Ballweber, & Dobie, 1985). Therefore, there are no extant norms against which patients' BICs can be

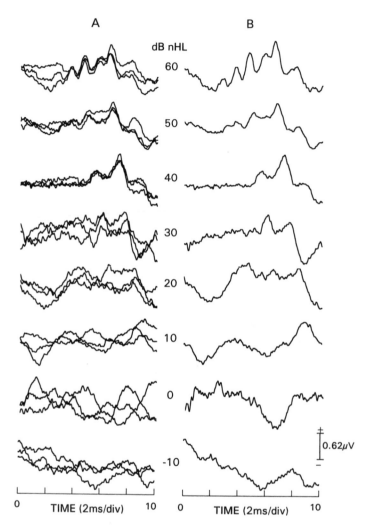

FIGURE 5-4 **Early potentials (EPs) from a normal-hearing woman as a function of click level. Click rate: 11.1/s. Filter passband: 30–3000 Hz. (A) Three replications with N per AEP = 800. (B) Composite AEP from the three replications in A. Clicks were barely audible to subject at 0 dB nHL; they were inaudible at –10 dB nHL.**

compared. If BIC is present in EPs, it is not robust. This is not surprising when one considers the probable generators of EPs. Generators for waves III, IV, and V of the EPs for the left side of the brain are only millimeters apart from the homologous generators on the right side of the brain. Remote far-field electrodes, therefore, probably are recording nearly as much activity from the contralateral generators as they are from the ipsilateral generators. The simultaneously recording from both sides during both monotic and diotic stimulation could obscure possible real differences between EPs from monotic and diotic stimulation.

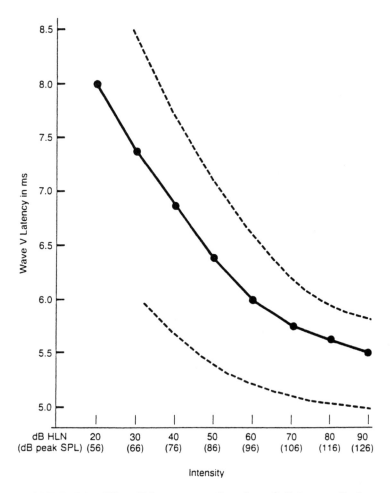

FIGURE 5-5   Wave V latency as a function of click magnitude. The solid line represents latency values for wave V for a normal-hearing subject. The broken lines mark the limits of ± 3 standard deviations from the clinic's normative latency values.

[Reprinted with permission from Hood & Berlin, *Auditory Evoked Potentials*, Pro-Ed, 1986.]

Subject Parameters

Age

EPs can be elicited from persons of any age, from neonates and young infants to adults in their ninth decade (Cone-Wesson, Ma, & Fowler, 1997; Hecox & Galambos, 1974; Oku & Hasegewa, 1997). EP latencies, amplitudes, and general configuration, however, do change with age. The EPs in Figure 5-6 exemplify those changes. They are in response to distinctly suprathreshold clicks.

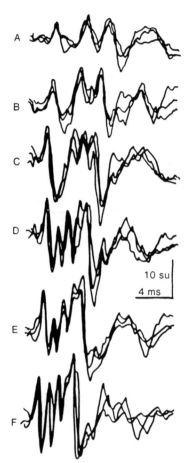

10 su
4 ms

FIGURE 5-6   Early potentials (EPs) to suprathreshold clicks as a function of age. Each set of traces is from a different individual in the following age groups: (A) preterm, 32 weeks conceptional age; (B) preterm, 35 weeks conceptional age; (C) full-term neonate; (D) 3 months; (E) 1 year; (F) 3 years.

[Reprinted with permission from Salamy, *Journal of Clinical Neurophysiology 1*:293–329, 1984.]

Notable is the decrease in peak latencies and increase in peak amplitudes from early infancy to young adulthood. Also, interwave intervals shorten with age. The most rapid changes occur within the first six months and EPs become nearly adult-like by 18 months.

The EPs in Figure 5-6 are from subjects whose ears, as well as brains, are normal or presumed to be normal. Normality, however, does not mean full maturity. Normal, full-term neonates may have normal ears, but the sensitivity of their ears is different from that of young adult subjects. Neonatal low-frequency sensitivity apparently is equivalent to that of adult sensitivity but *normal* neonatal high-frequency sensitivity is poorer (Sininger et al.,1997; Wolf & Goldstein, 1980). Therefore, some of the latency difference between neonatal and adult EPs is attributable to normal differences in high-frequency sensitivity. The longer neonatal interwave intervals can be attributed to differences in neural rather than cochlear maturation.

Changes in EPs with advancing age are small apart from sensitivity impairment (Oku & Hasegewa, 1997; Weber, 1992). Similarly, if the older person has not sustained damage to the central nervous system, age by itself has a small but significant effect on peak latencies and interwave intervals.

In older children and adults, clicks presented to one ear elicit similar EPs from both sides of the head (Figure 5-2). In neonates, however, the contralateral EP is smaller and less well-defined than the ipsilateral EP (Katbamma, Metz, Bennett, & Dokler, 1996). Neonatal ipsilateral-contralateral differences are at least as or even more distinct for MPs (Wolf & Goldstein, 1978). The clearer distinction for MPs probably is due in part to the wider separation of the principal ipsi- and contralateral generators. As pointed out earlier, the generators for waves III, IV, and V of the EPs for the left side of the brain are only millimeters apart from the homologous generators on the right side of the brain. The remote far-field electrodes, therefore, probably are recording nearly as much activity from the contralateral generators as they are from the ipsilateral generators.

Gender

Women have shorter EP latencies and larger EP amplitudes than men. Differences are small but they must be considered when establishing clinical norms (Elberling & Parbo, 1987; Watson, 1996). Comparing a patient's measures with the patient's gender norms is less likely to lead to clinical error than comparing with norms based on values taken from a mixed gender sample. The basis for the gender difference is not certain. Women, on the average, have smaller heads than men. Some investigators believe that head size rather than intrinsic gender differences account for the different latency values for men and women (Dempsey, Censoprano, & Mazor, 1986; Durrant, Sabo, & Hyre, 1990).

Head Size

As just mentioned, smaller head size has been implicated as a probable cause of intersubject differences in EP latencies. If head size is a significant factor, then one would expect latencies to become longer with age as head size increases. Figure 5-6, however, illustrates the common observation that the latency of wave V is longer in neonates than in adult subjects with larger heads. It is possible that the head-size effect in neonates is more than counterbalanced by the elongating effects of immature high-frequency sensitivity and of synaptic and, perhaps, axonic immaturity.

Temperature

As mentioned earlier, abnormally cold body temperature can lead to abnormal elongation of EP latencies. Whether slight differences in normal body temperatures influence normal latencies is not as certain. If body temperature does influence the range of latencies used as clinical norms, then patients' temperatures should be taken routinely before and during any EPA procedure for which EPs serve as the response index.

Race

Most reported latency and amplitude norms for EPs were obtained on white subjects. Whether these norms can be extrapolated to other racial groups is not certain. Also not certain is whether there are any interactions between race and gender, head size, or temperature that affect EP latency or amplitude norms.

$Chapter$ **6**

Signal-Related Potentials: Middle Potentials

We define middle-latency AEPs or **middle potentials (MPs)** as those replicable positive and negative peaks that occur between 10 and 50 ms after the onset of the eliciting signals. Characteristic MPs in response to clicks are shown in Figure 6-1. The earliest peaks in this time zone may begin before 10 ms and the latest peaks may end beyond 50 ms. A common designation of these potentials is **MLR** for **middle latency responses**.

Historic Background

MPs have generated much controversy and misunderstanding. We present the following historic background to help resolve some misconceptions that pervade the literature and to provide a framework for effective application of MPs, which are being used increasingly clinically.

MPs were the first AEPs studied systematically for audiometric purposes. Geisler and colleagues (Geisler, Frishkopf, & Rosenblith, 1958; Geisler & Rosenblith, 1962) showed that a positive peak (temporal referred to occipital electrodes) at about 30 ms in response to clicks diminished in amplitude and increased in latency as click level decreased (Figure 6-2). Threshold estimated from the AEPs corresponded closely to the subject's psychophysical threshold for those clicks. Geisler and colleagues speculated that the positive peak reflected activity of neurons in the primary auditory cortex.

Lowell and colleagues (Lowell, Troffer, Warburton, & Rushford,1960; Lowell, Williams, Ballinger, & Alvig,1961) began to use componentry within the first 50 ms after click onset in objective threshold assessment. Then, Bickford and colleagues (1964) challenged both the neurogenicity of the first 50 ms of recorded activity and its relation to cochlear stimulation. They claimed that this early activity came from postural muscles of the head and neck stimulated by acoustic activation of the vestibular system, not the cochlea. The sup-

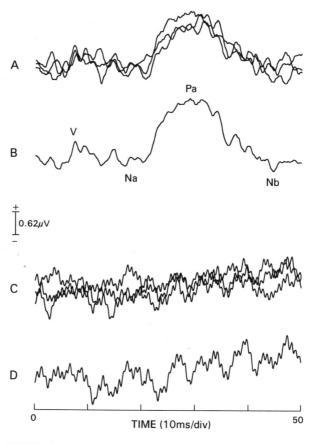

**FIGURE 6-1   Middle potentials (MPs) from a
normal-hearing woman. Filter passband: 5–1000 Hz.
(A) Clicks at 50 dB nHL; rate: 17.1/s. N per AEP:
500. (B) Composite AEP from the three replications
shown in A. (C) Clicks at –10 dB nHL, inaudible to
subject. (D) Composite AEP from the three replications shown in C.**

port for the myogenicity of what was then called the *early* or *fast* components of the AEP
was so strong (Borsanyi, 1964; Davis et al., 1964) that only a few investigators continued
to study this time zone for audiometric or other purposes (Goldstein & Rodman, 1967;
Ruhm, Walker, & Flanigin, 1967) . In time, however, the possibility of applying these components to tonal threshold audiometry stimulated increased interest in their properties.

Since the years during which the first 50 ms was called early or fast, a change occurred
in the latency-related designation of the AEP components. According to a scheme presented by Picton and colleagues (1974) (Figure 6-3), early components are those positive
and negative peaks occurring within the first 8 ms after the onset of a click at 60 dB nHL,

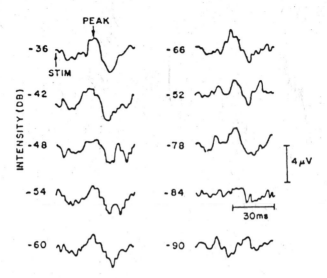

FIGURE 6-2   AEPs to monotic clicks at 15/s. N per AEP = 1000. Upward deflection indicates positivity of a scalp electrode over the right temporal area relative to an electrode on the midline in the occipital region. Intensity values are relative to the maximum voltage applied to the earphone. This subject's behavioral response threshold for the clicks was –88 dB.

[Reprinted with permission from Geisler & Rosenblith, "Average responses to clicks recorded from the human scalp." *Journal of the Acoustical Society of America, 34,* 125–127, 1962.]

middle components between 8 and 50 ms, and late components between 50 and 300 ms. Unfortunately, this convenient and popularly adopted time division engendered unanticipated confusion about response componentry. We already alluded to the confusion in the previous chapter and will be referring to it again in this and later chapters. Additional historic and technical facets are injected here to show why a clear-cut description of middle components is difficult.

Analysis Window

Most signal averagers with which AEPs were studied did not allow investigators to view the AEPs for just 8 ms, the edge of the early component time zone defined by Picton and colleagues (1974). However, an analysis window of 10 ms (or 10.24 ms) was possible. Therefore, by default but without formal declaration of the change, early components were regarded as any replicable activity in the 10 ms following signal onset. About the same time, investigators recognized that the most definable peaks in that early time zone arose from auditory-related

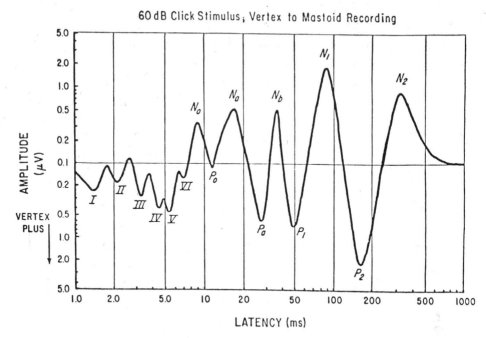

FIGURE 6-3 **Diagrammatic representation of the auditory averaged evoked potential (AEP) components plotted on logarithmic scales. Mean data from eight subjects.**

[From Picton, Hillyard, Krausz, & Galambos, "Human auditory evoked potentials. I. Evaluation of components," *Electroencephalography and Clinical Neurophysiology, 36,* 179–190, 1974. Reprinted with kind permission from Elsevier Science Ireland Ltd., Bay 15K, Shannon Industrial Estate, Co. Clare, Ireland.]

structures within the lower brainstem. Soon, it became more common to refer to that early activity as "brainstem responses" (ABR, BSER, and other initial designations).

A common observation during threshold audiometry was that wave V of the ABR was the only recognizable peak close to threshold. To many clinicians, wave V and ABR were synonymous. In adults, when the eliciting clicks are close to threshold, the latency of wave V is about 8 to 9 ms. For neonates, wave V at threshold usually is greater than 10 ms, that is, in the middle-latency time zone defined by Picton and colleagues (1974). When low-frequency tone bursts are the eliciting signals, wave V latency is greater than 10 ms for any patient even at most suprathreshold levels. Is wave V still an ABR or is it an MP? It is both. This is not a contradiction because the same activity is being described along two different dimensions, one *anatomic*, the other *temporal*. However, failure to recognize that it is the same phenomenon led to confusion about what constitutes EPs and MPs.

Some experimenters extended their boundaries to encompass large waves just beyond 50 ms with the expectation or hope that these large, later peaks would be useful for clinical or investigative purposes (Mendel & Goldstein, 1969; Suzuki, Kobayashi, Aoki, & Umegaki, 1992). This activity beyond 50 ms still was designated "middle" by some and "late" by others.

Because properties of this later activity differed in some ways from those within the first 50 ms, there was considerable uncertainty about what the MPs and their properties were.

When one records the middle latencies, defined with any time boundaries, one records earlier latency activity as well. Some activity that begins before 8 to 10 ms may not peak until the circumscribed middle-latency zone. At the other end of the analysis window, some activity that begins before 50 ms may peak in what has been delineated as the late-latency time zone.

Filters and Filter Passbands

When investigators returned to study this time zone after being diverted by the myogenicity contention, they had no clear guidelines for an appropriate filter passband. Several who had been studying the late AEPs used the same filters for studying the middle components that they had been using for late components, about 1–30 Hz. It is understandable that they could not record robust MPs because much of the spectral energy that best defines MP peaks lies above 30 Hz. Some investigators also used a notch filter to eliminate the 60 Hz artifact, further depleting the middle components of defining spectral components. The analog filters confused the situation in still another way because of the phase leads or lags that they induced. Comparing observations across laboratories was difficult, and often within the same laboratory, because the different types of filters and different passbands led to different apparent peak polarities, latencies, and amplitudes.

Use Made of MP Peaks

Some researchers and clinicians used the same amplification, filter, analysis window, and signal parameters for one purpose such as threshold audiometry, as well as for other purposes such as ascertaining the site and determining the nature of a lesion in the brain. Therefore, properties of MPs derived from one category of investigation have been generalized instead of being related to the particular circumstances of their elicitation and recording. The consequence, at times, has been contradictory conclusions.

Identification of Peak Generators

Some clinical applications require knowledge of the anatomic structure(s) responsible for the generation of particular peaks or at least knowledge of the region of the brain from which the peaks arise. This knowledge has been obtained about EPs or ABRs with reasonable certainty from laboratory studies on animals and clinical studies on human patients. Conclusions from these studies are compatible with the anatomy and function of auditory-related structures in the human brainstem and with the time of occurrences of the individual peaks of the EP. Investigators had equal expectations for MP peaks. Unfortunately, two circumstances thwarted those expectations.

Clinical observations from threshold audiometry and audiometrically related research on humans have provided more information about MPs than has come from careful laboratory studies directed specifically at generator sources. In the clinical studies, extensive bandpass filtering with its selective attenuation and with phase lags and phase leads often distorted the AEP waveform. Intentionally created distortion does not hamper the use of the distorted AEPs for threshold audiometry; the distortion usually enhances the AEP as an index for this purpose. However, it is nearly impossible to determine the actual peak latencies and amplitudes or even to be certain that some consistent peaks might not have been artifactually created. Thus, relating these peaks to generator sources had limited value.

A second source of frustration is that MP peaks hardly can be attributed to a single generator or to a restricted area of the brain. Those peaks, as they are ordinarily recorded, are the accidental algebraic addition of contributions from many generators at different brain levels and from different portions at each level. It is possible that one generator may dominate the peak addition but it is risky to assign the whole of one middle-latency peak to just one generator or to one small region of the brain. The assignation of individual peaks to specific generators is even more problematic for peaks later than 50 ms.

An unfortunate corollary consequence ensued from lack of certain knowledge of the MP generators. Some clinicians and researchers argued that lack of knowledge of the generators precluded the use of MPs as a response index for threshold audiometry. This was questionable reasoning. In conventional behavioral response threshold audiometry, a common indication of a response is the patient's pressing a button that lights a bulb on the audiometer. The exact neuromuscular generators of button-pushing can be determined. However, that information *never* is required for an audiologist to relate the lighting of the bulb to the reading on the hearing level dial or to the final estimate of the patient's threshold. All that is required is a consistent relation between the button pressing (and subsequent lighting of the bulb) and the level of the sound presented to the patient. MPs could have been used in the same way without any knowledge of their generators.

Characteristics of MPs

The long introduction was presented to explain why the following descriptions of MPs will not be clear-cut or unequivocal. The descriptors are derived from diverse laboratory and clinical reports with few common threads running through them.

Recording Parameters

Analysis Window or Recording Epoch

Despite our definition of MPs (replicable peaks between 10–50 ms), most recordings of MPs also will include the first 10 ms, or EPs. It is possible to delay some signal averagers until 10 ms after signal onset. However, the delay and exclusion of EPs serve little clinical purpose. At the other extreme, the window can be extended beyond 50 ms if the clinical answer sought warrants it. In short, the 10–50 ms definition of MPs given for intra- and interclinic comparisons should not inhibit expansion or contraction of the analysis window in actual clinical use.

Filters

McGee, Kraus, and Manfredi (1988) found the major concentration of energy in a 100 ms window to be between 3–300 Hz. Our own clinical and research experience affirms that the

3–300 Hz applies as well just to the first 50 ms, the boundary of our definition of MPs. Nevertheless, frequencies below 3 Hz also contribute to the definition of the positive and negative peaks, especially to their magnitude. In addition, frequencies above 300 Hz help to define the peaks, particularly their sharpness. The downside of extending the high-pass cutoff below 3 Hz is that large, lower-frequency activity is more state-dependent and hence is more variable than higher-frequency activity. Variability reduces the replicability of traces obtained with identical signal conditions. The downside of making the low-pass cut-off higher than 300 Hz is letting high-frequency activity unrelated to the response (e.g., muscle potentials, instrumental noise) enter the recording and superimpose itself on the signal-related peaks. The superimposition of what is essentially noise increases the difficulty of identifying peaks and measuring their latencies and magnitudes.

As pointed out in Chapter 3, analog filters not only attenuate spectral energy outside the filter passband, they also can cause phase lags and leads especially for those frequencies close to the high- and low-pass ends of the passband. These phase-shift distortions are of no consequence when MPs are used for threshold audiometry as long as the distorted patterns are replicable. Figure 6-4 shows the difference between the AEP to the same signal

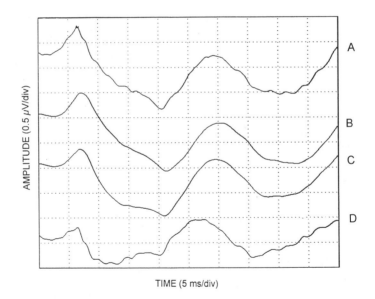

TIME (5 ms/div)

FIGURE 6-4   AEP to 50 dB nHL monotic clicks recorded simultaneously from a single electrode pair (Cz-M1) through four different filter passbands: (A) 3–500 Hz, a recommended filter passband; (B) 1–200 Hz; (C) 10–200 Hz; (D) 30–500 Hz. Differences in peak amplitudes and peak latencies are artifacts of the analog filters. An upward deflection represents positivity of the vertex electrode (Cz) relative to the mastoid electrode (M1). Subject: normal-hearing young man.

recorded simultaneously through different filter passbands. Figure 6-5 shows the extent of replicability in a filtered waveform (5–1000 Hz) and the consistent changes in latency and magnitude with decreases in signal level. Estimation of threshold sensitivity from these waveforms is practical, relatively easy, and valid even if filters may have distorted the waveform in some way.

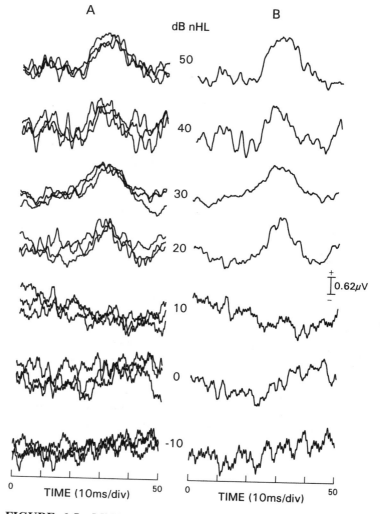

FIGURE 6-5 **Middle potentials (MPs) from a normal-hearing woman as a function of click level. Monotic clicks at 17.1/s. (A) Three replications with N per AEP = 500. (B) Composite AEP from the three replications in A. Clicks were audible to subject at 10 dB nHL but not at 0 or –10 dB nHL. Filter passband: 5–1000 Hz.**

Electrode Montage

Studies on optimal electrode placements for MPs have been reviewed by Hall (1992, pp. 200-202). Unfortunately, findings have not been conclusive enough to dictate specific recommendations either for otoneurologic diagnosis or for threshold audiometry. A suitable practice is to refer an electrode on the vertex (Cz) (or slightly anterior to it) to an electrode on the earlobe or mastoid (A1 or A2 or M1 or M2). This practice has the advantage of being favorable for recording EPs as well if simultaneous examination of both time zones is a goal.

Signal Parameters

Spectral Characteristics

Clicks elicit large and distinct MPs. When one uses MPs as an index for otoneurologic purposes, clicks can be the signal of choice. As pointed out in Chapter 3, clicks are broadband acoustic signals that stimulate the entire cochlea. If a patient being evaluated for otoneurologic purposes has a hearing loss, the patient may not show the expected waveform for a given suprathreshold click even if the patient's auditory system central to the cochlea is completely normal. Deviations from normal are more likely if the patient's loss either for the high or for the low frequencies is distinctly greater than for the remaining frequencies. Ideally, waveform norms for otoneurologic purposes should be established for narrow-spectrum signals so that patients can be tested at frequencies at which their threshold sensitivity is best. Such norms have not been established.

Clicks also serve as useful signals for threshold audiometry, especially when the audiologist just wants to obtain a crude overall estimate of the patient's auditory sensitivity. However, clicks cannot be used to obtain the equivalent or the parallel of a pure-tone audiogram without coarse judgments derived from the so-called latency-intensity function or without some sophisticated, time-consuming procedures based on selective masking (see Chapter 10). Fortunately, it is possible to approximate a pure-tone audiogram with narrow-spectrum tone bursts used in a simple, straightforward testing procedure (see Chapter 9).

The spectrum of a tone burst is not the single line of a pure tone. However, the longer the duration of a tone burst, the narrower is its spectrum (see Figure 4-4, Chapter 4). Unfortunately, the longer the duration, the more the signal invades the 50 ms analysis window. Long tone bursts have two disadvantages: (a) The most defining portion of the response may occur later than 50 ms, that is, outside the recording window, and (b) the electric artifact generated by strong tone bursts and picked up by the recording electrode may be larger than the response of interest and may obscure much of the response. Short tone bursts are not plagued by these problems but suffer from a spectrum that may be too broad to elicit MPs that can be used with confidence to estimate pure-tone thresholds. A reasonable compromise for threshold EPA is a tone burst whose total duration from onset to offset is about 10 ms.

Signal Rate

If the clinician uses a 50 ms analysis window, the maximum allowable signal rate is 20/s, that is, the reciprocal of the set period of 50 ms. If faster rates are used, a second signal occurs within the analysis window, interfering with the waveform elicited by the previous signal. Overlapping responses are generated intentionally when one wishes to observe the

40 Hz phenomenon (see Chapter 10). However, the time-amplitude configuration of MPs cannot be studied with rates faster than 20/s.

MPs recover rapidly in the mature brain. No significant changes in peak latencies or amplitudes occur with signal rates at least as fast as 16/s (McFarland et al., 1975). We recommend a rate of 17/s (or 17.1/s) to allow rapid data acquisition without risking amplitude reduction because of adaptation. The odd rate reduces the likelihood of accidentally locking on a fixed phase of a 60 Hz artifact. Randomly staggered rates around some fixed rate (e.g., 15.1–19.1/s) also reduce the likelihood of locking on a fixed phase of 60 Hz artifact or of some rhythmic EEG activity. Variable rates may also help to reduce habituation that can occur with monotonous repetitive stimulation.

Jerger, Chmiel, Glaze, and Frost (1987) reported that normal 2- to 6-month-old infants seldom showed a characteristic large positive peak close to 50 ms in response to 500 Hz tone bursts when signal presentation rate exceeded 4/s. They stated further that ". . . the MLR appears to be absent . . ." at stimulus rates exceeding 8 to 10/s. This report has raised concern with others (Mora, Expósito, Solís, & Barajas, 1990) who appeared to have generalized the conclusions of Jerger and colleagues to include any replicable activity in a defined MP time zone. The middle potential time zones defined by others since the Picton and colleagues (1974) publication fall within a fairly narrow range: 10–80 ms (Kraus, McGee, & Stein, 1994); 10–50 ms (Polich & Starr, 1983), or 12–50 ms (Davis, 1976; Hall, 1982, p.21). Given those common definitions, activity in the 10(or 12)–30 ms region can be considered MPs. A 20/s rate produced robust MPs in the 10–30 ms region from normal neonates in a study by Sininger and colleagues (1997). The discrepancy between the Jerger and colleagues and the Sininger and colleagues studies can be attributed as much to interpretation of what constitutes MPs as it can to actual experimental observations. As a general observation across subjects of all ages, the later the response component, the more it is degraded by rapid signal rates. Correspondingly, signal rate should be less when one is looking at later activity in a window than when one is examining earlier activity.

We have discussed the rate issue in some depth partly to emphasize a point made in the previous chapter about the advisability of comparing potentials along only one dimension. That dimension can be *time* (e.g., early vs late), *anatomy* (e.g., brainstem vs cerebral cortex), *spectrum* (e.g., low-frequency vs high-frequency), *psychologic function* (e.g., awareness vs comprehension), or something else. Cutting across dimensions (*ABR [anatomic]* vs *MP [temporal]*) for comparative purposes can be as confounding as trying to compare the mass of one object to the volume of another. A more reasonable comparison or foil for ABR would be something like TCR (for thalamo-cortical response).

Subject Parameters

Age

Although MPs can be elicited from persons of any age, peak latencies and amplitudes will vary with age, as will the overall waveform. Because there has been no uniformity in the way that MPs have been elicited and recorded, no age-related norms are available for clinical reference and comparison. Neonatal and adult MPs do differ in at least one critical way. If recordings from adults are made simultaneously from both sides of the brain (e.g., Cz-A1 and Cz-A2), and the left ear is stimulated with a moderate level signal (e.g., a click at 50 dB

HL), clear and nearly indistinguishable distinct MPs will be recorded from both sides of the head. The same is true for right-ear stimulation. With neonates, however, distinct MPs are recorded only from the side of the head ipsilateral to the stimulated ear, that is, Cz-A1 for left-ear stimulation and Cz-A2 for right-ear stimulation (Wolf & Goldstein, 1980).

Gender and Race
In one early study (Mendel & Goldstein, 1969), women showed shorter latencies and larger amplitudes for some MP peaks. In general, however, neither gender nor race have been explored systematically as factors in MP responses.

State
The state of patients tested under the same circumstances and for the same purposes may differ widely. Some patients attend closely to the test signals while others are in oblivious reverie. Some patients fall asleep and the state of sleep varies throughout the test session. Some patients have their level of attention influenced by drugs and drugs can induce varying levels of sleep. As with rate, sleep seems to diminish later activity in the 10–50 ms window more than it diminishes earlier activity (Suzuki et al., 1992). Some later response-related activity may even be eradicated.

The negative consequences of state effects depend upon the clinical question being addressed. If pattern comparisons are used for diagnostic clues in otoneurologic assessment, then norms must be established for each of the various patient states that are commonly encountered because usually it is difficult to control the patient's changing states. The clinician also must monitor the patient's state so that the proper normal template can be applied.

Drawbacks of variations with state are less consequential when MPs are used for threshold audiometry (Kupperman & Mendel, 1974). Although MP waveforms are modified by state, replicability within a given state is good (Kraus, McGee, & Comperatore, 1989). Therefore, replicability can be used as the principal indicator of response for audiometry. Furthermore, the earliest portions of the MP, that is, between 10–20 ms, vary little as a function of state and, thus, their configuration usually can be used as a response indicator (Mendel & Goldstein, 1969; Mendel & Kupperman, 1974).

Replicability

Much criticism has been leveled against the clinical practicality of MPs because of their presumed variability. However, the critics may not be distinguishing between *response* variability and *trace* variability. MP traces generally are more variable looking than EP (ABR) traces. The filter passband commonly used for EP is 100–3000 Hz. MPs are defined best when the recording filter passband is 3–500 Hz or 1–500 Hz, which, of course, allows considerably more low-frequency energy to enter the trace. Unfortunately, those generators most responsible for creating the low-frequency energy are more susceptible to patient state than are the generators responsible for the higher frequency energy. Some of the low-frequency energy is response-related but more of it is unrelated noise. Therefore, the changing noise from time to time can make successive traces appear variable. The response component is not as variable.

A procedure to reduce the noise components in MP traces (as well as in traces for EPs and LPs) is to make an average of several AEPs for example, three, obtained under identical signal and recording conditions. This **composite AEP** will be smoother than any of the three individual AEPs from which it is derived. Peaks of interest will be easier to identify and to measure than they are in the individual AEPs even when the three of them are superimposed (see Figure 6-5). The compositing procedure also shows that the actual response-related portions of the MPs are not nearly as variable as the literature generally implies.

Myogenic Potentials

Since the period when MPs were presumed to be completely or mostly myogenic (Bickford et al., 1964; Davis et al., 1964), others proved that MPs, obtained under clinically applicable circumstances, were primarily or exclusively neurogenic (Harker, Hosick, Voots, & Mendel, 1977; Horwitz, Larson, & Sances, 1966; Ruhm et al., 1967). Nevertheless, post-auricular muscles and other scalp muscles near or between the electrodes can be activated by acoustic signals, especially at levels greater than 70 dB HL. Even weaker signals can elicit myogenic potentials when post-auricular muscles are under tension. Myogenic potentials usually are most pronounced 10 to 20 ms after signal onset. Neurogenic potentials in that time zone ordinarily are about 1 μV or less, depending largely on signal level. Myogenic potentials often exceed 5 μV. Any MP component greater than 2 μV should be suspected of being contaminated with myogenic potentials. Comfortable positioning of the patient reduces the risk of myogenic contamination. When possible, the patient should lie supine on a bed, cot, or examining table, with the head resting on a soft pillow. A comfortable neck pillow that restricts the turning of a patient's head is desirable to reduce the probability of neck tension because of the turning of the head too far to one side.

Signal-Related Potentials: Late Potentials

We define late-latency AEPs or **late potentials (LPs)** as those replicable positive and negative peaks that occur between 50 and 500 ms after onset of the eliciting signals. Figure 7-1 shows a characteristic LP to a distinctly suprathreshold signal. The earliest peaks in this time zone may begin before 50 ms and the latest peaks may end beyond 500 ms. Other terms and initials have been used to designate LPs, the most common of which are *auditory late responses* or *ALRs, cortical potentials*, and *vertex potentials*.

Generators of the LPs are more difficult to ascertain than are the generators of the EPs and MPs. The later the occurrence of an electroencephalic phenomenon, the greater are the number and variety of generators contributing to its definition. Also, the later the electroencephalic activity, the more variable it is. These two properties have discouraged clinical use of LPs. On the positive side is the likelihood that LPs are more correlated with conscious perception than are EPs or MPs. Thus, the normal physiologic variability that plagues LPs in threshold audiometry and in neurologic diagnosis may be a virtue in helping to determine the perceptual intactness of the patient.

Situations that lead to the elicitation of event-related potentials (ERPs) (to be discussed in Chapter 8), also affect the LPs, qualifying them to be considered ERPs under some circumstances. However, in this chapter, concentration is on how properties of LPs relate to the physical properties of the eliciting signals, that is, LPs as signal-related potentials (SRPs).

Historic Background

Although the LPs were not the first AEPs to be studied or used clinically for audiologic purposes, they were the first components to receive intensive attention both clinically and experimentally. What had been called early or fast components, that is, 0–50 ms, had been

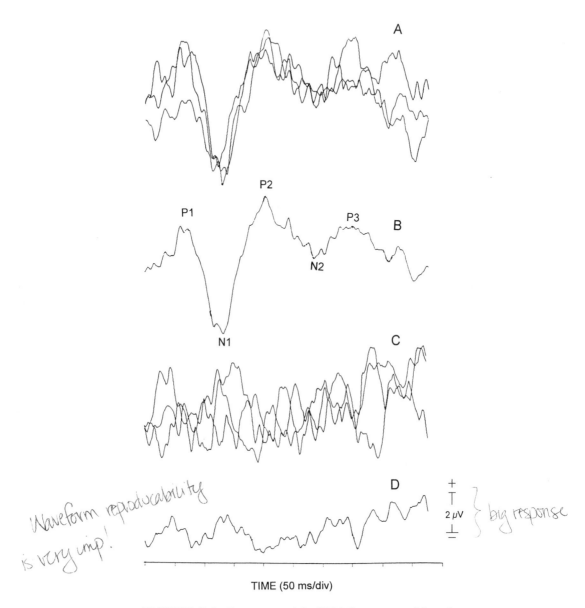

TIME (50 ms/div)

FIGURE 7-1 **Late potentials (LPs) from normal-hearing young woman. Filter passband: 1–70 Hz. (A) 1000 Hz tone burst (10 ms rise/fall time, 20 ms plateau) at 60 dB nHL; rate: 1.1/s. N per AEP= 90. (B) Composite AEP from the three replications shown in A. (C) Tone bursts at –10 dB nHL; inaudible to subject. (D) Composite AEP from the three replications shown in C.**

relegated to temporary oblivion because of their interpretation as being only myogenic. Enough evidence of LPs' neurogenicity spared them the stigma of myogenicity.

One commonly used temporal delineation of LPs, 50–300 ms, was that set out by Picton and colleagues (1974). Others have used a later starting point, for example, 75 ms. Still others have used an indefinite closure time, that is, their definition includes all activity after 50 ms (or after whatever late boundary that they placed on the MPs). By necessity, recording of the LPs also includes the first 50 ms of post-stimulus activity, that is, EPs and MPs, unless one sets the trigger of the signal averager to begin at 50 ms. However, because of the way that LPs usually are recorded (500 ms analysis window and a filter passband of about 1–30 Hz), much of the early and middle latency activity is filtered out. What remains is so crunched into the beginning of the analysis window to obscure definition of the component waves.

From about 1962 through 1972, LPs were exploited extensively both clinically and experimentally (Barnet & Lodge, 1967; Bogacz, Vanzulli, & Garcia-Austt, 1962; Davis, Hirsh, Shelnutt, & Bowers, 1967; McCandless & Rose, 1970) . However, audiologists and other clinicians gradually became disenchanted with LPs as a response index for threshold audiometry because of the dependency of the waveform on the ever-changing state of the patient. Neurologists were disappointed with LPs as an index of structural abnormality or of functional disorder because of the state dependency of the waveform and because of the complexities of the normal waveform. Then, publications on EPs and MPs diverted both clinicians' and experimenters' attention away from LPs. However, some limitations of the activity between 0–50 ms have caused clinicians to reconsider LPs as additional indices both for threshold audiometry and otoneurologic diagnosis.

LPs have two attributes that argue for their audiometric use. First, their amplitudes are large compared with amplitudes of EPs and MPs. Second, LPs can be elicited with longer-duration, narrower-spectrum signals than can be used in threshold EPA with EPs or MPs as the response index. In addition, LPs are not as variable as their bad press suggests, especially if the clinician attempts to keep patient state constant.

Characteristics of LPs

Recording Parameters

Analysis Window or Recording Epoch

As defined earlier, LPs are those replicable positive and negative peaks that occur between 50 and 500 ms after onset of the eliciting signals. Nevertheless, most recordings of LPs also include the first 50 ms, or EPs and MPs. However, as just mentioned, much of the early- and middle-latency activity is filtered out, and what remains is so squeezed into the beginning of the analysis window that definition of the component waves is obscured. Delaying some signal averagers until 50 ms post-signal-onset is possible but little purpose is served by excluding the first 50 ms either for audiometric or neurologic evaluation. At the other extreme, the window can be extended beyond 500 ms or reduced below 500 ms if the clinical answer being sought warrants the variation. In short, any definition of LPs established for intra- and interclinic comparisons should not inhibit expansion or contraction of the analysis window if a clinical situation warrants it.

Spectrum and Filters

Clinicians have reached no consensus on the best filter passband for recording LPs. The recommendation in this book is for a 1–70 Hz filter passband.

According to Hyde (1994), the major concentration of energy in the 50–500 ms time region is between 2–10 Hz. This is in accord with our own empiric observation that the major LP energy lies mainly between 2–7 Hz (Goldstein, 1973). In one study involving LPs (McRandle & Goldstein, 1973) we used a 1–12 Hz passband. Hyde contends that there is negligible LP energy below 1 Hz and above 12 Hz. However, we have noted during laboratory exercises that the energy below 2 Hz does contribute to the definition of the positive and negative peaks, especially to their magnitude. Frequencies above 12 Hz also help to define the peaks, particularly their sharpness. The downside of lowering the high-pass cut-off below 2 Hz is that the large, low-frequency activity is more state-dependent than the higher-frequency activity and hence is more variable. Variability reduces the replicability of AEP traces obtained with identical signals. The downside of extending the low-pass cut-off higher than 12 Hz is letting some high-frequency activity that is unrelated to the response superimpose itself on the signal-related peaks. Superimposition of what is essentially noise increases the difficulty of identifying peaks and measuring their latencies and magnitudes. Despite these unfavorable aspects of a wide passband, the clarity of LPs seems to be more enhanced than degraded by the energy below 2 Hz and above 12 Hz. The biggest noise troublemaker is 60 Hz. If 60 Hz cannot be reduced sufficiently during the averaging process, the low-pass cutoff can be dropped below 70 Hz (e.g., 30 Hz) without doing great violence to the LP waveform.

Analog filters not only attenuate spectral energy outside the filter passband, they also can cause phase lags and leads especially for those frequencies close to the high- and low-pass ends of the passband. These phase-shift distortions are of no consequence when LPs are used for threshold audiometry as long as the distorted patterns are replicable. Figure 7-2 shows the extent of waveform replicability and the consistent changes in latency and magnitude with decreases in signal level. Valid thresholds can be estimated from these waveforms.

Electrode Montage

Many topographic studies have been done to help identify the anatomic generators of LPs. Information from these studies may be used to try to relate abnormalities in LPs to the site of brain lesions or malfunctions. However, the studies are too extensive and diverse to be able to extrapolate from them the electrode montage that would be best for recording LPs clinically. The consensus for threshold audiometry, derived primarily through clinical experience, is that one recording electrode should be on or close to the vertex (Cz). Consensus about the second electrode of a pair is not clear. However, as with EPs and MPs, the most common placement for the other electrode has been either the earlobe or the mastoid (A1 or A2 or M1 or M2). Clinical questions about the site, extent, and nature of brain lesions or dysfunctions are too broad to justify recommending any one electrode montage for all clinical applications.

Signal Parameters

Signal Spectrum

Clicks elicit large and distinct LPs. Just as with the EPs and MPs, when one uses LPs for otoneurologic diagnostic purposes, clicks are the signals of choice. A patient with hearing

Major adv: ability to use long-duration tone bursts that are nearly pure-tone-audiometry-like + thus highly freq specific inc. low freqs)

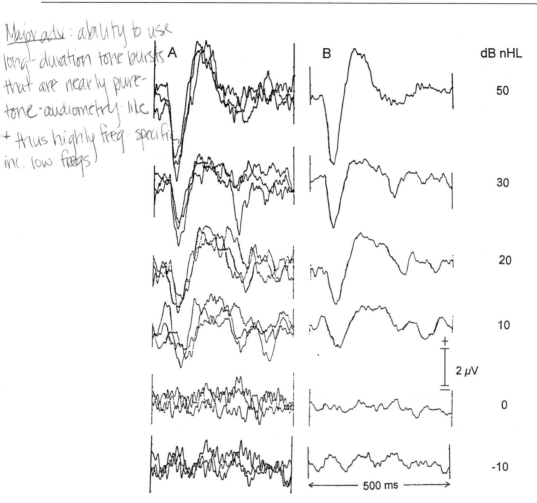

FIGURE 7-2   This is a reproduction of Figure 1-5. Late potentials (LPs) from a normal-hearing young woman as a function of signal level. Signals: 1000 Hz tone bursts (10 ms rise/fall time, 10 ms plateau) to right ear at 1/s. Tone bursts were inaudible at 0 and –10 dB nHL. Electrode montage: Cz-A1; filter passband: 1–70 Hz. (A) N per AEP = 90. (B) Composite AEPs of the three replications in A.

N1 shiftless

impairment being evaluated for neurologic purposes may not show the expected waveform for a given suprathreshold click even if the auditory system central to the cochlea is completely normal. This is especially true if the patient's loss either for high or for low frequencies is distinctly greater than for the remaining frequencies. However, the deviations from normal usually are not as pronounced as they may be when EPs and MPs are the response indices.

LPs can be used as response indices when clicks are used to obtain a crude estimate of the patient's auditory sensitivity. However, a major audiometric virtue of LPs, compared with EPs and MPs, is that they can be elicited by long-duration tone bursts (e.g., 50 ms) whose spectrum is nearly as narrow as those used in conventional behavioral response audiometry. Therefore, little correction has to be made for threshold as a function of signal duration for comparisons with or estimations of behavioral response thresholds. For LPs, just as with MPs, low-frequency tone bursts elicit AEPs with longer latencies and larger amplitudes than AEPs elicited by high-frequency tone bursts.

Another comparative advantage of LPs is their large magnitude. With suprathreshold response magnitudes often exceeding 2 μV, less amplification of the raw EEG is needed and, thus, less extraneous noise contaminates the AEP traces. Finally, because severe low-pass filtering can be used, much of the physiologic and instrumental noise that can contaminate MPs is reduced or eliminated.

The biggest disadvantage of LPs for threshold EPA is their dependency on patient state. When patient state is held constant, which often is possible with adults and older children, LPs are sufficiently replicable for reliable sensitivity measures. However, if the audiologist can control patient state for threshold EPA, odds are high that the audiologist could have assessed the patient's threshold more conveniently and cheaply by behavioral response audiometry. Controlling state in neonates and young infants for whom EPA may be most necessary is far more diffiult. Maintaining physical control over neonates and young infants is easy. However, the clinician usually cannot control *when* they will sleep, which is often, or the *level* of their sleep, which can vary widely during an evaluation. One can control state with drugs but different drugs can have deleterious effects on the LPs.

Signal Rate

If the clinician uses a 500 ms analysis window, the maximum allowable signal rate is 2/s, that is, the reciprocal of the set period of 500 ms. If faster rates are used, a second signal occurs within the analysis window. Amplitudes are larger when rates slower than 2/s are used. Complete recovery requires about a 10-second inter-signal interval (Davis et al., 1966), but rates as fast as 1/2s or even 1/s can evoke clinically usable LPs.

Subject Parameters

Age

LPs can be elicited from persons of any age but LPs vary as a function of age (Allison, Hume, Wood, & Goff, 1984; Barnet, Ohlrich, Weiss, & Shanks, 1975; Price, Rosenblüt, Goldstein, & Shepherd, 1966). LPs are earlier and larger in young adults than they are in infants. Latencies change little with further increases in age but amplitudes become slightly larger. Clinicians may have to consider age-related differences for neurologic interpretations. However, age-related differences can be ignored for assessment of threshold unless a fixed AEP configuration or template is used as an index of response.

Gender and Race

LPs are earlier and larger for women than for men (Buchsbaum, Henkin, & Christiansen, 1974; Price et al., 1966). They are also earlier and larger for European American than for

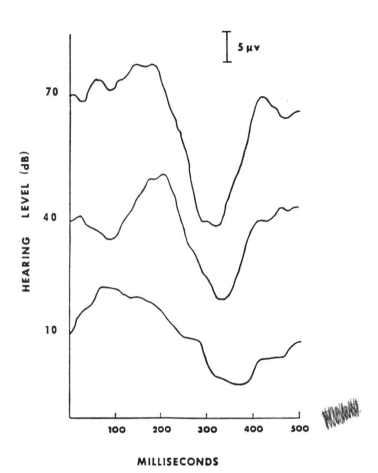

FIGURE 7-3   Late potentials (LPs) to clicks from 2½-year-old boy, asleep after having been medicated with Nembutal. Note the large negative deflection at and beyond 300 ms. Although the configuration of the AEPs differed from those from awake children and adults, the different pattern was consistent enough to determine that the boy's threshold for clicks was within the normal range.

[From Price & Goldstein, "Averaged evoked responses for measuring auditory sensitivity in children." *Journal of Speech and Hearing Disorders, 31,* 248-256, 1966. © American Speech-Language-Hearing Association. Reprinted by permission.]

African American persons (Price et al., 1966); however, a gender by race interaction clouds the certainty of this generality. Other racial groups have not been studied in sufficient numbers in comparative investigations to allow broad, conclusive statements to be made about the relation between ethnicity and LPs.

State

Experimental evidence (Becker & Shapiro, 1981; Davis, 1965; Jacobson, Calder, Newman, Peterson, Wharton, & Ahmad, 1996) as well as clinical observations support the contention that LPs vary widely with subject/patient state. LP amplitude in particular varies even when subjects are awake, depending on whether they attend to the test signals or ignore them, and on whether they are alert or drowsy. Even LP configuration changes during sleep, and differs with the stage of sleep. A marked change occurs during one stage of sleep when a small positive deflection at about 300 ms is replaced by a large negative deflection (Barnet et al., 1975; Williams, Tepas, & Morlock, 1962). REM sleep appears to obliterate LPs altogether or at least to render them unrecognizable as response-related deflections.

The shortcoming of state dependency diverted audiologist's efforts from trying to use LPs routinely on difficult-to-test patients. Nevertheless, this shortcoming can be lessened by attempts to keep the patient's state as uniform as clinical circumstances allow. LPs from a normal-hearing subject are shown in Figure 7-2. Replicability is sufficient for a clinician to affirm that the traces are or are not response related, and to estimate threshold from changes in the AEPs as a function of signal level. Even when LP configuration changes with sleep, as long as the state of sleep remains relatively constant, thresholds can be estimated with reasonable enough certainty for those patients for whom EPA is necessary (Price & Goldstein, 1966) (Figure 7-3).

Chapter 8

Event-Related Potentials

Event-related potentials (ERPs) are those components of AEPs that are related to the circumstances under which they are elicited rather than to the physical properties of the signals that elicit the AEPs. They could be labeled "circumstance-related potentials (CRPs)" but "event-related" is too entrenched to displace.

The word **exogenous** sometimes is used synonymously with "signal-related" or "stimulus-related," and the word **endogenous** with "event-related." An implication of these synonyms is that conditions external to the listener determine exogenous potentials and that conditions internal to the listener determine endogenous potentials. While this implication is broadly true, it clouds the interaction of the two effects. Circumstances internal to the listener do much to shape SRPs, and manipulation of conditions external to the listener are crucial for eliciting ERPs.

Cognitive potentials is another term commonly applied to ERPs. The term is not entirely appropriate because conscious awareness of target signals, which "cognitive" implies, is not always requisite for the elicitation of ERPs. Also, this term can confuse inter-potential comparison. Cognitive has a psychologic connotation. SRPs usually are described along temporal (e.g., middle potentials) or anatomic (e.g., brainstem) dimensions.

Terms commonly used for two early (<250 ms) ERPs are **processing negativity (PN)** and **mismatch negativity (MMN),** proposed by Näätänen and colleagues (Näätänen, 1982; Näätänen & Michie, 1979). These terms have psychophysiologic connotations that make them difficult to compare across other ERPs (e.g., P300, which has a temporal dimension), and across AEPs in general. Also, their negative polarity depends upon the electrode configuration used in their recording; with other modes of measuring and quantification, such as area-under-the-curve, "negativity" may be irrelevant.

Considering all of these terminologic alternatives, we chose the commonly used term, *event-related potentials,* and the initials ERP for general descriptions of relevant phenomena, and we use temporal descriptors (post-stimulus time of occurrence) to designate the phenomena under discussion. However, at times, we use other authors' terms when we discuss phenomena that they have described in their writings.

Auditory ERPs have been used widely in assessing psychiatric disorders. This is an important area in which audiologists and other clinicians can assist. However, we emphasize ERPs mainly for assessing hearing and language dysfunctions. ERPs are powerful indices for assessing a patient's capacity for language communication through hearing. In time, using ERPs may even be possible instead of SRPs to assess simpler conditions such as sensitivity impairment, loudness dysfunctions, binaural interaction, and so on. Until these additional uses are validated clinically, however, assessment of peripheral or central auditory dysfunction with ERPs should be preceded by assessment of basic auditory function and integrity through behavioral responses or through SRPs.

Many people think of ERPs only in terms of what has been called the oddball paradigm and the resulting P300. We, too, shall stress the oddball paradigm and the P300 and related ERPs because of their audiologic value. Nevertheless, there are other paradigms and other ERP manifestations that could and probably should be exploited. These will be summarized briefly later. They have not yet been exploited clinically to the extent that the oddball paradigm and the P300 have.

Historic Background

One can infer possible audiologic application of oddball ERPs from early psychophysiologic studies (Davis, 1964; Sutton, Braren, Zubin, & John, 1965). Reports of actual clinical audiologic applications, however, for which ERPs provided defining information not available from other test indices have been too sparse and recent to determine which studies have landmark significance. Nevertheless, the work of Näätänen and colleagues on early ERPs probably will be considered in retrospect to have launched particularly valuable audiologic clinical applications. Näätänen provides several extensive reviews of his work and the work of others on what he terms the PN and MMN (1990, 1995).

Oddball ERPs *Paradigm*

The simplest form of the oddball paradigm, from which ERPs are obtained, is one in which a signal (e.g., 1000 Hz tone bursts at 50 dB nHL) is presented to the listener at a regular rate (e.g., 1/s). This the frequent, standard, or expected signal. Randomly and infrequently (e.g., one in ten, or 10% of the time) a different signal (e.g., 2000 Hz tone burst equally as loud as the frequent 1000 Hz tone burst) is substituted for the 1000 Hz tone burst. The different signal is known variously as the infrequent, deviant, unexpected, rare, or oddball signal. The electroencephalic activity for a fixed period (e.g., 750 ms) following each frequent signal is stored in one memory bank of the signal averager; and activity following the oddball signal is stored in a separate memory bank. If 100 signals had been presented in this example, the resultant frequent AEP would be made up of 90 samples and the oddball AEP of 10 samples.

If the AEP for the 1000 and 2000 Hz tone bursts had been acquired by themselves in two separate test runs, they would resemble each other closely except for small signal-related differences in peak latencies and amplitudes (Figure 8-1). Acquired in the inter-

Compare 8.1 + 8.2
No difference

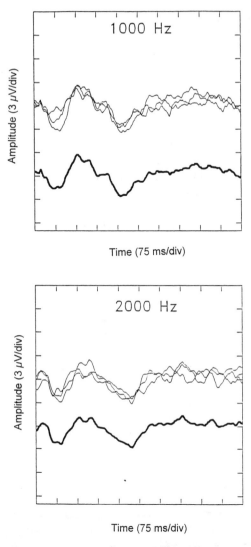

**FIGURE 8-1   Signal-related AEPs from
a 23-year-old normal-hearing woman.
Tone bursts: rise/fall time of 10 ms and a
plateau of 20 ms. Signal level: 85 dB
nHL. Presentation rate: 0.9/s. Superimposed traces: 90 sweeps each. Heavy
trace below, composite AEP: sum of three
individual traces divided by 3.**

mixed fashion described, they also have distinct differences as well as some similarities (see Figure 8-2, which is a reproduction of the upper portion of Figure 1-6). The AEP to the 2000 Hz oddball signal contains some activity not seen in response to the 1000 Hz frequent signal, the most prominent of which is a large positive deflection at or just beyond 300 ms. This prominent deflection often is referred to as P300. Other, differences also occur before and after 300 ms. All these differences in the oddball AEP are the event-related potentials or ERPs.

At times discerning the ERP differences between the oddball and the frequent AEPs is difficult. Those differences become more definable when the frequent AEP is digitally subtracted from the oddball AEP (see Figure 8-3, which is a reproduction of the lower portion of Figure 1-6). The difference trace contains the ERP and the difference in uncanceled noise between the oddball and the frequent AEPs. This noise difference can blur the ERP and can even lead to clinical misinterpretations.

The P300 is so prominent that often all differences between the frequent and oddball AEPs are genericized by many as P300. Even the paradigm by means of which the ERPs are elicited often is called the P300 paradigm. The generic P300 term is convenient but it

P300

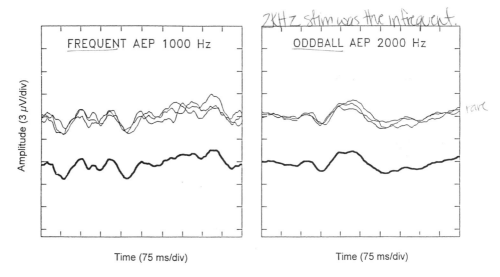

FREQUENT AEP 1000 Hz   ODDBALL AEP 2000 Hz

2KHz, stim was the infrequent.

Amplitude (3 μV/div)

rare

Time (75 ms/div)   Time (75 ms/div)

FIGURE 8-2   This is a reproduction of the top portion of Figure 1-6. AEPs from a 23-year-old normal-hearing woman. Frequent AEP: 1000 Hz tone burst at 85 dB nHL, probability 81%. Superimposed traces: 73 sweeps each. Heavy trace below, composite AEP: sum of the three individual traces divided by 3. Oddball AEP: 2000 Hz tone burst at 85 dB nHL, probability 19%. Superimposed traces: 17 sweeps each. Heavy trace below, composite AEP: sum of the three individual traces divided by 3. Subject kept mental count of number of oddball signals during each trial.

take difference b/w the deviant-
+ std-evoked responses

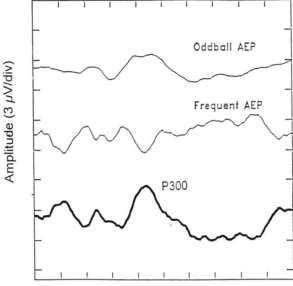

useful but unperfect

FIGURE 8-3   This is a reproduction of the lower portion of Figure 1-6. Oddball and frequent AEPs are the composite AEPs from Figure 8-2. The difference trace of which the P300 is part was obtained by subtracting the composite frequent AEP from the composite oddball AEP. Although P300 is the most prominent deflection in the heavy trace, other differences between oddball and frequency AEPs also are evident.

clouds other important ERP phenomena and diverts attention from other ways of eliciting clinically useful ERPs.

Recording Parameters

Analysis Window or Recording Epoch
No one recording epoch serves all purposes. If the observer concentrates on P300, the analysis window should be at least 500 ms to allow definition of the trailing edge of that large positive deflection. Wider or longer windows are necessary if one wishes to study the effects of semantic or syntactic differentials, instead of differentials in basic acoustic prop-

erties such as frequency or amplitude. ERP activity before 300 ms also can be observed with analysis windows wider than 300 ms. However, the wider the window, the more crunched together the earlier activity is and, thus, less definable. If one wishes to examine early activity (e.g., the first 250 ms) with precision, one should use a 250 ms recording epoch.

Window width interacts with signal repetition rate. If, for example, a clinician wants to examine 1 s (1000 ms) of post-signal activity, then signal rate is limited to a maximum of 1/s. Rate also is limited by the signal averager's need to do some of its own internal sorting and other housekeeping duties. Therefore, when the analysis window is 1000 ms, maximum rate usually is limited to less than 1/s.

Spectrum and Filters

For ERPs, just as with SRPs, the earlier the peak the higher is its spectral composition. However, even for the earliest ERP usually recorded (peak latency about 75 ms), energy above 40 Hz contributes little to the definition of the waveform. Low-frequency energy, by contrast, is contributory. Some ERP components are so gradual that they approach being direct current (DC). A DC high-pass, therefore, would be ideal. Unfortunately, DC coupling usually is not practical for most clinical electrophysiologic recordings. A high-pass of 0.1 Hz may be feasible but widely varying electrophysiologic noise between 0.1 and 1.0 Hz can contaminate recordings seriously. A recording bandpass of 1–70 Hz is a reasonable compromise for most clinical ERP recordings. Given the common filter roll-off of 12 dB/octave, some large, low-frequency activity that may contribute to the ERP waveform can still make some contribution; and all activity at least through 40 Hz will come through unattenuated.

Electrode Montage

Many different anatomic generators in the brain contribute to all components of the ERP. In addition, contributing generators will differ with the different circumstances under which ERPs are elicited. Therefore, one cannot specify one electrode montage, or sets of montages, for all ERP studies. The montage(s) of choice also depends on the clinical question asked of the ERPs. Site-of-lesion tests may require different electrode combinations than tests of functional integrity require. Nevertheless, at least for ERPs 300 ms and later, it usually is wise to place one electrode on the midline in the parietal area slightly posterior to the vertex.

ERPs are not stationary in time. Activity usually begins earliest frontally and moves posteriorly (Polich, Alexander, Bauer, Kuperman, Morzorati, O'Connor, Porjesz, Rohrbaugh, & Begleiter, 1997). Therefore, if time course of the ERP is crucial to the clinical question asked, then more than one set of electrodes is essential. Site-of-lesion tests also require multiple electrode pairs.

Electric activity resulting from eye movements synchronized with the eliciting signals can contaminate ERP recordings. Sometimes eye movements can be controlled or limited by instructing subjects or by diverting them with visual tasks. If eye movement contamination remains a problem, then additional electrodes have to be placed near the eyes to record the electrooptical or electroretinal potentials. This enables the clinician to determine which samples should be rejected from the averaged response.

Signal Parameters

Physical Characteristics

Selection of physical characteristics of the frequent and oddball signals depends entirely on the clinical question being asked. Whatever the clinical question, however, the frequent and oddball signals should differ only along one dimension. In the example given earlier (frequent = 1000 Hz; oddball = 2000 Hz), the clinician should be certain that loudness of the two signals is the same. Even for a person with normal hearing sensitivity, a 50 dB nHL signal at 2000 Hz does not necessarily have the same loudness as a 50 dB nHL signal at 1000 Hz. This issue is especially troublesome if thresholds for the two frequencies are different. If loudness does differ, then the patient's response to the oddball may contain ERPs to a loudness differential as well as to a pitch differential. Equal Sensation Levels (SL) do not assure equal loudness, especially if there is loudness recruitment at one frequency and not at the other. When the frequency differential is smaller (e.g., frequent = 1000 Hz; oddball = 1050 Hz), loudness differences for equal HLs or SLs are less likely.

Another simple differential is that of signal magnitude (e.g., 1000 Hz tone burst with frequent = 75 dB nHL; oddball = 60 dB nHL). Although pitch can change with a decrease in signal level (Stevens, 1935), that change most likely will be minuscule or nonexistent at moderate signal levels and not likely to introduce a pitch differential to confound the ERP evoked by the signal magnitude difference. If the oddball signal is an increase in magnitude compared with the frequent signal, it could evoke activity of unadapted neurons, thus introducing an additional response variable. An oddball signal that is a decrease in magnitude is not vexed by this problem.

Time is another dimension along which acoustic signals can be differentiated. It may be the most important dimension for assessing the brain's ability to process and to interpret speech and language messages. Temporal characteristics are more complex than those of magnitude and frequency (or spectrum). Examples of some temporal subdimensions are rise or onset time, duration, rate, and order. Temporality also interacts closely with pitch and loudness. Therefore, temporal oddballs have to be structured to counteract confounding pitch or loudness cues.

Localization in space is another physical dimension along which frequent/oddball differentials can be constructed. This dimension obviously involves binaurality. Magnitude, spectral, and temporal dimensions also can be structured to assess binaurality.

Of the acoustic dimensions discussed, magnitude differentials are the least likely to be contaminated by inadvertent cues from the other dimensions. Also, they may be the easiest to create instrumentally. On the other hand, assessment of the brain's capacity to process magnitude differentials may give the least insight into the brain's capacity for processing speech signals and speech messages. However, this apparent shortcoming of magnitude differentials may not be a serious limitation in the clinical assessment of the brain's ability to process signals along all of the basic acoustic dimensions. CANS structures responsible for elemental acoustic dimensions are clustered together in small structures. It is improbable that a tumor, stroke, or traumatic injury that caused dysfunction of magnitude processing would leave intact the ability to process spectral, temporal, or spatial dimensions of the same signals. In fact, it is likely that the neuronal systems that process magnitude properties of acoustic signals are involved to some extent in the processing of the other signal properties. Therefore, for those clinical situations in which spectral, temporal, and spatial processing capabilities cannot be assessed directly, some inference about their integrity might be drawn from the assessment of magnitude-processing capability.

When the brain expects to receive a frequent signal as part of a regularly repeated sequence, it reacts to the *absence* of an expected sound (Donchin & McCarthy, 1979; Sutton, Tueting, Zubin, & John, 1967). The resulting ERP sometimes is referred to as an **emitted potential.** Obviously, no SRP is associated with it. Use of emitted potentials can aid in the assessment of a patient's ability to sense or to appreciate a rhythmic pattern. Because there are no dimensions to the absent or omitted signal, no inadvertent acoustic differential is introduced into the oddball paradigm.

Clinicians and experimentalists are interested in going beyond simple acoustic differentials and in using ERPs to assess the brain's ability to process complex speech-like signals, actual speech differentials, and language differentials (Diniz, Mangabeira-Albernaz, Munhoz, & Fukuda, 1997; Hagoort, Brown, & Swaab, 1996; Hillyard, 1985). The acoustic as well as the procedural complexities are greater for higher-level differentials than for the simple acoustic differentials described earlier. It is impossible to anticipate and to catalog all the contingencies that clinicians may encounter. Nevertheless, the principles of the oddball paradigm still apply to the assessment of higher-level differentials.

Signal Rate

As pointed out earlier, there is an inverse relation between the width of the analysis window and the maximum achievable repetition rate. Fortunately, the brain's capacity to process simple acoustic differentials can be assessed with ERPs that occur within the first 250 ms of signal onset, as well as with later ERPs such as the P300. With an analysis window of 250 ms, signal repetition rate can approach 4/s. Amplitude of early ERPs tends to increase as signal rates increase (Näätänen, 1995), unlike the decrement noted in the amplitude of SRPs with increased rate. The effect of rate on ERPs later than 250 ms is not well established because the length of the analysis window, usually at least 500 ms, places its own restriction on signal repetition rate.

Display and Quantification of ERPs

ERPs elicited by the oddball signal are superimposed on or blended with the SRPs elicited by that signal in a complex AEP. Theoretically, the AEP elicited by the frequent signal is only an SRP. When the frequent and oddball AEPs are placed side by side, as in Figure 8-2, or are overlaid, differences between the two will be apparent if the ear and brain can distinguish the oddball from the frequent signal. Residue of the subtraction of the frequent AEP from the oddball, as in Figure 8-3, allows the ERP to be seen apart from the SRP portion of the AEPs. The subtraction, however, is not pure ERP unless the SRP portion of the frequent AEP and the oddball AEP are identical. The SRP portions should be nearly identical if the difference in the frequent and oddball signals is small (e.g., 1000 Hz vs 1050 Hz, 75 dB HL vs 73 dB HL). When the frequent/oddball differences are large, however, the differences in the SRP portions can contaminate the subtraction trace that is supposed to represent only the ERP.

Frequent and oddball AEPs often differ in another way. The oddball AEP usually has more residual noise because it is composed of fewer samples than the frequent AEP (e.g., 10 vs 90). Noise differences have to be accounted for or extracted before the ERP portion of the oddball AEP can be described or quantified.

Chertoff, Goldstein, and Mease (1988) reported a procedure to reduce both the SRP and the noise differences between the frequent and oddball AEPs. A mock or control condition is run in which both the frequent and oddball signals are identical to the oddball signals used in the experimental or test condition. For example, if the frequent signal (e.g., 90% probability) a 1000 Hz tone burst at 75 dB HL and the oddball (10% probability) is the same signal at 60 dB HL, then in the control condition, both the frequent and the oddball signals are 60 dB HL. Listeners just hear a steady repetition of tone bursts at 60 dB HL. However, the recording instrument randomly stores and averages 90% of the responses in one memory bank and 10% in a different memory bank. The 10% AEP becomes the control AEP. It is composed of the same number of samples as oddball AEP in the real test condition and, therefore, approximately the same residual noise. Also, the SRP portions of both should be about the same because the signals for both the test and control oddball AEPs are identical.

ERPs are most commonly analyzed by measures of peak latencies and peak-to-peak (or baseline-to-peak) amplitudes. The peak variabilities limit the clinical value of ERPs for individual patients even when latencies and amplitudes for patient groups are statistically different from those of normal controls.

Area-under-the-curve (AUTC), discussed later in Chapter 10 for quantifying SRPs, also can be used to quantify ERPs. AUTC is an indicator of the total power of a response. The measure obviates the need for subjective decisions about which of the recorded peaks constitute a response. In fact, no distinct peak need occur in the time zone(s) of interest. Limited experience suggests that AUTC measures of ERPs have less intra- and intersubject variability than peak latencies and amplitudes (Barrett, 1992; Doherty, Barrett, & Goldstein, 1991).

Subject Parameters

Interactions between subject (and patient) parameters, test parameters, and the particular differential of interest are so great that they blur clear distinctions between groups. Therefore, we present only the broadest generalities.

Age

Amplitude of peaks around 300 ms and their distinctness increase and peak latencies shorten with increasing age from infancy to young adulthood (Martin, Barajas, Fernandez, & Torres, 1988; Polich & Luckritz, 1995). Then, with further aging, latencies increase, amplitudes decrease, and variability across subjects increases. The effect of age on earlier ERPs is not yet well defined. However, early ERPs have been elicited from persons along the whole age spectrum: neonates (Cheour-Luhtanen, Alho, Kujala, Sainio, Reinikainen,

Renlund, Aaltonen, Eerola, & Näätänen, 1995), school-age children (Oades, Dittman-Balcar, Schepker, Eggers, & Zerbin, 1996), young adults (Chertoff et al., 1988), and old adults (Pekkonen, Jousmäki, Könönen, Reinikainen, & Partanen, 1994).

Gender and Race
Women appear to have larger late ERPs (300+ ms) than men but latencies do not seem to differ between sexes (Martin et al., 1988; Polich & Kok, 1995). Too few studies have been reported to be able to determine whether racial differences are apparent in ERPs or whether there is a gender by race interaction as there is for some SRPs.

State
The way in which oddball ERPs usually are elicited make state a crucial factor. A common procedure is to have the subject or patient count silently the number of oddball signals presented during a test trial. The listener is rewarded verbally or monetarily for the correctness of the count reported at the end of the trial. The subject obviously must be awake and attentive during the trial.

P300 and other late ERPs can be elicited from inattentive subjects who are not instructed to count the oddball. Resulting ERPs, however, are small or even indistinguishable in this **ignore condition** (Donchin & McCarthy, 1979; Ford, Roth, Dirks, & Kopell, 1973). An ignore condition is used by some researchers and clinicians to provide a baseline or control AEP against which the oddball AEP from the attend condition is compared. Because the test and the control oddball AEPs are obtained with identical stimulus and recording parameters, the difference between the two AEPs is regarded as entirely ERP.

ERPs occurring before 300 ms are less attention-dependent (Chertoff et al., 1988; Näätänen, 1995). More is said about the effects of state in the context of some specific test paradigms and of clinical concerns associated with them.

Test Parameters

Probability
The lower the probability of random occurrence of the oddball, the larger is the ERP in response to the oddball (Duncan-Johnson & Donchin, 1977; Polich, 1990). This dictum applies to both early and late ERPs. The most commonly reported probabilities range between 10 and 20%.

In a truly random series, several oddballs can occur in succession. If this happens, then the next frequent signal, in effect, becomes an oddball. This, then, blurs the difference between frequent and oddball AEPs. Possible solutions to this problem include (a) making the first several signals in a trial always be the frequent signal of the pair to prime the brain and (b) programming that does not allow two oddballs in succession (Chertoff et al., 1988). Unfortunately, these solutions require more internal housekeeping time and, therefore, put a lower cap on the fastest signal rate that can be used. With early ERPs, the faster the rate, the larger the amplitude.

Probability affects the signal-to-noise (S/N) ratio of the oddball AEP and of the ERP embedded in it. (As a reminder, *signal* here refers to the response portion of the trace, not to the eliciting sound.) For example, if the total test trial consists of 200 presentations and the oddball probability is 10%, then the frequent AEP will consist of 180 samples and the oddball AEP of 20 samples. The signal portion of the oddball AEP, and especially the ERP embedded in it, is large because of the low oddball probability. The noise portion also is large because of the small sample size. Sample size for the frequent AEP usually is large enough to produce an AEP with little noise. Probability only has a small effect on the amplitude of the frequent AEP, which is almost entirely an SRP. With an oddball probability of 20%, the noise portion of the oddball AEP is reduced because the sample size is now 40; however, the signal portion also is reduced because of the higher probability. Still higher oddball probabilities (e.g., 33%) result in less noisy oddball AEPs because of the correspondingly larger number of samples, but the S/N may remain unchanged because the signal portion also is smaller.

If a test trial were extended to 1000 signals, then even with only a 10% oddball probability, an oddball AEP of 100 samples should have a good S/N (Cohen & Polich, 1997). On the downside of an extended trial, the time needed to complete the trial increases. More than 8 minutes would be required if the signal rate were as fast as 2/s, about 16.5 minutes would be required for a slower rate of 1/s. Subjects and patients become restless over that period and their restlessness usually leads to increased noise in the recording. Additionally, keeping the subjects/patients attentive and keeping their state consistent during the procedure is difficult. Changes in attentiveness and in state lead to changes in the signal portion as well as in the noise portion of the AEPs.

A practical alternative to extending the number of signals per trial to 1000 is to have several shorter identical trials (e.g., five) with 200 signals each. Composite AEPs (average of the five separate AEPs) can be made. Compositing is justified because attentiveness and state can be kept relatively constant across the five shorter trials of less than 3.5 minutes at 1/s or less than 2 minutes at 2/s.

Size of Differential

The larger the difference between the frequent and oddball signal, the larger is the resulting ERP; as the difference approaches the perceptual difference limen, ERP latencies increase and amplitudes decrease (Alho, Töttölä, Reinikainen, Sams, & Näätänen, 1987; Polich, Howard, & Starr, 1985). These generalities, although broadly applicable, will vary with the nature of the differential (e.g., simple acoustic differences vs semantic differences) and with the portion of the ERP (i.e., early vs late).

Subject or Patient Task

As mentioned earlier, oddball protocols often call for the subject to attend to the target or oddball signal and to keep a silent count of the oddball signals. Sometimes the task is to press a response button each time the oddball is detected. ERPs later than 250 ms generally are distinctly larger and more definable with attention than when the subject is totally passive. Later ERPs are smaller when the subject is instructed to ignore the oddball signal, or when the attention is diverted from the oddball. Sometimes no ERP can be discerned under these conditions that often are broadly classified as *ignore*. ERPs earlier than 250 ms are less related to subject task or attention.

Clinical Limitations

Patient

A major factor in the clinical success of the oddball paradigm is the ability of the subject or patient to do the usual tasks required during data acquisition. Most older children and adults have the required ability. The intellectually, motorically, and emotionally capable patients, however, seldom have to be evaluated by any form of EPA. Behavioral response, acoustic-immittance, and otoacoustic emission measures coupled with good case histories and physical examinations usually provide sufficient information for confident diagnoses.

Examples of patients for whom evaluation with oddball or other ERP measures is most needed are neonates and young infants, persons of any age who are intellectually deficient, comatose persons, and persons whose aberrant emotional status prevents their full cooperation in other evaluations. Unfortunately, these are the patients who are least likely to be able to keep a running silent count of oddball signals or to press a response button when they detect an oddball signal.

Even capable and cooperative patients may have some difficulty with the ignore condition. If the ignore condition is first in the protocol and if the patient is given no instructions other than to sit or lie quietly, indifference to the oddball should lead to no difference between frequent and oddball AEPs other than for the stimulus-related differences between them. However, if the ignore condition is not first and attention is directed to the oddball, it is difficult for the patient to disregard the oddball during the later ignore condition. Also, if a patient is retested in a later session, disregarding the oddball during the ignore condition will be nearly impossible for the patient, even if that condition is first.

Some testers try to accomplish the effect of an ignore condition through some diversion or distraction from the oddball signals (e.g., engaging in a visual task, watching a silent slide show or movie). Unfortunately, most persons for whom this form of testing may be necessary cannot be distracted by diversionary ruses.

Interpretation

Professionals who refer their patients for evaluation with ERPs usually are concerned most about their patients' ability to process speech signals and language messages. The duration of the test signals and the time needed for high-level processing dictate that late ERPs be the response indices. If the patient's ERPs for the test signals are normal, it is safe to infer that preliminary acoustic processing also is normal. However, if the patient's late ERPs are abnormal, that information alone is insufficient for useful clinical conclusions. The patient's central processing problem could be only a high-level one, for example, some deficiency in semantic differentiation. On the other hand, the problem could be simpler or more basic. For example, if the patient cannot process the temporal properties of the acoustic make-up of the words for the semantic differential, then any subsequent higher level processing of the speech message will by necessity be faulty.

The clinician cannot automatically assume that a patient's problem is solely in the auditory domain even when ERPs indicate either basic-level or high-level auditory dysfunction. Visual and/or somatosensory ERPs must be assessed before a confident diagnosis can be made and appropriate remedial measures instituted. If visual and somatosensory

ERPs are normal, then abnormal auditory ERPs may be construed to reflect a modality-specific dysfunction. On the other hand, abnormal ERPs across all modalities tested suggest a broader or more pervasive dysfunction.

Response Stability

The later the component of any AEP, the more susceptible is that component to changes in patient state. This dictum, which has been discussed previously, applies to ERPs as well as to SRPs. Late ERPs, the most commonly used components for speech perception and language evaluations, are more labile than earlier ERPs and, therefore, more likely to be misinterpreted.

Strategy to Minimize Clinical Limitations

Clinicians should forego the temptation to evaluate a patient's speech perception and language capacities before they assess more fundamental capacities. The status of the peripheral auditory system must be determined first, and then of the brain's ability to transmit signals received from the periphery. For most patients for whom ERP testing is necessary, the status check probably has to be done by EPA in which SRPs are used as response indices. If the initial evaluation shows the periphery to be normal and central transmission to be normal, then any ERP abnormality noted later can be attributed safely to some CANS dysfunction. If either the periphery or the central transmission is faulty, then the effects of those faults must be accounted for if ERP abnormalities are noted.

The next step is to use early ERPs to evaluate the brain's ability to make simple differentiations along dimensions of frequency, magnitude, time, and/or space. If those differentiations are normal, then abnormalities noted in later ERPs can be attributed safely to higher order speech perception or language disorders. When simple differentiations are not normal, then the effects of basic abnormalities must be accounted for before ERP manifestations of higher order disorders can be interpreted.

Other Forms of ERPs

Contingent Negative Variation

Procedures

The **contingent negative variation (CNV)** results from a form of conditioning (Alexander, Binnie, & Margerison, 1971). For the example illustrated in Figure 8-4, a sound precedes a light flash by two seconds (Walter, Cooper, Aldridge, McCallum, & Winter, 1964). The listener has been instructed to press a switch when the light appears. Initially, the electric recording shows only the expected SRP after sound and after the light. However, after a few pairings of sound and light, an additional potential appears in the record following the SRP to the sound. This is the CNV. It is a large negative deflection whose time course is so slow as to suggest that it is a direct current (DC) shift. As a reminder, electroencephalographers and some electrophysiologists plot negativity as an upward deflection.

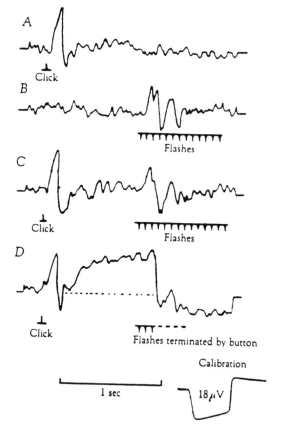

FIGURE 8-4   Elicitation of a contingent negative variation (CNV). Negativity is represented by an upward deflection. (A) AEP to clicks alone (N = 12 in this and other traces). (B) AEP to flickering light flashes alone. (C) AEP to click followed by AEP to flicker. (D) AEP to clicks followed by flicker terminated by the subject's pressing a button as instructed. The large, long negative deflection is the CNV.

[Reprinted with permission from Walter, Cooper, Aldridge, McCallum, & Winter, "Contingent negative variation: an electric sign of sensori-motor association and expectancy in the human brain." *Nature, 203*, 380-384, 1964. Copyright 1964 Macmillan Magazines Limited.]

The CNV might be interpreted as an anticipatory response in preparation for a motor reaction following the alerting or warning signal (Gaillard, 1977). However, a CNV can be generated by asking the subject to think about pressing the switch in anticipation of a light after the sound hearing the sound (Walter et al., 1964). CNV habituates rapidly. It is undetectable after several pairings of sound and light without a motor response, or without thinking about a motor response following the sound.

Signal order can be reversed if visual function instead of auditory function is being evaluated. Signals in other modalities (e.g., somatosensory) can be paired with sound. Also, two sounds can be paired; or two signals in other modalities, if other than auditory assessment is the goal of the procedure.

Clinical Applications
Routine clinical audiologic use of CNVs has not been reported. Patient cooperation is the most obvious drawback to CNVs. If the patient can attend and respond to the preparatory signal, that patient probably can be evaluated more thoroughly and definitively by behavioral response procedures. Therefore, clinical use of CNVs probably has to be restricted to those instances in which the subtleties of a patient's cognitive disorder cannot be dissected through behavioral procedures (Goto, Adachi, Utsunomiya, Nakano, & Chin, 1978; Michalewski & Weinberg, 1977) .

Steady-State Potential

In 1955, Köhler and Wegener described what appeared to be a DC shift in humans for the duration of an audible tone presented to the subject. Davis (1976) aptly named the phenomenon a "sustained cortical potential." Köhler did not exploit this phenomenon for experimental or clinical purposes. However, some other investigators since Köhler have explored the phenomeon further (Ebenbichler, Uhl, Lang, Lindinger, Egkher, & Deecke, 1997; Pihan, Altenmüller, & Ackermann, 1997). Although definitive clinical studies still remain to be done, we call attention to DC potentials because they may be directly related to the percept of the eliciting signal and may reveal aspects of auditory and language dysfunctions not obtainable through other ERPs.

We call attention to DC changes for an additional reason. Because they persist through the duration of the eliciting signals, they are truly steady-state potentials. This is in contrast to the overlapping of transient responses in the 40 Hz phenomenon that also has been labeled as a steady-state potential. The 40 Hz phenomenon is discussed further in Chapter 10.

Part IV

Applications

Chapter *9*

Threshold Audiometry:
Basic Principles

One major goal of evoked potential audiometry (EPA) is to predict or to estimate a patient's behavioral response audiogram from evoked potential data. Threshold EPA usually is done when obtaining a reliable behavioral response audiogram is impossible or impractical. It is also done sometimes for medical-legal purposes if validation of the behavioral response audiogram is required.

Threshold audiometry is a critical first step in the evaluation of communicative disorders, even those in which dysfunctional language or dysfunctional speech is the most prominent manifestation. Threshold audiometry also should precede other tests in which hearing measures are used in otoneurologic diagnosis.

An abnormal threshold audiogram says that a patient's auditory sensitivity is impaired, that is, a stronger test signal is necessary for the patient just to be able to detect a given signal one-half the times that signal is presented than is required for the average young adult listener upon whom audiometric norms are based. An air-conduction (AC) audiogram yields important information. It tells the audiologist something about the integrity of the peripheral auditory mechanism. If the audiogram is not normal, that is, if there is some manifestation of hypacusis, the audiologist infers that something (or several things) from the external auditory meatus to where the auditory nerve enters the brainstem is not functioning normally. If thresholds also are obtained by bone conduction (BC), similarities or differences in the AC and BC thresholds can tell the audiologist whether the patient's loss is conductive, sensorineural, or mixed.

For most patients, voluntary behavioral response audiometry is the least expensive and most definitive of all approaches to threshold audiometry. For some patients, however, thresholds can only be obtained with reasonable confidence through some form of electrophysiologic audiometry, with evoked potential audiometry (EPA) being the most effective form.

One should ask at least five broad questions when preparing to perform behavioral response audiometry: (1) What frequency range is to be used, how many frequencies are to

Durrant prefers ERA over EPA → used when real audiometry doesn't work or is otherwise impractical or medical-legal

TABLE 9-1   Questions to Be Asked and Answered Before Assessing a Patient's Threshold by Behavioral Response Audiometry or by EPA

1. What frequency range is to be used, how many frequencies are to be sampled, and how frequency-specific do the individual test frequencies have to be?
2. What signal magnitude range is to be used and how large should the magnitude steps be in this range?

How methods are applied

3. What response index is to be used and what can be done to insure that the responses are reliable?
4. What criterion (criteria) is (are) to be used to establish threshold on the basis of the responses?
5. How valid will the test results be in terms of the patient's actual auditory sensitivity?

be sampled, and how frequency-specific do the individual test frequencies have to be? (2) What signal magnitude range is to be used and how large should the magnitude steps be in this range? (3) What response index is to be used and what can be done to insure that the responses are reliable? (4) What criterion (criteria) is (are) to be used to establish threshold on the basis of the responses? (5) How valid will the test results be in terms of the patient's actual auditory sensitivity?

The prime clinical inquiry when threshold EPA is contemplated is "What would this patient's threshold audiogram have been had I been able to obtain it reliably by behavioral response audiometry?" Therefore, the audiologist should ask the same five questions of EPA and the answers to the questions should determine the test parameters and procedures. These questions are repeated in Table 9-1 for emphasis.

The most common form of threshold EPA uses broad-spectrum clicks as test signals and EPs as the response index. However, given the prime clinical question above, we present first various approaches to threshold EPA with narrow-spectrum tone bursts as test signals. Additional approaches with narrow-spectrum signals and with broad-spectrum clicks are discussed in the next chapter. Also, only air-conduction audiometry is discussed in this chapter. Bone-conduction audiometry will be discussed in the next chapter.

A discussion of those patients for whom EPA is the most appropriate precedes descriptions of threshold EPA. For EPA, the answers to the five questions above depend on the kinds of patients being evaluated and, therefore, influence or determine the actual signal, recording, and analysis procedures to be used.

Patient Selection

EPA is essential for neonates and probably is the threshold test of choice for infants less than three months old. Neonatal thresholds assessed by observing overt behavioral responses to test signals are, at best, tentative because behavioral responsivity is so state dependent and state is almost impossible to control. Also, the subjectivity of human observers adds large variance to the threshold estimations. Other approaches more objective than overt behavioral response observations (e.g., acoustic-immittance measures, otoacoustic emission measures) are useful as screening devices. They also provide valuable information about the integrity of the neonate's peripheral auditory mechanism. However, they do not yet provide direct measures of threshold sensitivity.

Another category of patients for whom EPA is a test of choice are those patients whose intellectual capacities are too severely impaired to allow them to be tested reliably by any behavioral response procedure. Test procedures that require overt voluntary responses may be impractical for some patients with severely restricted motor capabilities. EPA may be the test of choice for these patients as well. Patients whose emotional or psychologic set leads to erratic and unreliable voluntary responses may be evaluated more reliably by EPA. Finally, EPA may be necessary in cases where compensation is being sought for hearing loss caused by injury or by excessive occupational noise. Compensation commissioners and juries sometimes are skeptical of test results that depend on a patient's voluntary cooperation. Often they have more faith in the results of tests such as EPA with hard-copy evidence of hearing or hearing loss obtained without the patient's active cooperation. In other medical-legal cases, results of EPA may serve as corroborative data.

EPA also is done at times even when the results of behavioral response audiometry are reliable, precise, and unequivocal. For example, some parents are reluctant to believe the results of behavioral response audiometry, even when they witness their child's reactions (or lack of them) during the test procedure. Corroborative results from EPA may be necessary to convince the parents so that they will accept and participate in appropriate (re)habilitation for the child. Corroborative results also are needed at times to convince a referring physician or other professional whose view of the patient's hearing is distinctly different from what the audiologist reports as a result of behavioral response audiometry. Again, appropriate treatment or (re)habilitative measures may not be taken or prescribed until the referring professional is convinced of the correctness of the audiologist's contrary opinion.

Unfortunately, EPA often is done for one of three wrong reasons. (1) Some professionals believe that threshold audiograms obtained through EPA and through behavioral response audiometry are different and have different clinical implications. No evidence supports this contention. If an audiologist can obtain reliable thresholds by behavioral response audiometry, EPA is not necessary. (2) EPA is used inappropriately as a substitute for behavioral response audiometry by a clinician who is unskilled in working with young children or with other patients who, ordinarily, are difficult to test behaviorally. Rather than admit to ineptitude, the clinician turns to EPA, sometimes subjecting the patient to unwarranted sedation or anesthesia to accomplish the task. (3) Patients, patients' families, and third-party carriers are willing to pay more for EPA than they are for behavioral response audiometry even though the latter usually yields more definitive results. Therefore, EPA sometimes is ordered for revenue enhancement rather than because of clinical necessity.

Procedures

No single procedure for threshold audiometry can be used with all patients. The audiologist must consider the nature of the patient to be evaluated, the specific clinical information needed from the evaluation, the needed or desired precision of the test results, and other related factors in establishing the test protocol for a specific patient. What follows are procedural recommendations that should be applicable to most patients for whom threshold EPA is necessary. The recommendations are summarized in Table 9-2. However, in some examples presented later, the test and analysis conditions differ from the recommended

TABLE 9-2   Recommended Parameters for Coarse, Initial Threshold EPA on Patients for Whom No Pretest Estimation of Threshold Is Available

Signal
   configuration: rise/fall time = 5 ms
                          plateau = 1 ms
   central frequency: 500 Hz and 2000 (or 3000) Hz
   presentation rate: 17.1/s
   ear (monotic): right; left
   levels: 100, 60, 20 (or 90, 50, 10) dB nHL; silent control
   N per AEP: 500
   replications per condition: 3
   contralateral masking: none for intitial evaluation

Recording
   electrode montage: Cz-A1; Cz-A2 or Cz-M1; Cz-M2
   analysis window: 50 ms
   filter passband: 3–500 Hz

Criteria for Reponse
   replicability of three traces for each condition
   systematic change of peak latencies and amplitudes with changes in signal level
   difference between signal-related traces and silent-control traces

Criterion for Threshold
   midpoint between weakest response level and next lower level for which traces do not represent responses

---

conditions. In addition, some EPA systems may not allow the exact recommended conditions; close approximation of the recommended conditions should be satisfactory.

Signals

Ideally, EPA test signals should be the same as those most commonly used in behavioral response audiometry, that is, tones with linear rise/fall times of at least 20 ms and plateau durations of at least 150 ms (ANSI, 1989). Signals of this duration require analysis windows of 500–1000 ms, with the most definitive aspects of the AEP occurring beyond 250 ms. As pointed out in earlier chapters, this late activity usually is too state-dependent and variable to be used routinely as a response index for threshold audiometry.

The most reliable electroencephalic activity occurs within the first 50 ms after signal onset, that is, in the early- and middle-latency time zones. Short signals that are long enough to be considered narrow band (e.g., half-power bandwidth less than 200 Hz and all side bands at least 25 dB below the fundamental) still are too long for the 10 ms EP analysis window. However, they can be used with a 50 ms analysis window. Signals that have proved satisfactory clinically are those with a linear rise/fall time of 5 ms and a plateau of 1 ms. These signals have half-power bandwidths of about 100 ms and side bands that are at least 25 dB below the fundamental. The spectrum of a signal with 5 ms rise/fall time and no plateau is shown in Figure 3-3.

The initial discussion in this section centers around the use of what will be called 5–1–5 signals and an analysis window of 50 ms. Some recommendations offered concerning testing with narrow-spectrum signals are applicable to testing with other signals such as clicks.

The 5–1–5 tone bursts can be presented at any of the usual octave frequencies and at any desirable intermediate frequency. Transducers limit the extremes of frequencies that can be presented. For example, some insert earphones do not allow useful testing at frequencies above 4000 Hz.

Patient management difficulties and the time needed to obtain the AEPs with sufficient reliability and precision preclude testing in one EPA session at all of the frequencies that audiologists test in conventional voluntary behavioral response audiometry. Time constraints dictate only sampling of frequencies in any one EPA session. The clinician usually is limited to determining threshold only at a representative low frequency (e.g., 500 Hz) and a representative high frequency (e.g., 2000 or 3000 Hz). Sometimes it is possible to estimate the remainder of the audiogram from the thresholds at these two frequencies with sufficient accuracy for initial diagnostic or (re)habilitation purposes. If clinical management requires greater precision, the patient should be rescheduled for testing at other frequencies.

Signal rate of 17.1/s allows rapid data accumulation without taxing either instrumental capability or the recovery rate of the principal response generators. Rates up to 20/s can be used if the test instrument permit them. Rates that are subharmonics of 60 Hz should be avoided to reduce the likelihood of accidentally locking in on artifactual 60 Hz components picked up by the recording electrodes. As pointed out in Chapter 6, random jittering of a rate around a center rate (e.g., 15.1–19.1/s around 17.1/s) further reduces the probability of locking in on a rhythmic artifact.

Level increments in dB are small during a threshold search in voluntary behavioral response audiometry, especially in the 5-up-10-down stage close to threshold. Given the usual time constraints, 5 dB increments/decrements and even 10 dB steps are impractical in a single EPA session. Therefore, level sampling becomes just as desirable as frequency sampling.

Sometimes level sampling must be coarse. As an example, a 2-year-old child is referred for EPA because prior attempts at behavioral response audiometry yielded no estimate of threshold that the referring person could use with confidence for guidance in establishing a program of auditory habilitation and early education. The most that an audiologist could hope to determine in an initial EPA is a coarse estimate of threshold in each ear for a representative low and high frequency. It is wise for the audiologist in this instance to obtain AEPs at widely separated levels of 90, 50, and 10 dB HL (or 100, 60, and 20 dB HL if the higher output is available). Table 9-3 presents the findings in this hypothetic case. No AEP obtained at any level for a 2000 Hz signal to the right ear could be identified as a response. For the 500 Hz signals, response-related AEPs were obtained at 100 dB HL but not at 60 or 20 dB HL. For the left ear, response-related AEPs were obtained for the 500 Hz signals at 100 and 60 dB HL but not at 20 dB HL. For the 2000 Hz signals, response-related AEPs were obtained only at 100 dB HL.

The information in Table 9-3 is not precise but it is accurate and may give the referring professional enough information for diagnosis and initial remedial steps. If the precision is insufficient for these purposes, the child can be retested with smaller level separations. For

TABLE 9-3   Results of Threshold EPA on Hypothetic Patient (Test signals were tone bursts of 50 Hz and 2000 Hz. + = response; – = no response)

(handwritten note: 20 dB steps, or reduce as time permits)

	Left		Right	
	500 Hz	2000 Hz	500 Hz	2000 Hz
100 dB HL	+	+	+	–
60 db HL	+	–	–	–
20 db HL	–	–	–	–

example, 500 Hz in the right ear can be tested at levels of 95, 80, and 65 dB HL to ascertain where within the range of 60–100 dB the child's threshold lies. Similar steps can be used to get a more precise measure of the sensitivity of the left ear. Additional test sessions may be necessary to assess the child's air-conduction thresholds at other frequencies and to assess the child's bone-conduction thresholds.

Clinicans should eschew the temptation to get all the necessary information in a single test session. To do so limits the number of replications of individual test conditions, which in turn limits the accuracy of the threshold estimations and the confidence with which the audiologist can report test results. More will be said shortly about the value of replicating test conditions. Clinicians must weigh the relative values of precision, accuracy, and validity, especially when testing young children. The few extra hours or even days required for increasingly refined testing must be balanced against a possible lifetime of negative consequences of misjudgments made because of overconcern with a few hours or a few dollars.

The sampling of test conditions can be more precise to begin with if history, physical examinations, and other kinds of hearing tests give usable guides to where the child's thresholds may lie. If, for example, there is strong presumptive evidence of profound hearing loss that could not be confirmed behaviorally, the initial sampling levels can be restricted to 60, 80, and 100 dB HL. On the other hand, if prior information suggests normal or nearly normal sensitivity, sampling levels can be 10, 30, and 50 dB HL. Seldom is it necessary to determine the exact levels if sensitivity approaches normal. If response-related AEPs can be elicited at 10 dB HL, it is unlikely that a child's communication dysfunction can be attributed to a significant sensitivity impairment.

Recording Parameters

One electrode should be attached at the vertex (Cz) or slightly forward of the vertex, and two others attached to the earlobes (A1 or A2) or mastoid (M1 or M2). The ground electrode can be on the forehead.

The analysis window should be 50 ms and the filter passband should be 3–500 Hz. If the resulting AEP is too noisy and if the signal-averaging equipment permits, digital post-averaging filtering can be done with narrower passbands. Another way of ridding the AEP trace of high-frequency noise is through post-averaging 3-point (or more) smoothing. If all pretest attempts to reduce disturbing high-frequency noise are inadequate, the low-pass of the filter may have to be dropped to 400 Hz or 300 Hz. Similarly, if all pretest attempts do not keep low-frequency noise from being too disrupting, the high-pass end of the filter pass-band may have to be raised to 5 Hz or even 10 Hz.

Differentiating between response-related AEPs and AEPs that represent just unaveraged electroencephalic noise will be discussed more fully later. One differentiating criterion, the replicability of AEP traces obtained under identical conditions, influences the number of replications for each signal condition. Many clinicians are content with examining two overlapping or superimposed AEPs. Three or more superimposed traces, however, give the examiner substantially more confidence in the replicability or in the variability, especially at weak signal levels. Also when composites or averages of averages are made, noise reduction is considerably better when three or more replications are averaged.

When signals are distinctly suprathreshold, two replicated AEPs usually are sufficiently similar to dissuade most clinicians from running a third replication. As mentioned, close to what may be threshold, additional replications do provide the needed confidence to judge whether the AEP traces are response related. Therefore, some audiologists recommend that only two replications be made when strong signals are presented and three or more replications be made for weaker signals. This recommendation is questionable on two accounts: (1) the demand for immediate on-line judgment whether an acquired pair of traces represents a response; and (2) lack of uniformity of data acquisition reduces the value of later comparison across conditions. It is more desirable to decide in advance which signal conditions are going to be used during the EPA, settle on the number of replications per trial and the number of trials per condition, and make conclusive judgments **off-line** about the presence or absence of response at the conclusion of the EPA.

Work with the EPs has conditioned clinicians to obtain samples to at least 1000 signals per AEP (N=1000); 2000 signals often are recommended. For the recording and signal conditions outlined above, an N of 500, and perhaps less, suffices. The signal-to-noise ratio improves little beyond 500 samples. In fact, the noise part of the AEP may increase at times beyond 500 samples because of the restlessness of the patient. This observation argues against a common recommendation to increase the N per AEP with successively weaker signal presentations. Also, as with varying the number of trials as a function of level, different Ns at different signal levels reduce the ease of cross-condition comparisons both for the superimposed replications and for the composite AEPs made by averaging the replications. A better practice is to have the same N per AEP trial (e.g., 500) and the same number of trials per test condition (e.g., 3).

As a digression, texts (Coats, 1983; Hall, 1992, p. 217) often state that residual noise decreases in proportion to the square root of the number of samples taken for an AEP. That dictum, however, is valid only if the background noise is random and unchanging . Neither condition holds true during EPA (although Hyde [1994a] contends that normality of distribution of the background noise is all that is essential for the square root principle to apply). First, EEG, the main background noise, does not have a random spectrum; certain frequencies dominate most recordings. Randomness is violated further by filtering of the background activity. Second, changes in patient state change the spectrum of the EEG and movement can introduce other noise, especially large voltage muscle potentials. These conditions probably disrupt the normality of noise distribution as well.

After the completion of the actual test procedure, AEPs are examined in terms of replicability, configuration, and systematic changes in both as a function of signal frequency and level. Even after this examination, the clinician often has questions, particularly about AEPs associated with weak-level signals. Do the small amplitude AEPs represent responses or just the uncanceled background electric activity? Do the AEPs for any signal level represent responses or do the observed positive and negative peaks represent accidental averaging of electric artifacts picked up by the recording electrodes? For these reasons, obtaining some traces without any signals presented to the patient is important. These **silent controls** provide baseline AEPs against which the signal-related AEPs are compared. If signal-related AEPs do not differ appreciably from the silent-control AEPs, then they are unlikely to represent responses.

Adding silent-control conditions adds to the total test time unless fewer signal conditions are included. The improved accuracy and validity of the EPA warrant the sacrifice of some signal conditions. Accuracy is of greater benefit to the patient than questionable results obtained for the sake of greater precision. As pointed out before, if the clinician requires greater precision, additional EPA sessions should be scheduled.

Throughout, the recommendation has been for the clinican to examine not only the superimposed replications of three or more AEPs for each signal condition but also the composites or average of the averages of the replications. One can argue that it takes less time and is more convenient to run a single trial of 1500 samples than to take three separate trials of 500 samples and then to make a composite of the three separate AEPs. However, the composite AEP ($AEP_1 + AEP_2 + AEP_3$ divided by 3) almost always is more noise-free, that is, smoother or cleaner, than a single AEP of 1500 consecutive samples. The most likely explanation for the difference is that the noise background for the three separate AEPs is different enough in phase and possibly character to be reduced even further overall when added algebraically in the compositing and averaging process. Also, as pointed out earlier, the shorter trial runs allow time for more trials for replication comparisons, and they do not force the patient to be restrained as long per trial during which noise could increase rather than decrease.

Criteria for Response

The most common practice is to use some aspect of the time-amplitude configuration of the AEP trace as a response index. Said differently, the clinician asks "Does the waveform represent a response or does it just represent the residue of uncanceled noise?" How can the clinician answer this question? In what way(s) can the AEP waveform answer the response/no response question?

Clinicians often look for a characteristic waveform or pattern to allow them to say this AEP is (or is not) a response. They are conditioned to do so largely because of their experience with click-elicited EPs. There are some characteristic positive and negative peaks in response to tone bursts with the recommended recording and signal parameters. However, they are inconsistent enough to diminish the value of AEP configuration as the prime index of response. Even among completely normal subjects there are some differences attributable to age, state, possibly gender, and the fundamental frequency of the tone burst. Differences in the kind of filter used can make small differences in resulting waveforms. If changes have to be made in the filter passband or filter slope because of the exigencies of a given clinical situation, then still more changes can occur in the expected pattern. When testing patients with abnormal brains, a common clinical situation when threshold EPA is necessary, even larger and less predictable deviations from expected patterns may be anticipated. Comparison with silent-control AEPs is especially important in these cases.

It is possible in theory for silent-control AEPs (*control AEPs* henceforth for brevity) to be straight lines. In practice, however, control AEPs rarely are straight or flat. Uncanceled background noise gives most control AEPs some positive and negative deflections. Sometimes these deflections occur with the same latency as the deflections in signal-related AEPs. How often do characteristic positive and negative peaks appear in signal-related AEPs compared with their appearance in control AEPs? The answer helps to determine if a signal-related AEP represents a response or if the eliciting signal is below threshold and the resulting AEP just represents the residual uncanceled noise.

Even if the time-amplitude configuration of the AEP per se cannot be used as the primary criterion for response, it can be used indirectly in several ways as a response index for threshold audiometry. First, the latency of the peaks can be expected to increase and peak amplitudes can be expected to decrease as the eliciting signals become weaker. Systematic changes in latency and amplitude can be followed with successively weaker signals until the peaks are small and bear no apparent relation to the peaks in AEPs elicited by stronger signals. The clinician then concludes that threshold has been reached. As mentioned earlier, certain time-amplitude configurations are common across most patients, but sometimes a patient's waveform is not typical for the recording and test circumstances. Nevertheless, the peaks that do occur for that patient will show the same systematic increase in latency and decrease in amplitude with decreasing signal levels.

Peak latencies are slightly longer and amplitudes are slightly larger for low-frequency tone bursts than they are for high-frequency tone bursts. Therefore, if characteristic AEP configuration is used as a response criterion, slightly different configurations must be expected at each of the test frequencies.

Another characteristic that the clinician looks for is the similarity of AEP traces obtained under identical test circumstances. Whatever their configuration, two or three AEPs obtained under identical conditions should resemble each other closely. Similarities are best seen when the traces are superimposed (see Figure 9-1A and C).

Replicability at a given signal level argues that the eliciting signals were suprathreshold. Signal levels are lowered until the superimposed traces no longer are replicable. The clinician then infers that threshold has been reached.

In the example shown in Figure 9-1, using the criteria of replicability and systematic changes, EPA thresholds for both the 500 Hz and 4000 Hz tone bursts would have been 10 dB greater (poorer) than the subject's behavioral response threshold. This would not have been a consequential error for either diagnostic or management purposes had the traces come from an actual clinical patient.

One way to circumvent inter- and even intra-patient differences in AEP configuration is to measure the total energy or power of the response. This can be done easily and quickly with some signal averagers as a total area-under-the-curve (AUTC) measure (Anthony, Durrett, Pulec, & Hartstone, 1979; Maeda, Morita, Kawamura, & Nakazawa, 1996). The measure may be expressed as microvolt-millisecond (μV-ms) or millisecond-microvolt (ms-μV) because of the dimensions of the AEP trace.

Area-under-the-curve measure has two distinct advantages over time-amplitude configuration in setting criteria for response in threshold audiometry. First, it does away with subjective peak-picking, which is particularly troublesome for AEPs to weak signals. Second, it allows the clinician to establish an objective, quantitative criterion for response vs no-response based on inferential statistics. Baseline area measures are made on control

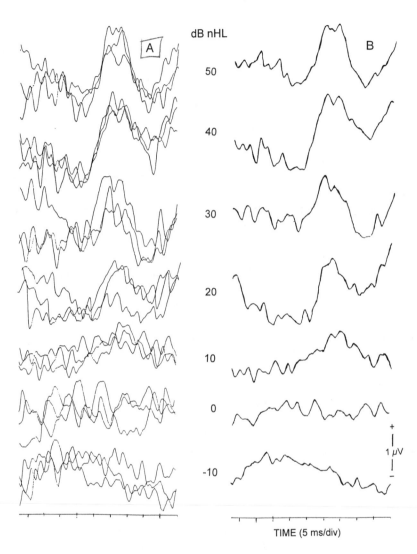

FIGURE 9-1   Middle potentials (MPs) from a normal-hearing young man. Filter passband: 3–500 Hz. (A) 500 Hz tone burst (5 ms rise/fall time, 1 ms plateau) at 17.1/s. N per AEP = 500. Signal was audible at 0 dB nHL but not at −10 dB nHL. (B) Composite AEPs from the three replications shown in A.

AEPs and outside limits of no-response are established based on area variances (e.g., ±2.5 standard deviations). A third advantage of AUTC measures is that they can be made quickly and inexpensively even by persons who have little experience making judgments based on time-amplitude configurations.

Most clinicians judge **on-line** whether a given AEP (or superimpositions of several AEPs obtained for identical test conditions) is or is not a response. Then, based on this decision, they either raise or lower the next set of signals as part of the threshold search. This

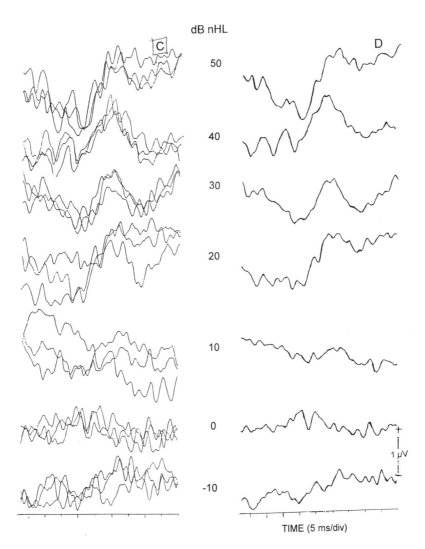

(C) Three replications of middle potentials (MPs) to 4000 Hz tone bursts (5 ms rise/fall time, 1 ms plateau). Signal was audible at 10 dB nHL but not at 0 or –10 dB nHL. (D) Composite AEPs from the three replications shown in C.

practice allows clinicians to obtain a relatively precise estimation of threshold without having to reschedule a patient for more refined testing. The practice is partially defensible if a clinician tries to obtain thresholds for clicks and uses EPs as the response index. Also, it may be defensible for a quick-and-dirty initial screening procedure. On-line analysis, however, is subject to many clinical errors, especially when thresholds for narrow-spectrum signals are being sought with the 50 ms AEP as the response index. Clinicians seldom can remain objective when they decide if the small wiggles in a trace represent a response or just noise residue. For example, if the patient is a child referred because of suspicion of profound hearing loss, those wiggles are likely to be discounted as accidental. Conversely, if the child is suspected of having good auditory sensitivity despite an apparent hearing difficulty, the identical wiggles are apt to be considered a response.

Off-line or after-the-test analysis is slower and usually leads to less precise threshold estimates than can be achieved with on-line judgments. Nevertheless, off-line analysis is the procedure of choice in any form of threshold EPA. It frees the clinician or technical assistant from making hasty and often questionable on-line judgments. Off-line analysis allows the clinician to examine waveforms and their replicability without the pressure of deciding what the next set of test signals should be. It allows the clinician time to make composite AEPs from the replications without extending the time for keeping the patient quiet or sedated. It allows time to stack AEPs as a function of signal level (see Figure 9-1) and to examine and to measure changes in peak latencies and amplitudes with changes in signal level. It allows time to refilter data digitally to obtain peaks that are more distinguishable from random noise, and to analyze the AEP in different ways (e.g., AUTC) for measures that make estimation of threshold more secure. Finally, off-line analysis allows others to assist in judgments of response/no response in those instances when judgments are difficult.

Criteria for Threshold

Conventional voluntary behavioral response audiometry uses a 50% criterion for threshold, that is, threshold is considered the weakest signal level at which the patient responds at least three of the minimum of six times that signal is presented (American Speech and Hearing Association, 1978). Signal levels are varied in steps of 5 and 10 dB and the certainty of the reported threshold is given as ±5 dB. Time constraints in EPA limit the number of signal levels that can be used and the number of times AEPs can be obtained at each signal level, even when the operator tries to bracket threshold with on-line judgments. Therefore, clinicians often report as threshold the weakest signal level at which the elicited AEP is considered response-related. When EPA and voluntary behavioral response audiometry can be done on the same patient, the result usually is that EPA thresholds are reported as being poorer than psychophysical thresholds. This is because the signal-to-noise ratio is poorer for AEPs than for the motor responses in behavioral response audiometry and because different criteria for threshold are use for the two procedures. Unfortunately, however, readers of the reports infer that patients do have different thresholds when measured with two different response indices and that these thresholds have different clinical implications. The reality of the differences is that they merely reflect the clinician's inability to assess the threshold with equal certainty or precision by two different methods.

As an illustration of the similarity of psychophysical and EPA thresholds, the threshold resulting from a psychophysical test on a patient is 40 ±5 dB. EPA threshold for the identical test signal is 50 ±15 dB. (The confidence range for EPA almost always is greater than for psychophysical measures when the two can be done on the same patient.) Do the two thresholds differ by 10 dB? The real psychophysical threshold can range between 40–50 dB HL; the real EPA threshold can range between 35–65 dB HL. Given the extensive overlap between the two ranges, the two thresholds cannot be considered different. The clinical literature contains no examples of patients whose psychophysical and EPA thresholds are clearly and consistently different. When both thresholds are obtained for the identical test signals, are ascertained with the same criterion or criteria, and both are obtained with equal confidence (although not necessarily with the same precision), the two thresholds will be the same with the limits of confidence for the two separate threshold measures.

Validity and Utility of EPA Thresholds

EPA and behavioral response thresholds for 5–1–5 tone bursts are the same but how closely do these thresholds correspond with 20–150–20 thresholds, that is, with behavioral response thresholds obtained with tones used in conventional voluntary behavioral response audiometry? On the basis of the time-intensity trading relation (Plomp & Bouman, 1959; Watson & Gengel, 1969), tone burst thresholds should be about 10 dB higher (poorer) than thresholds for the longer duration signals. The exact difference will differ with frequency and with the particular temporal configuration of the tone bursts that one chooses to use for EPA. If the clinician wishes to predict the conventional tone audiogram from the EPA thresholds, the clinician can establish the differences psychophysically on a jury of normal-hearing listeners as well as on juries of hearing-impaired listeners with various well-defined peripheral impairments.

Often, for the patients for whom threshold EPA is most needed, a clinical question to be asked is how does the EPA threshold compare with psychophysically established norms for the tone bursts that are used. That comparison usually provides insight and sufficient information for the diagnostic or for the management question for the patient who is being tested by EPA. However, for some patients, closer approximation to a conventional pure-tone audiogram is needed.

How well do EPA or behavioral response thresholds for tone bursts predict or how well do they parallel the audiogram obtained with tones whose temporal properties are at least as long as 20–150–20? Predictability or the parallelism is close for persons with normal sensitivity and for patients with conductive hearing impairments. They are also close for many patients with presumed cochlear impairments, and cochlear impairments probably are the bases for most sensorineural hearing losses. Insufficient data are available to assess predictability and parallelism in patients with hearing losses that are exclusively or primarily neural. Similarly, insufficient data are available to know the effects of central nervous system lesions on either predictability or parallelism.

Predictability and parallelism are poorer in patients with severely sloping high-frequency sensorineural hearing losses. Even when 5–1–5 tone bursts are close to what is the true threshold for a high-frequency signal (e.g., 4000 Hz), the lower-frequency side-bands may be sufficiently above the threshold for the patient's lower-frequency sensitivity to elicit behavioral or evoked-potential responses to a frequency or frequencies other than the 4000 Hz center frequency. Too few real-life clinical reports are available to know how often, if ever, the discrepancies from the tone burst thresholds have led to incorrect diagnostic or management decisions.

Poor low-frequency sensitivity in the presence of normal or nearly normal high-frequency sensitivity can be more consequential clinically. Patients with this hearing profile often will respond to the high-frequency sidebands of low-frequency tone bursts.

Therefore, inappropriate judgments often are made about the patients' low-frequency sensitivity, which in turn may lead to incorrect diagnostic or management decisions. However, these same misjudgments can occur even with tones with temporal dimensions of or greater than 20–150–20 (Goldstein et al., 1983).

Predictability and parallelism of thresholds determined with 5–1–5 tone bursts are good enough in most patients to preclude major diagnostic or management errors. In cases where greater certainty is required, EPA can be repeated with tone bursts more nearly resembling the temporal configuration of tones used in conventional behavioral response threshold audiometry. When this is done, longer analysis windows (e.g., 500–1000 ms) are needed, the low- and high-pass ends of the filter passband have to be lowered, and more control has to be exercised to keep patient state consistent.

Sometimes patients give no EPs that can be interpreted as responses. One of two probable explanations for response absence can be invoked if instrument failure or procedural errors cannot be blamed. A simple explanation is that the patient is totally deaf, that is, has no auditory sensitivity at the test frequencies. A more complex explanation is that the patient's brain is incapable of organizing recognizable AEP waveforms. Therefore, before rendering a diagnosis of deafness, the clinician should examine the patient's AEPs to visual or somatosensory signals or both. If the patient gives replicable AEPs in other modalities, that provides presumptive evidence of deafness for the failure to obtain replicable AEPs to sound. If, however, the patient is unresponsive in all sensory modalities, the failure to respond to sound cannot be used as evidence either for or against deafness.

Other Approaches to Determining Thresholds

All of the preceding discussion relates to current practices and to most of the relatively inexpensive evoked potential systems currently in use. Technologic capabilities already are available for other approaches to threshold audiometry that may be simpler, quicker, and more objective than those discussed above. Two alternative procedures are described briefly now with the expectation that instrumentation for them may become inexpensive enough to warrant common clinical use. Although they are described for the 5–1–5 tone bursts and a 50 ms analysis window, they can be adapted easily for other test signals and recording epochs.

One alternative is analogous to the psychophysical method of constant stimuli. The sequence of presentation of signals is programmed in advance. The program is quasi-random with respect to ear, center frequency, level, and silent control. No two identical signals (frequency, level, ear, control) are presented in succession. The electroencephalic activity following each combination of conditions is stored in different memory banks of the signal averager. For example, activity following 500 Hz in the right ear at 70 dB HL is stored in one bank; 500 Hz in the right ear at 50 dB HL (or whatever the set differences between levels) stored in a different bank; activity during controls stored in still a different bank, and so on. A fixed number of samples per condition (e.g., 200) is presented until all conditions are equally represented. The whole process is repeated once, twice, or three times, whatever the number of replications the clinician decides is necessary.

At the completion of the data acquisition, the replications of the AEPs for each ear and frequency are displayed or plotted in descending signal levels. Control AEPs also are displayed. Composite AEPs for each condition can be displayed or traced alongside the corresponding set of replications. Judgments of threshold level are made from the displays, either by eyeball or by some form of machine scoring (e.g., the level at which area-under-the-curve first differs significantly from the area for the controls). Human judgments or machine scorings are done without the pressure of immediate on-line decision processes that are necessary if on-line judgments dictate the next signal level to be chosen. Consequently, the off-line judgments of response/no response and of threshold level are made more objectively and, probably, more accurately.

The programmed approach just described has other advantages over the more common approaches now practiced in addition to those of greater objectivity and greater accuracy. One of these is that because of the quasi-random signal presentations, the background noise levels for all AEPs will be nearly identical. With uniform noise background, differences in AEPs can be attributed almost exclusively to difference in the response portions of the AEPs. A second advantage is that the quasi-random signal presentation minimizes the response-reducing effects of adaptation and habituation. These effects are small for the generators of response activity within the first 50 ms. Nevertheless, a small increase in response magnitude can enhance the response portion and, therefore, improve the signal-to-noise ratio of the AEPs. A third advantage is cost because after the initial instrumental investment, clinical data acquisition can be done by well-trained technical assistants. A simpler form of this procedure has been applied successfully to EPs to tone bursts in mice by Mitchell, Kempton, Creedon, and Trune (1996). They claim that the test procedure is faster than the characteristic way of obtaining averaged responses as a function of frequency and level, one averaged EP at a time.

A second alternative to the more conventional approaches to threshold EPA is the equivalent to Bekesy or semi-automatic audiometry, although in this case the procedure is totally automatic. The procedure depends on automatic instrumental response recognition and automatic adjustment of signal level. Real-time response recognition is feasible (John, Chabot, Prichep, Ransohoff, Epstein, & Berenstein, 1989), and an approximation to the proposed procedure already has been achieved (Özdamar, Delgado, Eilers, & Urbano, 1994).

In this alternative approach, one frequency is tested at a time separately for each ear. Presentation for an individual frequency (e.g., 250 Hz) begins at a preselected level (e.g., 50 dB HL). After a preselected number of presentations (e.g., N=200), the acquired AEP is evaluated by a machine-scoring program in terms of response/no response. The evaluation program can be based on time-amplitude configuration, AUTC, or on other criteria that may be superior to either. If the machine-scoring decision is *response*, the level of the next set of signals drops by a preselected amount (e.g., 10 dB) and the process repeats until *no response* is registered. Threshold is then judged to be between the weakest response level and the first no-response level. For greater certainty, the process can be repeated until the same threshold is reached for a preselected (e.g., 3) number of times. The program then changes the test frequency (e.g., to 500 Hz) and the process repeats until testing at the preselected frequencies is complete. Then the process is repeated for the other ear. If, at the first presentation level, the machine does not identify the AEP as a response, the program raises the signal level until a response is identified but the automatic process for evaluating threshold will still be the same.

Alternatives other than the two discussed above also should be considered as new hardware and software become available and as clinical research shows that the alternatives are clinically feasible.

Chapter 10

Sensitivity Assessment: Special Considerations

The basic principles of threshold evoked potential audiometry (EPA) presented in the previous chapter apply to most patients referred for sensitivity assessment. Those basics were discussed in terms of air-conduction testing without masking, and in terms of what is generally available instrumentally and technically. We address two additional basic principles in this chapter: bone-conduction (BC) audiometry and masking. Then we present approaches to tonal threshold audiometry other than those already discussed. Finally, the chapter covers popular forms of threshold EPA in which broad-spectrum clicks are the test signals.

Bone-Conduction EPA

The test signals recommended for use in air-conduction (AC) EPA (tone bursts with 5 ms rise/fall time and 1 ms plateau) also can be used in bone-conduction (BC) EPA. BC vibrators transduce the electric 5–1–5 pattern at weak and moderate levels with little distortion. Distortion is greater at strong levels, just as it is with 20–150–20 (or longer) signals when they are at or beyond the maximum permissible level on standard audiometers.

A drawback to using 5–1–5 signals for BC EPA is the large voltage needed to drive the vibrators at suprathreshold levels and, consequently, the large electric artifact picked up by the recording electrodes. The artifact usually renders the first 10 to 12 ms of a 50 ms analysis window unusable, especially with strong-level signals at 500 Hz or lower. Nevertheless, activity in the remainder of the window is free from the large signal artifact and can be used successfully.

No report on the systematic study of BC EPA with 5–1–5 signals or their equivalent has been published. However, the findings from several unpublished studies support their clinical feasibility. Figure 10-1 shows the AEPs from a representative subject in one study (Block, 1984) and Figure 10-2 shows the grand-composite AEPs from the 20 normal sub-

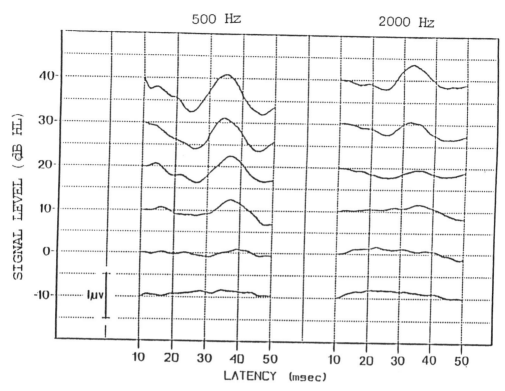

FIGURE 10-1   Middle potentials (MPs) from a normal-hearing young adult to bone-conducted tone bursts (5 ms rise/fall time, 1 ms plateau) presented at 17/s. Filter passband: 1–150 Hz. Each trace is a composite AEP (8 replications of 1000 tone bursts). The first 10 ms of the resultant AEPs was not used because of large signal artifacts in that time zone, especially for the 40 dB HL signal.

[Reprinted with permission from Block, Tonal bone-conduction thresholds by electroencephalic audiometry. Master's thesis, University of Wisconsin-Madison, 1984.]

jects in the study. The first 10 ms were not plotted because of the large artifact, especially for 500 Hz for the two strongest levels. Three factors account for the smoothness of the traces: (1) a filter passband of 1–150 Hz, (2) the large number of trials per condition [8] and samples [1000 per trial] for each subject, and (3) digitizing the hard-copy traces with a graphics tablet that eliminated some of the small, high-frequency noise. Nevertheless, the configuration of the 10 to 50 ms portion of the AEPs closely resembles equivalent portions of AEPs elicited by AC signals. Furthermore, the frequency dependency is the same: Low-frequency BC signals elicit larger peaks with longer latencies than are elicited by high-frequency signals.

Cone-Wesson and Ramirez (1997) used clicks and short tone bursts to elicit EPs and MPs from neonates and from adults. They, too, found that low-frequency signals evoke larger and later responses than are evoked by high-frequency signals.

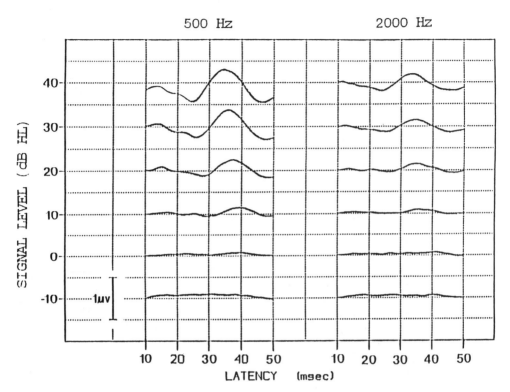

FIGURE 10-2   Grand-composite middle potentials (MPs) to bone-conducted tone bursts from 20 normal-hearing young adults (N per trace = 160,000). Signal and recording conditions the same as for Figure 10-1.

[Reprinted with permission from Block, Tonal bone-conduction thresholds by electroencephalic audiometry. Master's thesis, University of Wisconsin-Madison, 1984.]

Masking

Whatever is valid for masking in behavioral response audiometry is valid for AC and BC EPA as well. This simple dictum is true whether EPs (Humes & Ochs, 1982; Wu & Stapells, 1994), MPs (Gutnick & Goldstein, 1978; Smith & Goldstein, 1973) or LPs (Cheuden, 1972; Davis, Bower, & Hirsh, 1968) are used as the response index. All of the clinical phenomena discussed so far can be explained or rationalized with considerable security from what is known about the anatomy, function, and dysfunction of the auditory and associated systems. The basis for the undeniable parallelism of masking in behavioral response and evoked potential audiometry, however, is not patently evident.

In voluntary behavioral response audiometry, the audiologist can calculate the appropriate levels of contralateral masking for valid AC and BC measures from the initial unmasked thresholds. This luxury usually is denied in EPA because patients referred for threshold EPA are referred because little is certain about their unmasked thresholds. If threshold AC EPA reveals large differences between the ears, *and if patient management demands more precise knowledge of hearing in the poorer ear*, the audiologist can retest the poorer ear with estimated effective masking noise in the better ear.

Unmasked BC thresholds give the audiologist some insight into the integrity of the sensorineural mechanism, at least in the better ear. Usually these data, along with history, physical examination, acoustic-immittance measures, and otoacoustic emission measures suffice for diagnosis and management. The audiologist can repeat BC EPA with estimated effective masking in the contralateral ear if more precise information is needed about BC thresholds in each ear.

Different Approaches to Tonal Threshold EPA

The approach to tonal threshold EPA described in Chapter 9 is direct and uncomplicated and is sufficient for most patients referred for threshold EPA. Nevertheless, other approaches have been attempted. Their exploration was prompted partially by the desire to find even simpler, more objective, and, presumably, more valid procedures than the one already described. We now describe three alternative approaches. Other less direct approaches will be described later in the section on threshold EPA with broad-spectrum clicks as test signals.

Frequency-Following Response (FFR)

When long tone bursts of frequencies below 1000 Hz are presented, activity from the brain can be recorded with the same frequency as the test signal (see Figure 10-3). The periodic activity is called the **frequency-following response** or **FFR** (Clark, Moushegian, & Rupert, 1997; Marsh, Worden, & Smith, 1970). The electroencephalic activity is neither electric artifact nor volume-conducted cochlear microphonic. Reduction in the signal level leads to reduction in FFR amplitude. This makes the FFR an attractive candidate for a response index for tonal threshold EPA.

Two shortcomings limit clinical application of FFR. First, its application is restricted to assessment of low-frequency sensitivity. High-frequency FFR is too small to distinguish confidently from the background electroencephalic noise. Second, even for low-frequency signals, the FFR often becomes so small with reductions in signal levels to be indistinguishable from background noise below 30–40 dB HL. EPA with FFR as a response index never flourished. Nevertheless, it might be revived with sensitive spectrum analysis instruments that could help distinguish response from noise at weaker signal levels and at frequencies above 1000 Hz.

40 Hz Phenomenon

The phenomenon to be discussed is better known by its original designation "40 Hz ERP" (Galambos, Makeig, & Talmachoff, 1981), by a later term "steady-state evoked potential" (Jerger, Chmiel, Frost, & Coker, 1986), or by "steady state response" (Suzuki, Kobayashi, &

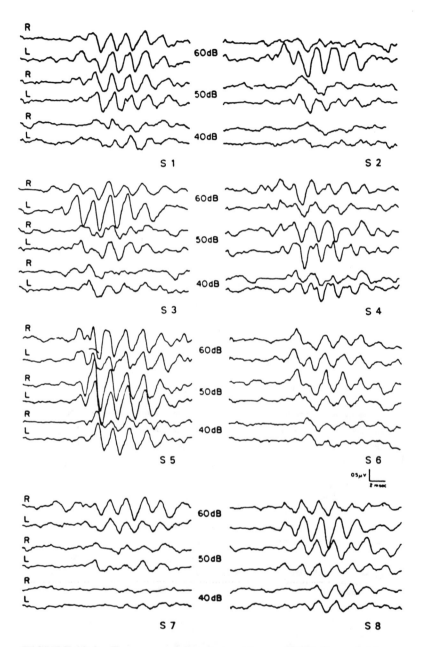

FIGURE 10-3   Frequency-following responses (FFR) from eight normal-hearing young women to monaural right and left 500 Hz tone bursts at 60, 50, and 40 dB Sensation Level.

[Reprinted with permission from Ballachanda BB, Rupert A, Moushegian G. Asymmetric frequency-following responses. *J Am Acad Audiol* 1994; 5:135.]

Umegaki, 1994). Names given to phenomena or to procedures usually are of little clinical consequence. In this instance, however, the names continue to cause confusion among readers who do not have sufficient background to realize the true nature of the phenomenon as a simple superimposition of middle-latency components. Literature searches for writings on event-related potentials (ERPs) based on keywords find articles on the "40 Hz ERP" that, to the consternation of the searchers, turn out not to be about ERPs.

The term "steady state potentials" is equally troublesome because it implies that the eliciting signal is on constantly or that the evoked potential is steady or unchanging, or both. The reality is that the signals are rapidly repeated (40 times per second) short-duration sounds, and the response to each signal is a *transient*, not steady-state, evoked potential. One consequence of this incorrect term is that it diverts interest from a true steady-state potential (Köhler & Wegener, 1955; Pihan et al., 1997) to a continuous tone. The real steady-state potential probably bears a close relation to the actual percept of the signal and is a phenomenon that deserves careful clinical research. Also, the initials SSEP, used at times as an abbreviation for steady-state evoked potentials, can be confusing because they are used commonly to designate averaged AEPs to somatosensory stimulation (American EEG Society, 1994b; Romani, Bergamaschi, Versino, Zilioli, Sartori, Callieco, Montomoli, & Cosi, 1996).

Criticisms of its designation, however, should not detract from the possible clinical applications of the **40 Hz phenomenon**. Its attractive features include simplicity of administration and the objectivity with which presence/absence of response can be assessed.

Peaks that occur in a 50–100 ms analysis window for signals presented at a slow rate (e.g., 10/s) are separated by about 25 ms. Given this near periodicity, their fundamental frequency is about 40 Hz. When test signals are presented at 40/s, the response to more than one signal will occur in a 50–100 ms analysis window. Overlapping peaks will distort or cancel each other if their phases are not coincident. At 40/s for many subjects, response peaks are coincident and, as a result, reinforce each other. Figure 10-4 illustrates the process and shows why the resultant response looks like a sine wave with a periodicity of 25 ms. Not everyone has middle-latency AEPs whose peaks have a periodicity of 25 ms. Prior to the threshold search, the patient should be tested with one suprathreshold condition over a range of signal rates to find the one rate near 40 Hz for which the response amplitude is largest.

As signal level is reduced, the resulting response becomes smaller and the latency of the corresponding waves increases (Figure 10-5). No periodic ripple is expected in the recorded trace when eliciting signals are below the threshold of audibility. Presence/absence of response may be judged by eyeball because all the operator needs to look for is some definable periodic ripple that is different from background noise. Unfortunately, this mode of analysis is prone to the same kinds of subjective errors that plague any eyeball procedure. However, instrumental spectral analysis of both amplitude and phase can bring objectivity to response identification and are comparatively easy and inexpensive to implement (Jerger et al. 1986; Lins, Picton, Boucher, Durieux-Smith, Champagne, Moran, Perez-Abalo, Martin, & Savio, 1996).

The 40 Hz phenomenon has been touted as superior to looking at the ordinary time-amplitude configuration of the middle-latency components, especially for low-frequency threshold assessment (Dauman, Szyfter, Charlet de Sauvage, & Cazals, 1984; Jerger et al.,

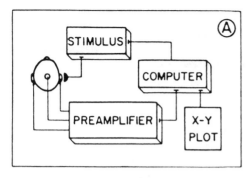

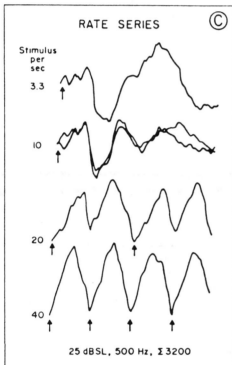

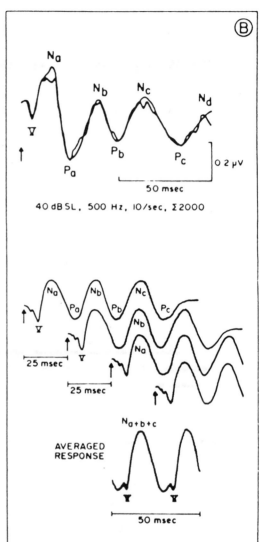

FIGURE 10-4   The process of eliciting and recording the 40 Hz phenomenon. Note that negativity of the vertex electrode relative to the ear electrode is plotted as an upward deflection.

[Reprinted with permission from Galambos, Makeig, & Talmachoff, "A 40-Hz auditory potential recorded from the human scalp." *Proceedings of the National Academy of Science of the United States of America, 76,* 2643-2647, 1981.]

Dynamics of Response

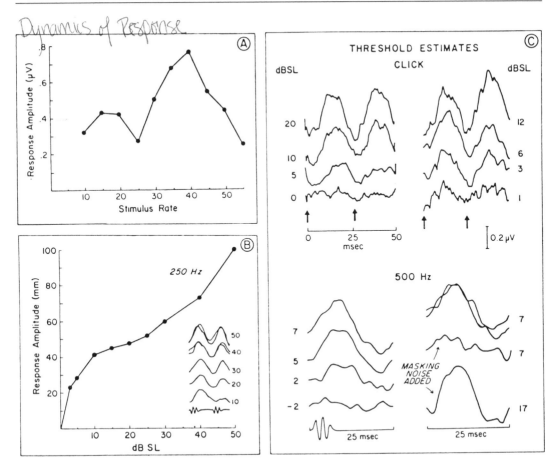

FIGURE 10-5   Three features of the 40 Hz phenomenon are illustrated in this figure. (A) Effect of signal rate on amplitude. (B) Effect of signal magnitude on response amplitude. (C) Efficacy of threshold assessment.

[Reprinted with permission from Galambos, Makeig, & Talmachoff "A 40-Hz auditory potential recorded from the human scalp." *Proceedings of the National Academy of Science of the United States of America*, 76, 2643-2647, 1981.]

1986). However, no study has been reported in which the 40 Hz phenomenon and the straight middle-latency AEPs as described in the previous chapter have been compared on the same patients. In one unequal comparison, Fowler and Swanson (1989) found no clear difference in the efficacy of the 40 Hz phenomenon and SN_{10} [described below] in threshold determination. SN_{10} is, in fact, an early part of the MP. In our own exploratory work, we found no advantage of the 40 Hz phenomenon over our recommended procedure for threshold assessment. One disadvantage of the simplicity of the 40 Hz phenomenon is that it eradicates any information that might be obtained from the time-amplitude configuration either for threshold assessment or for insights into other auditory functions or dysfunctions.

SN_{10}

In 1979, Davis and Hirsh described a phenomenon that they dubbed the SN_{10} for a slow negative deflection that peaks at or beyond 10 ms following signal onset. Typical of other AEP phenomena, the SN_{10} is smaller and occurs later with decreasing signal level. Close to threshold, therefore, the peak of the SN_{10} occurs well beyond 10 ms. Obviously, the recording requires an analysis window greater than the 10 ms commonly used for EPs. The recording also requires a high-pass cut-off lower than the typical 100 Hz for EPs to accommodate to the lower-frequency spectrum of the SN_{10}. Davis and Hirsh recommended a filter passband of 40–3000 Hz. Figure 10-6 illustrates the use of SN_{10} to assess threshold for a signal with a narrower spectrum than that of a click.

Davis and Hirsh (1979) believed that SN_{10} would be superior to EPs and MPs as an index for tonal threshold audiometry. The reality, however, is that SN_{10} is the trailing edge of wave V of the EP (ABR) and also may be part of what has been designated as Na of the MP. SN_{10} differs from the usual EP recording because of the 20 ms instead of the 10 ms analysis window and the lower high-pass end of the bandpass filter. It differs from MPs mainly because MPs usually are recorded with a 50 ms analysis window.

Using a 20 ms analysis window and a filter passband of 40–3000 Hz has some advantage over the usual EP recording conditions for measuring thresholds for a broad range of frequencies. It also has two advantages over a 50 ms analysis window: It allows a faster rate of signal presentation for quicker accumulation of clinical data and it capitalizes on the most stable components of the MPs. However, the 20 ms analysis window compels the use of short tone bursts with broad spectra and high sidebands. When the whole 50 ms analysis window is viewed, longer tone bursts with narrower spectra and lower sidebands can be used.

Threshold Audiometry with Clicks

Measures of Threshold for Clicks

A common EPA threshold procedure uses clicks as the test signals. Most commonly, the clicks are generated by delivering a 100 μs electric rectangular pulse to the transducer. The most common response analysis window is 10 ms and the most common filter passband is 100–3000 Hz. The most common index of response is wave V of the EPs. Click rates usually vary between 10 and 40/s.

Presence/absence of response is judged from waveform replicability and on predictable wave V latency increases with decreases in signal level. Figure 10-7 illustrates both the close replicability of AEPs obtained under the same signal and recording conditions, as well as the small but distinct changes in peak latency and amplitude with systematic signal level changes.

Response replicability, a desirable attribute for any form of threshold audiometry, is a major virtue of EPs to clicks. Another virtue is the systematic change with signal level, especially in the latency of wave V. Still another virtue is the independence of EPs from even major changes in patient state. Small changes do occur with natural and induced changes in state. However, for purposes of response identification for threshold EPA, these

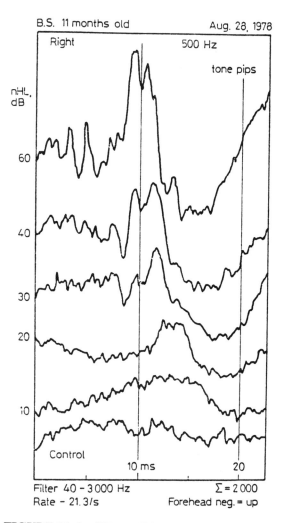

FIGURE 10-6   **SN$_{10}$ to 500 Hz tone pips as a function of signal level. Negativity of the forehead relative to the earlobe is plotted as an upward deflection. That deflection is identifiable even at 10 dB nHL. Most of the energy of the SN$_{10}$ occurs beyond 10 ms into the middle potential time zone, especially for the weaker signals.**

[Reprinted with permission from Davis H, Hirsh SK. *Audiology 18*:445-461, 1979.]

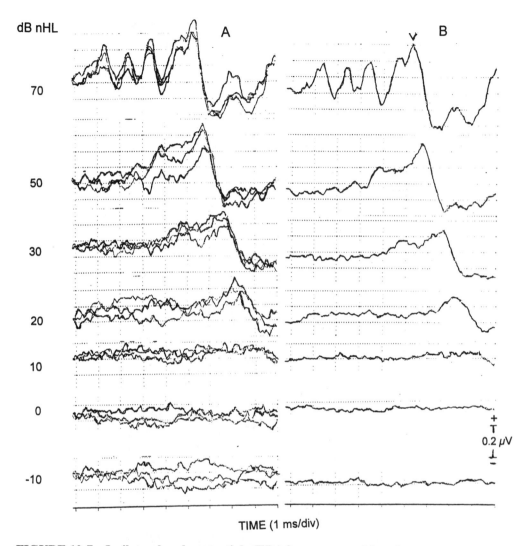

dB nHL

TIME (1 ms/div)

FIGURE 10-7   Ipsilateral early potentials (EPs) from a normal-hearing young man as a function of click magnitude. Filter passband: 100–3000 Hz. (A) Three replications (N = 800). (B) Composite AEPs of the three replications. Clicks were inaudible at 0 and –10 dB nHL. Note the progressive lengthening of the latency of wave V with decreasing signal magnitude.

changes are negligible even when a patient is comatose. Finally, although EPs vary with age, especially with the extremes of age, no age-related changes negate the use of EPs for threshold audiometry. This property makes EPs particularly valuable for assessing hearing sensitivity in neonates, even premature babies.

Given all of the virtues of click-evoked EPs, it is easy to understand why they became popular as an index for threshold EPA. Nevertheless, some important shortcomings limit their universal applicability. One of these is the poor signal-to-noise ratio close to threshold in some patients. Even at levels exceeding 70 dB HL, wave V, the largest component of EPs, is only about 0.5 to 0.6 μV. Nevertheless, this is sufficiently large to stand out distinctly against the noise floor. Closer to threshold, however, the response portion of the AEP trace may be too small to be distinguishable from the noise (although in Figure 10-7 one can identify wave V at the lowest level of audibility). As a consequence, EPA thresholds often are reported as higher (poorer) than behavioral response thresholds for the same clicks, when both forms of audiometry can be performed reliably on the same patients. A simple correction factor cannot be applied uniformly to all patients (e.g., true sensitivity is always 10 dB better than the EPA threshold) because signal-to-noise ratio varies between patients and sometimes even in the same patient from test to test. In other words, a simple linear extrapolation to threshold for all patients is hazardous because both the amplitude of the signal (i.e., the response portion of the AEP) and especially the noise floor of the AEP vary considerably between patients.

A second shortcoming of EPs is the risk either of overestimating or underestimating the extent of hearing loss. Steep high-frequency losses often are judged to be more severe overall even when low-frequency sensitivity is relatively good (Bauch, Rose, & Harner, 1980; Fowler & Mikami, 1992). On the other hand, significant low-frequency hearing losses may be overlooked when high-frequency sensitivity is good (Goldstein et al., 1983; Stapells, 1994). A related shortcoming is the lack of frequency specificity. The click has a broad spectrum, even though the recording conditions favor the response to the high-frequency components of the click. Therefore, click thresholds established with EPs give a good general view of the patient's auditory sensitivity, but they give little information about the patient's sensitivity as a function of frequency.

Little can be done to overcome the errors engendered by severe high-frequency or low-frequency hearing losses when clicks are the test signals. However, the problem of overestimation of hearing loss can be minimized by enlarging the analysis window at least to 20 ms and by lowering the high-pass end of the bandpass filter to 30 Hz or lower.

In many clinical instances when threshold assessment is the goal, it is impractical to keep the patient under test long enough to establish threshold sensitivity with the desired precision or confidence. This is especially true for squirmy infants and young children. One way to circumvent the time limitation is to plot what usually is termed a latency-intensity function, such as that shown in Chapter 5, Figure 5-5. In that figure, the latency of wave V to clicks is plotted as a function of increasing signal level. Unfortunately, the unit along the abscissa in most plots is designated as *intensity* even though the signal level usually is given in dB nHL or, occasionally, in dB SPL or in dB SL. The proper units of intensity are watt/cm^2 or watt/m^2.

Not all persons with normal peripheral function give identical wave V latencies for the identical signal level. The area between the broken lines in Figure 5-5 gives a range of normal values. In that figure, the range is ±3.0 standard deviations. Those clinicians who choose to be less conservative about what they call abnormal use a range of ±2.5 or even ±2.0 standard deviations. Each clinic must establish its own latency-magnitude function and range of normality because each clinic differs slightly with regard to recording filter characteristics, transducers, criteria for judging presence/absence of wave V, and so on. Despite these differences, agreement in values between clinics is close.

When a patient's threshold is assessed, latency of wave V is plotted as a function of signal magnitude for the signal levels that can be used. If all values fall within the established normal range, the clinician assumes that the patient's sensitivity for clicks is normal even if available time limits the establishment of threshold by a more precise bracketing measure. If a patient's latencies do not fall within the normal range, the extent of displacement of values along the abscissa provides an estimate of the patient's abnormal hearing level.

Clinicians have used the shape and slope of the latency-magnitude function to derive some insight into the possible nature of the patient's hearing impairment, for example, conductive, sensorineural, and if sensorineural is it likely to reflect a cochlear or a neural lesion (Galambos & Hecox, 1978; van der Drift, Brocaar, & van Zanten, 1988). By way of example, if a patient has a conductive hearing loss, the slope is expected to be normal and the whole function is expected to be displaced along the abscissa by the amount of the hearing loss (see Figure 10-8). As another example, if a patient has a sensorineural hearing loss because of a cochlear impairment, the slope of the latency-magnitude function is expected to be steeper than normal. For weak signals, the function is displaced by the extent of the hearing loss but at strong signal levels, wave V latencies are within the normal range.

Despite the commonness with which the latency-magnitude function is written about and discussed, some question exists about how often the function is used clinically to assess threshold compared to how often the eyeball technic discussed earlier is used. Also, how often it is used to diagnose the hearing loss measured by the function is not certain.

An important shortcoming limits the value of the latency-magnitude function for threshold assessment or for diagnosis, the number of points (i.e., wave V latency values) to which the curve must be fit. Even a crude estimation of any function requires a minimum of three points; four or more points are preferable. If the latency-magnitude function has to be used for threshold assessment, it is probable that time limitations prevented using other approaches. The same time limitation can preclude obtaining enough wave V latency values for a confident definition of the function.

Aaron R.Thornton and colleagues (personal observation) developed a probability approach to determining whether a series of clicks at some designated level elicits activity significantly different from background electroencephalic or other noise. An electronic template is built into the instrument for expected positive and negative voltages at fixed latency points. An internal count is made of how many concurrences and non-concurrences there are with these expected voltages for a fixed click level. Statistical probabilities are calculated. If the concurrences exceed a set probability criterion, a *response* is reported by the instrument; if the statistical criterion has not been met, then *refer* [for further testing] is reported.

The statistical approach just discussed has an advantage over most other procedures in that it is totally objective. It calls for no yes/no decisions based on waveforms. Also, because no special interpretative expertise is required, the test procedure can be managed by competent technicians. So far, this approach has been applied primarily to neonates and only for screening, not threshold, audiometry.

Signals resulting from delivering 100 μs rectangular electric pulses to bone-conduction vibrators have been used to assess bone-conduction thresholds with EPs as response indices (Collet, Chanal, Hellal, Gartner, & Morgan, 1989; Schwartz et al.,1985). Latency of wave V was reported to be later for the bone-conducted signal than for an air-conducted signal of

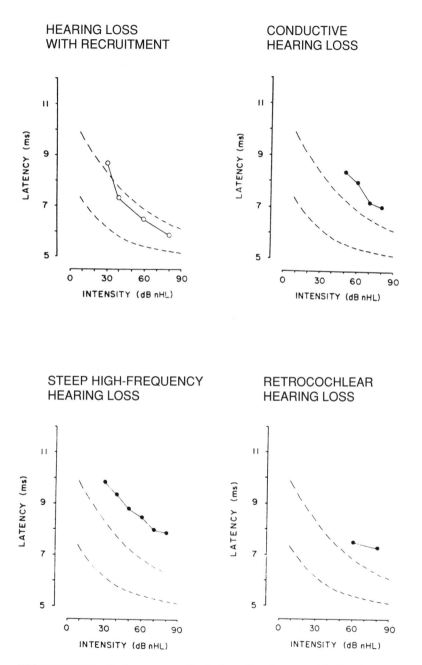

FIGURE 10-8   Latency-magnitude function for wave V of early potentials (EPs) to clicks for different kinds of hearing loss.

[Adapted and reproduced with permission from Stapells et al., in J. T. Jacobson (Ed.), *The auditory brainstem response*, Allyn & Bacon, 1985.]

the same Hearing Level. The likely difference was attributed to the low-pass filtering effect by the mechanical vibrator on the short-duration electric pulse. Latencies for low-frequency signals are longer than for high-frequency signals. On the other hand, when AC and BC clicks were of equal Sensation Levels, EPs elicited by them were more nearly alike (Durrant, Nozza, Hyre, & Sabo, 1989). Whatever limitations click-elicited BC responses may have, thresholds obtained with these signals still can give at least a crude estimate of a patient's air-bone gap.

Estimation of Pure-Tone Audiogram from Thresholds to Clicks

Although the click has a broad spectrum, techniques have been used to estimate thresholds as a function of frequency *range* from responses to clicks. One technique, usually called the **derived response** procedure (Burkard & Hecox, 1983; Don, Eggermont, & Brackmann, 1979), calls for first obtaining a patient's EPs for suprathreshold clicks as described above. Next, the patient's EPs are obtained in the presence of high-pass masking noise with a high low-pass cut-off, for example, 4000 Hz. Then the EP for the masked condition is subtracted from the EP for the unmasked condition. The difference between the two represents the contribution to the raw EP from stimulation by frequencies above 4000 Hz. The next step is to lower the noise filter cut-off to 2000 Hz and to obtain an EP to the click in the presence of noise at and below 2000 Hz. This EP is subtracted from the EP obtained with the 4000 Hz low-pass masking noise. The difference between the two EPs represents the contribution resulting from stimulation by the portions of the click between 2000 and 4000 Hz. These steps are repeated with successively lower low-pass noise filter cut-offs until contributions from each conventional audiometric frequency range have been sampled. An example of this technique is shown in Figure 10-9. Note that the analysis window is 20 ms covering both EPs and the early part of MPs. The technique just described defines the suprathreshold contributions to EPs from the different frequency regions. The procedure is repeated at successively weaker click levels until threshold for each frequency band has been determined. Figure 10-10 illustrates the results of a threshold-seeking procedure. A positive attribute of the derived-response technique is that in recording with the usual EP recording conditions (10–20 ms analysis window and filter passband of 100–3000 Hz), the most stable portion of the AEP is used in threshold determination. However, the technique suffers two clinical shortcomings. First, with a high-pass filter cut-off of 100 Hz, the contributions of the click's low-frequency components are unrealistically diminished. Second, the time to obtain thresholds is uneconomically long.

A second technique for estimating tonal thresholds from responses to clicks uses notched noise as a masker (Beattie, Garcia, & Johnson, 1996; Folsom & Wynne, 1986) . For example, to obtain thresholds for the spectral components of the click in a narrow band around 500 Hz, a quiet bite around 500 Hz is taken out of a broad-band masking noise. Therefore, the EP that is recorded presumably was elicited by the 500 Hz energy region of the click (see Figure 10-11). Click level is reduced until no definable activity is recorded. This, then, is the patient's threshold for the region of 500 Hz. Different frequency bands are notched in the noise until thresholds are obtained for each desired frequency range.

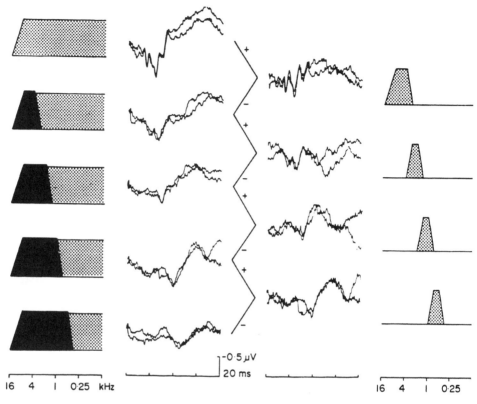

FIGURE 10-9   Example of derived responses of early potentials (EPs) and middle potentials (MPs) to clicks. Traces on the left are AEPs to 70 dB nHL clicks presented at 39/s alone (top trace) or in the presence of high-pass masking noise with cutoff settings at 4000, 2000, 1000, and 500 Hz. Each trace is the average of 2000 samples recorded with a vertex to mastoid montage; negativity of vertex relative to mastoid is represented by an upward deflection. Diagrams to the left of the traces represent the spectra of the clicks (dotted area) and the masking noise (black area). Traces on the right are the derived responses obtained by sequential subtraction of the responses elicited with successively lower filter settings for the high-pass noise. On the far right are diagrams of the narrow-band frequency regions that are presumed to have elicited the derived responses.

[Reprinted with permission from Stapells, Picton, & Durieux-Smith in J. T. Jacobson (Ed.), *Principles and applications in auditory evoked potentials*, Allyn & Bacon, 1994.]

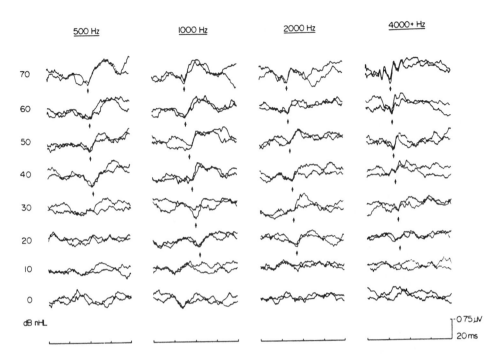

FIGURE 10-10   Derived response waveforms obtained with procedure described in the text and illustrated in Figure 10-9. The arrows point to wave V of the early potentials (EPs), which for 1000 Hz at weak signal levels and for all levels for 500 Hz occur as middle potentials (MPs). Negativity of the vertex relative to the mastoid is plotted as an upward deflection.

[Reprinted with permission from Stapells, Picton, & Durieux-Smith in J. T. Jacobson (Ed.), *Principles and applications in auditory evoked potentials*, Allyn & Bacon, 1994.]

The notched noise procedure has the same advantage as the derived response procedure in that it uses the most stable portion of AEPs. However, it is simpler and faster than the derived-band procedure. On the downside, as with the derived response technique, the initial recording filter passband of 100–3000 Hz can lead to an overestimation of hearing levels for the low-frequency bands. Also, the noise notch has a wider spectral spread than the 5–1–5 tone bursts that can be used in a more direct estimate of threshold as described in the previous chapter.

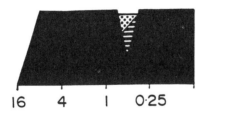

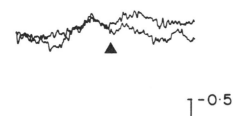

FIGURE 10-11   AEP waveforms obtained with notched noise procedure described in the text. The test signal was a 60 dB nHL click presented at 39/s. N per trace = 2000. Negativity of the vertex relative to the mastoid is plotted as an upward deflection. The solid black area represents the masking noise. The dotted area of the notch represents the effective spectrum (centered around 500 Hz) of the unmasked portion of the stimulating click; the area shaded by horizontal bars represents the spread of masking into the notch from its low-frequency edge. The solid triangle under the traces points to wave V, which falls in the middle potentials (MP) time zone. For threshold assessment, the click level is reduced until wave V no longer can be identified.

[Reprinted with permission from Stapells, Picton, & Durieux-Smith in J. T. Jacobson (Ed.), *Principles and applications in auditory evoked potentials*, Allyn & Bacon, 1994.]

Other Methods of Response Acquisition

Throughout this and the previous chapter, stress has been placed on getting a good AEP that is readily identified from the background noise in which it is embedded and on the practical matter of obtaining clinically useful responses as rapidly as possible. Future instrumental approaches, such as those discussed at the end of Chapter 9, may be able to achieve these goals more expeditiously than is currently possible. However, given the technologic capabilities of most contemporary evoked potential systems, we believe that programming all signal conditions, including the number of samples for each AEP, in advance of any testing, and then off-line analysis is a favorable way to attain these goals. Others are more secure with on-line decisions about response/no response judgments and immediate manipulation of subsequent signal conditions. However, they, too, are concerned about speed of response acquisition, and about when to continue and when to suspend a test run. Experimenters have developed two different procedures to help cope with these practical issues. So far, the procedures have been applied mainly to EPs (or ABRs) to clicks. We discuss them briefly without the technical bases or background.

The first of these was reported by Elberling and Don in 1984. The procedure often is identified by the initials F_{sp}, where F is a statistic representing a distribution or variance estimate of noise, and "sp" represents a single point in the analysis window whose measured noise over many sweeps determines the F value. The quality of the response to the eliciting signal, or the F_{sp}, is determined by a ratio of the variance of the response portion of the total recording to variance of the background noise. A test run is terminated when F_{sp} reaches a predetermined acceptable value. Obviously, F_{sp} will be achieved with fewer sweeps with stronger than with weaker signal levels. Elberling and Don have continued to refine their initial approach to improve the certainty and the speed with which their procedure can identify a response (1987, 1994, 1996). Whether their procedure can be extrapolated fruitfully to MPs and LPs is not clear.

A second procedure to speed data acquisition often is identified by the initials **MLS** for **maximum length sequences**. It was first proposed in the audiologic literature by Eysholdt and Schreiner (1982). The procedure calls for fast signal presentation rates that cause several responses to occur within the analysis window. However, a pseudo-random sequence of signal and no signal conditions allows the target AEP (EP, LP, or LP) to be separated from other activity and to be identified and measured. Burkard, Shi, and Hecox (1990) found little difference in form between EPs obtained with the fast MLS procedure and those obtained more slowly through conventional averaging. Picton, Champagne, and Kellett (1992) were able to collect EPs and MPs successfully at a rapid rate but found little advantage for LPs over a conventional averaging procedure. On the other hand, Weber and Roush (1995) found little advantage of the MLS procedure over standard averaging when testing neonates. Similarly, Musiek and Lee (1997) found no clear diagnostic advantage of MLS over standard averaging in the evaluation of MPs in patients with CNS lesions. As with the F_{sp}, the jury is still out with maximum length sequences as a significant way of speeding up or otherwise improving clinical procedures.

Chapter *11*

Neonatal Hearing Screening and Evaluation

Neonate implies a newborn baby, but the age at which that baby ceases to be a neonate and becomes another category of baby differs among writers. Our definition of neonate is a baby from birth to the end of the tenth post-delivery day. The definition applies whether the baby is full term or premature. We define **infant** as a baby between the ages of 11 days and 18 months. Neonatal hearing screening and threshold assessment by EPA are the emphases of this chapter.

The first section of the chapter, after the historic background, covers the principles of screening programs and then technical aspects of neonatal hearing screening. The next section deals with accessory aspects of neonatal hearing screening such as management feasibility, incidence of congenital hearing impairment, and the influence of economics on the directions that neonatal hearing screening has taken. Parental emotions also have played a determining role. Logically, discussion of these and related issues should precede the details of screening. These less tangible issues, however, may not be fully appreciated apart from the technical background on screening. The chapter concludes with the technical aspects of hearing evaluation as follow-up to hearing screening. It will become apparent that hearing screening and threshold assessment, technical and nontechnical issues, money and emotion, all are inextricably interwoven because each facet affects all the others. The facets are artificially separated in this chapter only to facilitate their exposition.

Historic Background

Prior to World War II, only sporadic attempts were made to screen or to assess neonatal hearing. It was generally assumed that educational measures for severely hearing-impaired children had to wait until the children were of school age. Clinicians and researchers who believed that hearing-impaired babies could benefit from early habilitative measures were thwarted in their attempts at neonatal hearing assessment by inadequate technical capabilities.

During and shortly after World War II, significant advances were made in electrophysiologic approaches to measuring thresholds in military personnel who complained of service-incurred hearing loss (Knapp, 1948; Michels & Randt, 1947). Some electrophysiologic approaches were adapted for testing neonates and infants (Bordley & Hardy, 1949; Hardy & Pauls,1952). Unfortunately, the adaptations had little success and could not be applied routinely for neonatal hearing assessment or screening.

Contemporary interest in neonatal hearing screening and threshold assessment began in the 1960s with the efforts of Marion Downs and others who shared her views (Downs & Sterritt, 1964, 1967). Downs called attention to instances of severely hearing-impaired children not having their impairments detected and diagnosed until they were two years old or older. The impairments could not be blamed on post-natal illness, toxins, or other extrinsic causes. Therefore, in retrospect, those children were judged to have been born with the impairments, that is, they were congenitally hearing-impaired. An extension of this observation was that if the impairments had been detected at birth, habilitative measures would have advanced the children's communicative, educational, and emotional well-being. Downs contended that neonatal hearing screening was feasible through observations of behavioral responses to controlled sounds. Her form of screening was adopted by some hospitals in the United States and elsewhere.

Downs' arguments and screening procedure had appeal and some validity but they were seriously flawed (Goldstein & Tait, 1971). Nevertheless, Downs' arguments and enthusiasm had a profound *positive* effect on neonatal hearing screening and evaluation. Interest in electrophysiologic and other test procedures was rekindled. Eventually, valid and feasible EPA procedures emerged. Some of the most influential early work was done by Galambos and Hecox (Galambos & Hecox, 1978; Hecox & Galambos, 1974) on neonatal AEPs to clicks. McRandle and colleagues (1974) added neonatal studies also with clicks as test signals, and Wolf and Goldstein (1978) used narrow-spectrum tone bursts as test signals.

Not all professionals and laypersons subscribed to routine neonatal hearing screening. Some arguments for and against EPA, and screening procedures in general are discussed later in this chapter.

Concept of Hearing Screening

Screening implies placing members of a target population in one of two piles: *likely* to have the problem for which the population is being screened, or *unlikely* to have the problem. In the case of neonatal hearing screening, it means identifying those newborn babies whose hearing *may* be impaired and whose threshold sensitivity should be measured.

Passing or failing a screening test cannot be interpreted as normal or abnormal. Screening is a game of odds. On follow-up evaluation, one should find a higher percentage of babies in the likely pile than in the unlikely pile to have confirmed hearing loss. Even if follow-up is done only on the likely pile, a higher incidence of hearing loss should be found than the incidence in the total baby population estimated from various prevalence studies of large populations of unselected infants and children.

One should not infer cause, nature, or severity of a possible hearing loss from failure to pass a sensitivity screening. Some guesswork may be justified if the screening instrument targets specific kinds of hearing loss (e.g., sensorineural). However, such specific targeting usually cannot be justified. Some screening programs target middle-ear disease or dysfunction. However, in these cases, one can infer little about hearing sensitivity even among those neonates who do not pass the screening.

Comparison between hearing screening and a window screen helps explain some compromises in neonatal hearing screening protocols. A window screen can be fine enough to keep out the smallest bugs and dirt particles. The cost of such fine screening is extreme restriction on the desired airflow and sunlight. At the other extreme, a screen mesh wide enough for maximum airflow and sunlight keeps out only birds and massive-sized insects. Most window screens compromise by having interwire spaces small enough to keep out all but tiny gnats and fine dirt particles, but large enough to allow acceptable airflow and light. Said differently, in the compromise, some unwanted insects and dirt are allowed through the screen and some restrictions are placed on desirable airflow and light.

Compromises shape specific screening procedures for detecting neonatal hearing problems. Ideally, neonatal hearing screening by EPA should sift out any hearing impairment that can interfere with communication development or that indicates a health-related problem. Such a fine screen, however, is not practical. Among the important compromise factors that determine the fineness (or coarseness) of a screen are: feasibility of complementary or substitute screening procedures, ability to provide follow-up evaluative and remedial services, consequences of false negatives, time available for screening, instrumental capabilities, financial resources, and community acceptance of the goals of neonatal screening. These factors and some of their interdependent corollaries are expanded later.

Screening Protocols and Parameters

We raise no arguments in this section on the wisdom of neonatal EPA screening, on alternative screening strategies, or on related issues. These matters are covered later. The assumption in this section is that neonatal screening by EPA is warranted and that technical resources are available and adequate.

Establishment of Follow-up Resources and Procedures

Establishment of follow-up programs should be the first step in any screening program for any disorder or problem, for any population—neonates at risk for hearing impairment, maintenance personnel in nuclear plants at risk for radiation poisoning, health workers at risk for contracting tuberculosis, and so on. If no helpful follow-up is available (e.g., full hearing evaluation, counseling, remedial services), neonatal hearing screening is futile and perhaps even detrimental because parents are left in a frustrating lurch.

The nature and extent of follow-up services influence the nature and extent of screening. For example, if physicians are the only follow-up personnel available, then screening procedures will be slanted toward finding those babies with medically or surgically correctable hearing impairments. If educators with their psychology and social work colleagues are on hand, then screening can emphasize finding any degree of congenital hearing impairment that is likely to interfere with communication and learning through hearing. These are only sample situations. Other settings may require different emphases or orientations. The main point of these examples is to underscore that EPA screening should be designed and implemented on the basis of the nature and extent of follow-up facilities and services, and only after the follow-up services are in securely in place. This point cannot be overstressed. Do not start the screening process until follow-up is operational.

Test Environment

Quick discharge of mothers and babies from hospitals poses an obstacle to in-hospital EPA screening. Nevertheless, at present, hospitals provide the most practical settings for hearing screening. Nursery rooms—intensive care or well baby—in which babies are housed often are too noisy acoustically and electrically for EPA screening. Quieter areas near the nursery may be available for screening. Screening should be done as closely as possible to the main nursery to minimize disruption of nursery routine and the risk of infection. However, even nearby areas may be too noisy acoustically. Also, they may be too close to equipment (e.g., x-ray machines, life-support systems) whose radiated electric power introduces obscuring noise in the recording electrodes. In some hospitals, transporting babies to a quiet test suite in a different part of the hospital may be necessary, if removal from the nursery is permitted.

Measures can be taken to cut down electric noise to a suitable level in an area adjacent to the nursery if it is not overwhelmingly powerful. Low inter-electrode impedances (not easily achieved with neonates) and careful grounding of both the EPA equipment and other nearby equipment reduces electric interference. If the room size and room use permit, testing could be done within a carefully grounded wire-screen cage.

Secure transducer coupling to the baby's ear does eliminate some acoustic noise in the test environment. If the transducer coupling cannot attenuate ambient acoustic noise sufficiently, small acoustic chambers should be considered. In our early work before convenient earphone coupling was available, McRandle devised a test chamber with a transparent lid (Goldstein & McRandle,1976). It was constructed from a commercial iced table serviette. The ventilated chamber provided about 15 dB of attenuation in the 500–4000 Hz range. More effective commercial chambers may be available now or chambers that provide electric as well as acoustic isolation can be constructed inexpensively.

Hearing screening in an intensive care unit (ICU) is debatable. The environment is hostile electrically as well as acoustically. Also, babies in an ICU usually are encumbered with electrodes that are monitoring life functions and with other equipment helping to sustain life. EPA hearing screening of ICU babies should wait until risk for survival passes and they have been transferred to an intermediate care nursery or, preferably, to a well-baby nursery.

Management

Neonates sleep most of the day. However, when they sleep and the length and depth of sleep are not predictable. Also, sleep may be disrupted by the handling in preparation for screening. Sleep is not mandatory when the AEP time-amplitude configuration is the response index but quietness and stillness are advantageous. A few minutes after feeding and burping may be the most propitious time for screening. A baby may awake and squirm and may cry when the scalp is prepared and electrodes and earphones are applied. The baby then must be comforted and quieted before screening begins.

Electrodes

Disposable electrodes are desirable to minimize risk of transferring infection from one neonate to another. The contact surface of a disposable electrode is covered with a paper or plastic protector that is removed just before electrode application. Part of the greater cost of single-use versus reusable electrodes is recovered in time saved by the operator in cleaning, sterilizing, and storing reusable electrodes. Nevertheless, conventional silver or gold disc electrodes can be used if proper attention is given to their maintenance.

Some disposable electrodes contain their own electrolyte to promote low-impedance contact between electrode and skin surfaces. Other disposable and all non-disposable electrodes require electrolyte application from a separate tube or jar. A baby's skin is sensitive. Electrolyte concentration should not be great enough to cause chemical burn. Some babies react adversely to the electrolyte and even to the electrode material, despite all precautions and care. These reactions seldom are serious but immediate attention should be given to them when screening is completed.

Low inter-electrode impedance is more difficult to achieve with neonates than with older children and adults. Neonatal impedance is higher to begin with (Hall, 1992, p. 493) and aggressive abrading of the skin done with adults is not feasible with neonates. Nevertheless, preapplication abrading can be done with coarse gauze, with or without gritty fluid or gel. There are also some commercially available pads with fine abrasive surfaces made specifically for use with neonates. Try to bring inter-electrode impedance below 10,000 Ω before beginning EPA screening.

Transducers

Technical improvements in transducers occur steadily. Thus, it is difficult to cite individual transducers that are best for neonatal hearing screening. Whatever transducer is used, it should be able to be coupled to the ear with minimal discomfort to the baby and with minimal opportunity for either acoustic leaks or ear canal collapse. These conditions can be contradictory and may require some compromise that does no violence to either. It would be advantageous if coupling of the transducer to the ear were firm enough to reduce masking by ambient noise. However, the operator should depend less on attenuation provided by the transducer and more on providing a quiet test environment.

An insert-type transducer such as the Etymotic ER-3A described in Chapter 3 satisfies the transducer criteria to a considerable extent. Another satisfactory transducer/coupler arrangement, at least for weak to moderate level signals, is the one that comes with the ALGO™ systems (Natus Medical) screeners. A soft plastic ring can be attached with its own adhesive to the baby's face, and fit securely around the baby's pinna. Sound is introduced into this ring through a tube inserted through a hole in its upper part.

Test Parameters

Two approaches to EPA screening have gained popularity. One is based on measures or judgments of response from the time-amplitude configuration of the AEP for a preset signal level. The other is based on automatic instrumental determination of response from an electronic template built into the screener. That approach is discussed later. The following recommendations are based on the assumption that the time-amplitude configuration of the AEP is used as the response index.

Recording

An Fpz-M1 (or M2) electrode array is recommended with the inverting electrode on the mastoid *ipsilateral* to the ear being screened. The contralateral mastoid lead can serve as the reference or ground electrode. The earlobes (A1 or A2) are used by some clinicians instead of the mastoid for placement of the inverting electrode. However, with many babies, the earlobes can be too small and too flaccid for secure electrode attachment. Although the vertex (Cz) may be a good placement for the non-inverting electrode for adults, in neonates the vertex is at a soft fontanelle where the cranial bones have not yet fused. The care necessary to prepare the vertex for electrode attachment deters most clinicians from using that placement.

An analysis window of 20 ms and a filter passband of 10–500 Hz are recommended. The low-pass cutoff could be raised to 1000 Hz or even 2000 Hz if the clinician prefers to have more sharply defined peaks. With these parameters (and the signal parameters below), the most prominent feature of the AEP will be wave V whose peak may lie in the EP time zone but whose defining trailing edge usually falls within the MP time zone. The recording conditions favor the most stable portion of the AEP, the portion least influenced by the effects of state, which are nearly impossible to control during the brief time available for screening.

Signals

Clicks should be the test signals with the understanding that the observed response is largely to the low-frequency portions of the click. The screening level should be no greater than 40 dB nHL (re: normal adult threshold as determined by voluntary behavioral responses to those clicks). If the acoustic and electric environment is sufficiently quiet, 35 dB nHL or even 30 dB nHL can be used. In noisier acoustic and electric environments, a screening level of 40 dB nHL is desirable to minimize the cost and emotional trauma of too many false positives. Screening should not be done in any environment in which a 40 dB nHL criterion is not feasible.

Despite some concern about neonatal recovery rate, we recommend a non-integer signal rate between 21 and 25 clicks per second. Two-hundred-fifty (or 300) samples free of major artifact should make up each AEP and at least three (preferably four) AEPs should be obtained for each ear. Presence or absence of response (i.e., pass/fail) should be based on AEP trace replicability and on the certainty of a wave V in the waveform.

ALGO Automated Screening Systems

Much of the initial and subsequent work leading to the ALGO systems (Natus Medical) was done by Aaron R.Thornton and colleagues (personal observation). Herrmann, Thornton, and Joseph (1995) provide much of the developmental history of and rationale for the automatic screening unit. Response recognition is based on probability rather than on time-amplitude waveform replicability and peak latencies and amplitudes. Test signals are clicks that are at 35 dB nHL, presented at 37/s. The analysis window is 25 ms, which includes both EPs and MPs. The recommended electrode montage is vertex to nape with a forehead ground.

Following each click, 25 ms of the raw EEG is examined for polarity at nine different latencies. From a time-amplitude waveform template derived from normal neonates, positive or negative deflections are expected at each of the nine time points. This is the response portion riding on the raw EEG. Raw EEG, which does not have a random spectrum, is, nevertheless, random with respect to signal onset time. Regardless of the polarity of the raw EEG at each of the nine preselected points, the response portion makes the EEG more positive at the positive points on the template and more negative at the corresponding negative points.

Because of the randomness of the EEG, sometimes at one positive point the large raw EEG is so negative that the small superimposed positive deflection still leaves that point negative. Similarly, at an expected negative point, the raw EEG may be too positive for the small superimposed negativity to result in a net negativity. Nevertheless, the superimposed positive and negative response-related voltage increases the probability that the net voltage will be positive where expected or negative where expected. It is not necessary to have 100% positive or negative deflections where expected to register a *pass*. An internal program of the instrument calculates the statistical probability of occurrence of positive and negative deflections. If the probability of response exceeds a criterion value after sufficient samples are taken, the machine stops, indicates *pass*, and similar testing continues on the other ear. If the probability does not exceed the criterion value, clicks continue until *pass* is registered or until 15,000 clicks have been presented at which time it registers *refer*, indicating that further testing is necessary.

The ALGO systems have some distinct advantages over the procedure described earlier. First, because they use automated statistical probability to read through background noise, they bypass the subjectivity of distinguishing the time-amplitude waveform from noise. The yes/no (or pass/fail) decision is totally objective. Second, it is faster because of the automation and the simplicity of its application. Third, because of its automation, it can be operated by persons whose salaries may be less than that for persons needed to operate a more conventional EPA system. In a screening study in which reasonable follow-up testing was done, the ALGO-1 proved to be "a viable alternative to conventional ABR instrumentation" for neonatal hearing screening (Jacobson, Jacobson, & Spahr, 1990).

Several shortcomings, however, diminish the comparative advantage of the ALGO systems. First is their relative inflexibility. The system algorithm cannot be altered easily or inexpensively. The more conventional EPA systems can be adapted more easily if parameters different from the standard ones prove to be more efficacious. Second, the system can be used for only one purpose—hearing screening only with clicks at one rate and, ordinarily, one level. Third, its sophisticated and effective artifact reject programs require more stillness (and, preferably, sleep) than may be required for conventional averaging. This demand can increase the overall test time. Finally, the age range of children on whom the system can be used is limited. Additional equipment is needed for follow-up EPA or for the use of AEPs (auditory and others) for audiologic or for neurologic purposes. Thus, total equipment cost is greater than that of more versatile EPA equipment, which can serve more purposes than just screening.

Issues in Neonatal Hearing Screening

EPA test equipment, parameters, and protocols for neonatal hearing screening depend largely upon the audiologist's stand on the non-instrumental and non-biologic issues of screening. We discuss some of these issues now. The purpose of this section is to provide general guidance toward planning of hearing screening programs for specific purposes and environments. Others have written extensively and well about the points to be discussed (Herrmann, 1994; Mencher & Mencher, 1993; Parving & Salomon, 1996; Tharpe & Clayton, 1997). It will be evident that issues are not independent but intertwine considerably with each other. The order in which they are discussed is no indication of their priority or importance.

Evaluating the Success of Screening

No practical hearing screening procedure has 100% sensitivity or specificity. Success of a procedure usually is assessed in terms of false positives and false negatives. A coarse screen leads to a low false positive rate. A coarse screen is justified if the purpose is to identify only neonates with severe enough bilateral sensitivity impairment to make them deaf by communication and education criteria. However, audiologists and educators place increasing emphasis on finding babies with less severe bilateral impairments and with unilateral impairments even when the other ear has normal sensitivity. We do not argue for one extreme or the other or for target goals in between. We simply point out that one consequence of a fine screen is a high false-positive rate.

One virtue of high false positives is that not many babies with any consequential hearing impairment will escape detection. A negative feature of high false positives is the attendant cost of follow-up, especially because follow-up threshold audiometry must be done by EPA. In addition, parents must face monetary and emotional costs and inconvenience until sensitivity impairment can be ruled out. Parental anxiety is not trivial.

Little is known about the rate of false negatives with EPA when applied to low-risk as well as high-risk babies and little is written about the negative consequences of false negatives. If a false negative occurs because the screen was not fine enough, the impairment may not be severe enough to be a major detriment to a child and eventually it may be detected in other ways. However, through technical error, a baby who is the false negative may have slipped through the screen despite a severe impairment. As a corollary, a false sense of security ensues and parents may ignore some clues to which, ordinarily, they would have been more attentive. When a child later manifests a communication problem, the problem may be misdiagnosed and mistreated because hearing impairment is not suspected. These errors are more likely to occur if there has been no intervening illness or trauma since birth to account for the communication problem. Now, inappropriate therapy because of misdiagnosis superimposes an iatrogenic problem on the undetected hearing loss. Iatrogenic problems are even more likely to occur with less severe hearing impairment because there are fewer behavioral clues to suggest that the communication difficulty stems from hearing impairment.

These comments on false positives and false negatives are not intended to argue for or against a coarse or a fine screen. They are presented as issues to be weighed in setting pass/fail criteria for EPA.

Degenerative Hearing Loss

A common estimate of severe bilateral congenital hearing impairment is 1 in 1000 births (NIH, 1993). Insufficient data are available for a confident estimate of the incidence of less severe hearing impairment or of unilateral impairments. The basis for the estimate of incidence of severe congenital hearing impairment is not strong. In screening programs, the hit rate for detection is much higher in those neonates who are already screened by the much-maligned high-risk register (Barsky-Firkser & Sun, 1997). This point has to be factored into success figures from any instrumental screening procedure.

The 1:1000 *incidence* estimate may be based largely on the *prevalence* of severe hearing impairment in infants and young children who did not suffer illness or accidents since their birth to which the hearing impairments could be attributed. Degeneration of hearing from time of birth to time of discovery of the impairment may confound comparisons of incidence and prevalence figures.

Heredo-degenerative hearing loss, especially pigmentary related loss, occurs more commonly than usually suspected. Degeneration can begin in days, weeks, months, and even years. The rate at which the loss progresses varies but, usually, the later it begins, the more slowly it progresses. The frequency range of greatest progression and loss varies as well. Although losses may be more apparent when they are high frequency, low-frequency degeneration also can occur.

Implications of heredo-degenerative loss for EPA screening are important. Hospital stay is brief and screening probably has to be done within 24 to 48 hours after birth. Degeneration may not be great enough at that time to be detected even with a fine screening criterion. Affected babies who slip through the screen technically may not be false negatives; they did not suffer their losses at the time of screening. Nevertheless, the consequences are equivalent to the real false negatives with later misdiagnosis and iatrogenic problems superimposed on their real hearing loss. Ironically, these may be the very babies discussed in the historic background who were the catalyst for initiating neonatal hearing screening—the fish that got away and were not seen for hearing evaluation until they were at least two years old. No early neonatal hearing screening procedure is immune from the problem. We highlight the problem as a factor for audiologists and others to consider in planning *when* EPA hearing screening should be done.

Time

One time element has just been discussed: If EPA screening is done within the first 24 to 48 hours of life, heredo-degenerative loss may be missed. Another time element is that of test administration. Test time per baby may be shorter with the ALGO systems than with using the time-amplitude configuration of the AEP as the response index. Regardless of the screening approach, less time is spent in the screening procedure itself than in the attendant logistics: bringing the baby into the test environment, preparing the skin for electrode attachment, electrode attachment and impedance check, removal of electrodes and cleaning the baby's skin, returning the baby to the nursery, and recording the results of the screening and, if necessary, recommendations for follow-up.

Time of stay in the hospital is another element of concern. When we did our early studies on neonatal hearing evaluation, babies remained in the hospital for 5 to 7 days. We had the luxury of waiting at least 24 hours before doing EPA. This gave babies a chance to stabilize and to resorb middle-ear fluid if there was any. Also, it allowed time for potential problems (e.g., hyperbilirubinemia) to manifest themselves. Currently, delivery and discharge approach drive-through speed. Healthy babies are discharged within 24 to 48 hours. Thus, despite legislative mandates for predischarge hearing screening, time available for stabilization and hearing screening may be impractically short. In addition, other things must be done for and to the babies during that same brief period. Some of the other things often have higher priority in the minds of hospital care givers.

Neonates who are at risk for survival have longer hospital stays but they spend much of that time in intensive care and intermediate care units. These are neither times nor places for hearing screening, except for medical purposes, and not only because of the hostile acoustic and electric environments. Most babies who are at risk for survival are intubated. Intubation can cause eustachian tube irritation with subsequent middle-ear problems. Fortunately, the middle-ear problems usually are transient. However, these babies may be screened by EPA in the well-baby nursery before the middle-ear dysfunction has resolved itself. Although the screening failures that occur are not false positives, the effect is the same as if referrals for follow-up were based on a false-positive test results.

Follow-up

At the risk of irritation we repeat—follow-up must be in place before the hearing screening process itself begins. In any screening program for any dysfunction, an important early step is to rescreen by the same procedure those persons who failed the initial screening. Can this be done for neonates who fail the EPA screen? Is there sufficient predischarge time for EPA rescreening? Will the cost of rescreening be prohibitive? On the other hand, given the reported rates of false positives with EPA and the cost of necessary evaluative follow-up, will not rescreening save money by reducing the number of unnecessary referrals?

The next two steps, which should be done as soon as possible following confirmed screening failure, are parental counseling and threshold EPA. Where should counseling and threshold EPA be done? A common argument for hospital-based neonatal hearing screening is that this is the only place and time when all babies are available for screening. The argument continues that if screening were not done in the hospital, many babies—perhaps a majority of them—never would be screened. Reports to parents and physicians about the results of the screening provide motivation for follow through with evaluation and counseling.

The compelling argument for hospital-based hearing screening loses some of its punch with the realization that time constraints (dictated mainly by financial constraints) make it difficult to squeeze in hearing screening during the 24- to 48-hour hospital stay. Assuming that hearing screening can be done prior to discharge, it is improbable that follow-up evaluation and thoughtful counseling also can be completed prior to discharge. Now, with the time gap between screening and follow-up, attrition will continue to be high, perhaps not quite as high it would be without the hospital screening.

Time constraints in hospital nurseries argue for considering physicians' offices or well-baby clinics with associated audiologic services as venues both for initial screening and for immediate follow-up. Attrition between screening and follow-up would be reduced. Also, the interval between birth and initial complete medical check-up would allow resolution of transient middle-ear conditions, thus reducing the number of follow-up referrals. Some of those babies born outside the hospital, and obviously not put through an in-hospital screen, would be put through the hearing screening during the first medical check-up. Babies born outside hospitals should have at least as high incidence of congenital hearing loss as babies born in hospitals. It is probable that little would be lost in terms of communication remediation by a delay of a few weeks. Such delays usually are inevitable anyway when hearing screening is done in the hospital nursery and follow-up is done after discharge. As an aside, Oudesluys-Murphy and Harlaar (1997) showed the feasibility of an at-home screening program with the ALGO-1 system.

Role of Emotion in Establishing and Conducting EPA Hearing Screening

Most laypersons and professionals consider hearing impairment to be a potential or actual handicapping condition. How and when are parents helped with their emotions when they learn that their baby has failed the EPA hearing screen? A full answer to these related questions is beyond the purview of this book. Nevertheless, we discuss some of the cogent issues because they influence the design of an EPA hearing screening program. The discussion is largely in the form of questions.

Ideally, parents should be counseled and guided immediately after screening. Will sensitivity and specificity be high enough so that it is safe *not* to give any counsel to parents of babies who pass through the screening? Should any counseling be done before follow-up is completed and hearing impairment is confirmed and quantified? That is, should only guidance for follow-up be given? Is there enough time during the hospital stay to provide adequate counseling? Will parental anxiety be heightened if counseling cannot be given at once? We said that most layperpersons and professionals consider congenital hearing impairment to be a serious problem. However, do these persons give it a high enough priority *vis à vis* other health concerns to allow enough time for adequate counseling before hospital discharge?

Familial hearing loss is the first item in most high-risk registers for congenital hearing impairment. Do all families with hearing impairment consider that impairment to be a handicap? Do all such families want to have congenital hearing impairment identified 1 to 2 days after birth or might some families be offended by attention to what they do not regard as a handicap?

Which Neonates Should Be Screened by EPA?

During the period of behavioral response hearing screening as proposed by Downs, most hospitals in which screening was done screened all neonates. With the advent of other screening procedures, and especially EPA, attention was focused on those neonates at risk for congenital hearing loss according to one or more criteria on the high-risk register. EPA hearing screening was time-consuming and expensive. Therefore, it was restricted to the population for which the hit rate was expected to be high. Gradually, professionals and laypersons became increasingly concerned about missing hearing loss in neonates who were not identified through the high-risk register and about the efficacy of the register itself. Consequently, support grew again for hearing screening for all neonates. Some states enacted legislation mandating predischarge hearing screening of all neonates.

Money continues to dominate clinical decisions. The number of at-risk babies is smaller than the number of non-risk babies. Why not concentrate one's financial, technical, and personal resources on the smaller group where the incidence of congenital hearing loss will be higher? One counterargument to this direction is that babies who are at risk for congenital hearing loss already have been screened out by the high-risk register. Many of them still will be followed up even if they pass a second screen, that is, the EPA screen (Barsky-Firsker & Sun, 1997). Follow-up is especially crucial if the baby is at risk because of familial hearing loss. Passing an EPA screen at 24 to 48 hours is no assurance that early degenerative hearing loss will not occur.

At least two arguments have been made against routine in-hospital EPA hearing screening of all those healthy neonates that are not screened out by the high-risk register: The cost is too high in terms of the expected low hit-rate and not enough time is available before the babies are discharged. However, audiologists should re-examine both arguments before eliminating the non-risk babies from a screening program. Insufficient data are available to allow realistic prediction of the hit-rate in the non-risk babies. This is especially true for unilateral impairments and less-than-profound bilateral impairments. The time factor also may be more manageable if automated procedures are instituted and if clinicans will test during late evenings and early mornings when they will interfere less with routine nursery care and when the test environment is more likely to be quiet. Also, if they do not have to rescreen those babies who have already been screened by the high-risk register, audiologists will have more time to screen the non-risk neonates.

Should EPA Be Abandoned in Favor of Other Screening Procedures?

Transient evoked otoacoustic emissions (TEOAE) have gained prominence as indices for neonatal hearing screening (Watkin, 1996; Welch, Greville, Thorne, & Purdy, 1996). While the superiority of TEOAE over EPA has yet to be established (Dirckx, Daemers, Somers, Offeciers, & Govaerts, 1996; Psarommatis, Tsakanikos, Kontorgianni, Ntouniadakis, &

Apostolopolous, 1997), it is clear that it is faster, cheaper, and less disruptive than EPA. Should EPA be used only for follow-up of those neonates who did not pass the TEOAE screening? Are there still other procedures that could become cheaper or more effective than either EPA or TEOAE screening? Although these questions have no unequivocal answers, they must be considered in planning a neonatal hearing screening program.

Reassessment of EPA Hearing Screening

The discussion of the interdependent issues surrounding EPA hearing screening makes it clear that no one easy solution exists for the problems attendant to establishing a screening program. Money is a dominant issue throughout but other factors also have to be weighed before a program is instituted. We hope that our focus on some of the major issues will provide direction for audiologists and other clinicians for their specific environments and circumstances.

Neonatal Auditory Threshold Assessment

The assumption for this section is that the neonates to be tested have already been identified by one or several screening procedures as patients whose auditory threshold sensitivity should be evaluated or assessed. A second assumption is that threshold assessment will be done by EPA.

The question asked about threshold EPA in Chapter 9 should be asked here as well: "What would this neonate's or young infant's threshold audiogram have been had I been able to obtain it reliably by behavioral response audiometry?" Therefore, the audiologist should ask the same of EPA and the answers to the questions should determine the test parameters and procedures (see Figure 9-1). Most of the signal and recording parameters recommended for screening EPA apply as well to threshold EPA. Therefore, the material that follows focuses mainly on the conditions and parameters peculiar to threshold EPA.

Test Signals

Spectrum: Narrow-Spectrum Signals

Audiologists can use tone bursts with rise/fall times of 5 ms and plateau duration of 1 ms (5–1–5) with neonates as well as with older children and adults. Likewise, a 50 ms analysis window recommended for mature patients also is recommended for neonates. With these signal and recording conditions, the most prominent portions of the AEP occur in the middle potential (MP) time zone.

When low-frequency tone bursts (e.g., 500 Hz) are used to test full-term, normal neonates, response-related MPs can be identified near or at the level of adult voluntary behavioral response thresholds for those same tone bursts. This observation on neonates (Frye-Osier, 1983; Wolf & Goldstein, 1980) was made in a less than ideal acoustic environment where masking of low-frequency signals often was possible. By contrast, high-frequency (e.g., 4000 Hz) tone bursts do not elicit what could be judged confidently as response-related MPs until the signals are about 30 dB HL (re: normal adult threshold). An example of these findings is shown in Figure 11-1 (Frye-Osier, 1983). The traces are grand composite AEPs across 10 babies tested at each frequency; a different set of 10 babies was tested for each frequency. That the grand-composite AEPs are truly representative is attested in Figure 11-2 in which the 50 dB nHL composite AEPs for all of the babies are displayed. The findings suggest that *normal* neonatal auditory sensitivity is adult-like for low frequencies but not for high frequencies. They also point to the necessity of determining normal neonatal thresholds across a range of usual audiometric frequencies. Results of other electrophysiologic (Folsom, 1985; Sininger et al., 1997) and behavioral response studies (Eisenberg, 1970; Franklin, 1983) support the contention that normal neonates and young infants have better sensitivity for low- than for high-frequency sounds.

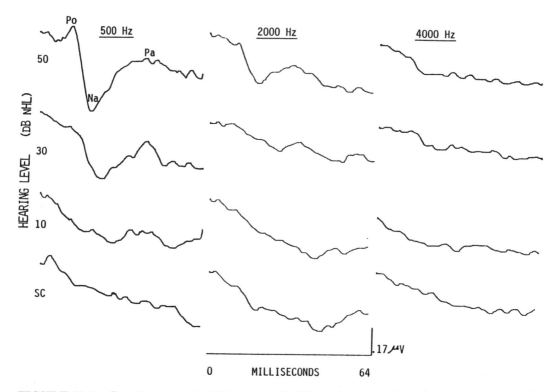

FIGURE 11-1   Grand-composite AEPs across 10 different neonates for each test frequency (N per trace = 20,000). See Figure 11-2 for the individual 50 dB nHL composite AEPs for each of the 30 neonates used in the study. Signals were tone bursts with linear 5 ms rise/fall time and no plateau presented at 5.4/s. 0 dB nHL was determined by voluntary behavioral response audiometry on normal-hearing adults in the same acoustic environment in which EPA was performed on the neonates. SC = silent control. The peak labeled Po is the same as wave V of brainstem response but with its peak falling in the middle potential time zone.

[Reprinted with permission from Frye-Osier, Simultaneous early- and middle-components of the averaged electroencephalic response elicited from neonates by narrow-spectrum signals. Doctoral dissertation, University of Wisconsin-Madison, 1983.]

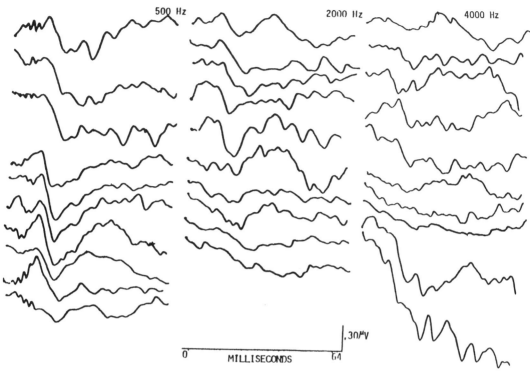

FIGURE 11-2 **Composite AEPs (2 replications of 1000 ÷ 2) for each of 30 neonates for 50 dB nHL tone bursts. These traces formed the 50 dB nHL grand composite EPS in Figure 11-1.**

[Reprinted with permission from Frye-Osier, Simultaneous early- and middle-components of the averaged electroencephalic response elicited from neonates by narrow-spectrum signals. Doctoral dissertation, University of Wisconsin-Madison, 1983.]

Spectrum: Broad-Spectrum Clicks

Clicks have been the most routinely used test signals for neonatal hearing evaluation. Latency of wave V for a given click level is longer in neonates than in older children and adults. The most common explanation for the longer latency is immaturity of synaptic transmission and axonic conduction. However, some of the neonate-adult latency difference should be counterbalanced by the neonates' smaller head size. A more probable basis for the longer neonatal wave V latency is that less of wave V is elicited by the high-frequency than by low-frequency components of the click. Adults with normal low-frequency thresholds but with distinct high-frequency hearing loss also show longer than normal latencies for a given signal level.

Signal Presentation Rate

Rapid data acquisition is important for neonatal testing because of the brevity of the hospital stay. During that brief stay, many things must be done for both mother and baby. Hearing screening and follow-up threshold EPA are only two of those things, and often their priorities are low. The faster that test signals are presented, the more rapidly EPA can be completed.

MP amplitude and clarity in neonates as a function of rate was discussed in Chapter 6. Because the exact nature of rate on neonatal MPs remains to be clarified, a non-integer rate of less than 10/s probably should be used. However, the signal rate of 17.1/s, which is favorable for recording adult MPs, possibly can be used with neonates as well.

Signal Number per AEP

We had recommended that in EPA for adults at least three AEPs of 500 samples each be collected for each signal condition. Collecting 500 samples at 17.1/s takes about one-half minute, assuming no time lost because of artifact rejection. The test run is longer with signal rates less than 10/s. Sometimes maintaining a neonate in a constant quiet state that long is hard, and artifact reject delays because of squirming and crying can extend collection time. Collecting four samples of 250 or 300 each may be preferable. The shorter collection time improves chances for a quiet and constant state for each trial, and the fourth trial provides another trace for replication comparison. It also improves chances for a less noisy composite AEP.

Signal Levels

Available time during a single test session rarely allows titration of threshold to the closest 5 dB or even to the closest 10 dB. Precision of threshold EPA should be based primarily on the short-term follow-up needs, for example, guidance for medical or surgical treatment, need for amplification, parental counseling. Level sampling is important for neonates just as it is for more mature patients. Level brackets should be wide, for example, 30–40 dB, and AEP trace analysis should be done off-line. If it is needed, greater precision can be achieved in follow-up EPA.

Level steps can be smaller and more targeted if preliminary other observations suggest a probable threshold region. For example, for a neonate who never reacts to soft sounds but does react overtly to sudden, strong sounds in the nursery, level brackets could be 50, 70, and 90 dB HL. By contrast, for a neonate who always stirs to soft sounds when in light sleep despite having failed screening, the level brackets could be 15, 35, and 55 dB HL.

Transducers

Transducer considerations discussed under hearing screening apply to threshold EPA as well. However, additional criteria have to be considered for threshold EPA. (1) The frequency range should be broad enough for the most important test frequencies and frequency-response curve within that range should be flat. (2) Signal magnitude range should be broad enough to sample at least near normal sensitivity to near total absence of hearing. For clicks and short tone bursts, it may be difficult to find a transducer whose output can exceed 90 dB nHL without producing disturbing distortion or without exceeding the linearity range of the attenuator. This upper limit seldom is a serious drawback in an initial evaluation for immediate management purposes. An insert-type transducer such as the Etymotic ER-3A satisfies most needs for threshold EPA to a considerable extent.

Recording Parameters

Analysis Window

A 50 ms recording epoch is desirable if 5–1–5 tone bursts are the test signals, and it is desirable even when the test signals are clicks. Regardless of signal characteristics and filter passband, the analysis window should be no shorter than 20 ms.

Filter Passband

The 3–500 Hz passband recommended for adults is applicable to neonates as well. The high-pass cutoff may have to be raised 10 Hz or the low-pass dropped to 300 Hz if low- or high-frequency noise interferes too much with response identification.

Electrode Montage

The montage recommended for EPA screening is desirable for threshold EPA as well. However, if the skull bones have fused by the time of follow-up threshold EPA, the clinician should consider moving the noninverting electrode closer to the vertex. For some insert-type transducers, the insert tube is terminated with an electrolyte-impregnated plug that acts as a recording electrode. It could substitute for the mastoid or earlobe electrode.

Chapter *12*

Otoneurologic Assessment

In this chapter we describe the use of auditory averaged evoked potentials (AEPs) to assess the organic integrity of the ear and brain. Often, this application is capsulized as **site-of-lesion testing**. Assessment, however, usually is more encompassing. Clinicians try to find out something about the extent and nature of lesions as well as their location or site. The term *brain lesion* ordinarily conjures up a picture of discrete damage to what had been a normal brain structure. However, lesion also may imply generalized brain malfunction due to some biochemical abnormality or it may imply maldevelopment without any additional acute or chronic damage.

Auditory dysfunction may not be the primary manifestation of a brain lesion under investigation. For example, paresthesia or a visual dysfunction often is the primary complaint of a patient with multiple sclerosis (MS). Nevertheless, aberrations in auditory AEPs provide valuable confirmatory evidence that MS is causing the patient's complaint.

Clinical emphasis in previous chapters has been on measures of auditory sensitivity. Knowledge of AEP generators is not crucial for these measures. In otoneurologic diagnosis, a fundamental assumption is that structural lesions and other pathologic conditions disrupt normal functioning of the structures that give rise to components of auditory AEPs. Therefore, for otoneurologic diagnosis, it is important to know which structures in the ear and brain are most responsible for the various components of auditory AEPs. In Chapter 5, we mentioned coarse correlations between component waves and probable generators. In Chapter 16 we expound further on the relations between components of auditory AEPs, probable generators, and possible functional significance of the component waves.

From this point on *auditory* will be omitted as a modifier of AEP. Except where other modalities are specifically indicated, AEP implies auditory AEP. The use of visual and somatosensory AEPs in peripheral and central assessment is covered in Chapter 14.

Historic Background

Clinicians have used AEPs in two complementary ways: (1) to assess the nature, site, and extent of lesions of the ear or brain; and (2) to assess and quantify auditory dysfunctions resulting from the lesions. We have already provided historic background in previous chapters on the latter use of AEPs. Now, we cover some stages in the use of AEPs to assess the nature, site, and extent of ear and brain lesions.

The work of Geisler and colleagues (Geisler et al., 1958; Geisler & Rosenblith, 1962) on what had been called the early components to clicks (0–50 ms) provided hope that functional integrity of the primary auditory projection system could be studied with extracranial electrodes. Unfortunately, the myogenic-neurogenic controversy about the generators of these early potentials derailed this promising avenue for otoneurologic investigation, just as it derailed attempts to use the potentials for threshold assessment. Clinical investigators then turned to late AEP components as possible indices for otoneurologic assessment. Some correlations were found between aberrations in late AEPs and nature, site, and extent of brain lesions (Barnet & Lodge, 1967; Bertolini & Dubini, 1969). Enthusiasm for late AEPs was short lived, however. They were so state-dependent that state-determined variations clouded the clinical value of differences in AEPs between patient and normal control populations. Clinical investigations diminished and confidence in AEPs waned.

Work on the first 10 ms of the AEP (now called early potentials) revived optimism and confidence in AEPs as indices for otoneurologic assessment. As pointed out in Chapter 5, the parallel work of Jewett and colleagues (Jewett, 1970; Jewett et al., 1970) and of Sohmer and Feinmesser (1967, 1970) marked the turning point. Replicability of early AEPs, or EPs, and their resistance to most changes in state were their principal assets. Although differences in EPs between patients and normal subjects were small, their clinical value was not obscured by intra- and intersubject variances, which were smaller. A virtual explosion of normative and of otoneurologic studies occurred in the years following the initial reports. Confidence in the efficacy of AEPs in otoneurology returned.

The return of confidence in early AEPs also revived interest in both middle and late signal-related AEPs. Contemporaneously, increased attention to event-related potentials (ERPs) for assessment of psychiatric disorders led to using ERPs in site-of-lesion testing. The power of various imaging techniques in finding and describing brain lesions and even peripheral lesions diverted some interest from AEPs. However, the alternate approaches to otoneurologic assessment have not displaced AEPs as described briefly earlier in this book and as expounded further in this chapter.

Parameters for Otoneurologic Assessment

Emphasis in this chapter is on EPs (early AEPs, brainstem responses) to clicks. No other signal-related or event-related potential has been explored nearly as extensively and, thus, has not yielded as many clinical correlations. Use of other SRPs and of ERPs in otoneurologic assessment are discussed only briefly at the end of the chapter.

Most reports of relations between otoneurologic lesions and EP abnormalities are based on the time-amplitude plot of the EPs. Characteristic traces are shown in Figure 12-1, which

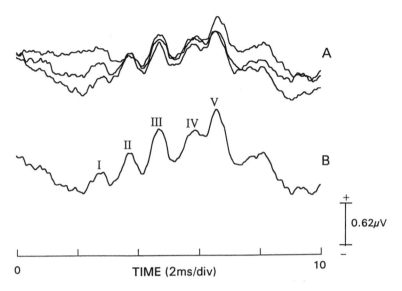

FIGURE 12-1   This is a reproduction of the top portion of Figure 5-1. Early potentials (EPs) from normal-hearing young woman. Filter passband 30–3000 Hz. (A) Clicks at 60 dB nHL; rate = 11.1/s; N per AEP = 800. (B) Composite AEP from the three replications shown in A. Roman numerals designate the five successive peaks commonly observed and measured for otoneurologic diagnosis.

is a reproduction of the top portion of Figure 5-1. Comparison of the patient's AEP waveform (time-amplitude configuration) with expected waveforms gives some indication of normality or abnormality. The most useful criteria for abnormalities derive mainly from peak latencies. Peak amplitudes have not been nearly so effective for identifying abnormalities.

Recommended initial recording and signal parameters are presented in Figure 12-2. The following discussion provides our rationale for the recommendations.

Recording Parameters

Electrode Montage
The noninverting electrode is placed on the vertex (Cz). Inverting electrodes are placed on each mastoid (M1 and M2) or on each earlobe (A1 and A2). The two-channel montage is Cz-M1 and Cz-M2. The ground or common-mode electrode is most conveniently placed on the forehead. We recommend two-channel recording because the usually clearer separation of waves IV and V in the contralateral recording helps in the identification of these waves in the ipsilateral recording. Also, one possible criterion for abnormality is based on the difference between ipsilateral and contralateral early AEPs with monotic stimulation.

Recording

Electrode placements: Cz, M1, M2, Fpz
Electrode montage: Cz-M1, Cz-M2, Fpz as ground or common-mode
Analysis window: 10 ms
Filter passband: 100–3000 Hz

Signal

Duration of triggering electric pulse: 100 μs
Polarity: rarefaction
Rate: 11.1/s
Level: 70 dB nHL
N per replication: 800
Number of replications: 3

FIGURE 12-2   Recommended initial recording and signal parameters for use of EPs (ABR) as response index for otoneurologic assessment.

Hair on the vertex often makes it difficult to obtain low interelectrode impedances and to maintain scalp attachment. Thus, some clinicians favor placing the noninverting electrode on the high forehead just below the hairline (Fpz). On the other hand, EP waves usually are better defined with the vertex placement. If the noninverting electrode is placed on the forehead, the ground electrode sometimes is placed elsewhere on the head other than Cz or elsewhere on the body (e.g., sternum), that is, a **noncephalic lead**.

At times identifying wave I with the Cz-M1 and Cz-M2 montages is difficult. Some investigators (Hall, Morgan, Mackey-Hagadine, Aguilar, & Jahrsdoerfer, 1984; Starr & Squires, 1982) suggest an M1-M2 or A1-A2 montage to obtain a better defined wave I in these cases. Others (Ruth, Hildebrand, & Cantrell, 1982) report no distinct improvement in wave I identification with this **horizontal montage**. An electrode deep in the ear canal, either as a separate electrode or combined with an insert earphone, is closer to the source of wave I. It may yield a better defined wave I than is usually obtained with earlobe or mastoid electrodes.

Analysis Window

By our definition, early AEPs (EPs) occur within 10 ms after signal onset. Therefore, 10 ms is an appropriate analysis window that suffices for most patients. With some pathologic conditions, however, wave V is delayed enough so that its trailing edge is not sufficiently long to help define the peak of wave V. Extending the window helps to define the peak. The American EEG Society (now the American Clinical Neurophysiology Society) (1994a) recommends that the analysis window be at least 15 ms.

Analysis window and signal rate interact. With a 10 ms window, click rate can approach 100/s without having responses to two successive clicks fall within the same window. With a 15 ms window, maximum signal rate is limited to about 66/s. One criterion for abnormality is based on changes in wave V latency as a function of click rate. If a clinic's criterion is based on rates faster than 66/s, then a window shorter than 15 ms is necessary.

Filter Passband

A filter passband of 100–3000 Hz is satisfactory for most patients. The low-pass setting can be lowered to 2000 Hz to obtain less noisy recordings but with the sacrifice of sharpness of peaks of interest. When children younger than 18 months are tested, a high-pass setting of 40 Hz is preferable to 100 Hz. The clinician has to establish age-related norms with the 40–3000 Hz passband.

Signal Parameters

Click Polarity

Clicks are generated by delivering a rectangular electric wave of 0.1 ms (100 μs) duration a transducer. The acoustic output, as described in Chapter 3, is a series of condensation and rarefaction waves lasting about 1.5 ms at levels ordinarily used. Clicks usually are described as rarefaction or condensation depending on the initial deflection of the transducer's diaphragm. That initial deflection is determined by the polarity of the rectangular electric wave delivered to the transducer. Manufacturers determine the electric/acoustic polarities at their factories and mark their instrument prompts (often RARE and COND) accordingly. Clinicians should affirm the validity of the prompts (see Chapter 3) before establishing their own norms. Also, they should reaffirm the polarities if any changes are made in the wiring to the transducer or in any internal instrumental controls.

We suggest starting with a rarefaction click. For most patients, click polarity does not affect diagnostic conclusions. If the EP configuration for the rarefaction click appears normal, continue to use that polarity. For a few patients, however, the two polarities evoke distinctly different EPs. Therefore, if the rarefaction click does not elicit a normal-looking EP configuration, retest with a condensation click. If the condensation configuration appears normal, then obtain EPs separately with rarefaction and condensation clicks for each test condition. If initial examination shows negligible difference between rarefaction and condensation EPs, then, for purposes of consistency, use only rarefaction clicks for the remainder of the examination. If a signal artifact interferes with identification and measurement of wave I for any patient, use an alternating rarefaction and condensation click to reduce the interfering effect of the artifact.

Spectrum

The spectrum of the click is broad. It is, essentially, the frequency-response curve of the transducer as long as the transducer is operating within its linear range. Thus, each transducer produces its own click spectrum. Fortunately, all transducers of the same basic design have similar spectra. Transducers of distinctly different designs will produce spectra that may lead to small differences in the properties of EPs. Because these small differences could affect diagnostic conclusions with some patients, it is important to establish norms for the particular transducer used in a clinic. Transducer properties can change over time, most often because of inadvertent physical abuse or because of extremes of temperature or humidity. Therefore, periodic rechecks of transducer spectra and reconfirmation of clinic norms are desirable.

Spectra also differ with the duration of the electric signal delivered to the transducer. The rationale for recommending a 100 μs duration as the triggering electric signal is its wide use, even though no clinical justification ever was offered for that duration before 100 μs became nearly universal.

Finally, spectra will vary, even for the same transducer, when operating levels are high or strong enough to produce amplitude distortion. Unfortunately, clinicians often do use distortingly high levels without cognizance of the effect of these levels on the click spectrum.

Click Level

Otoneurologic assessment is feasible only if peaks are large and discrete enough to allow confident measures of latency and amplitude. This clinical necessity dictates that clicks be distinctly suprathreshold. Initial click level should be consistent to allow patient-normal comparisons, as well as intra- and interpatient comparisons. Additional levels may be necessary or desirable *after* the set protocol level is used.

Level specification is not a simple or a uniformly agreed upon matter. Should level be specified as Sensation Level, Hearing Level, Peak Sound Pressure Level, Peak Equivalent Sound Pressure Level, or some other psychophysical or acoustic measure? Whatever the measure, how strong should the protocol level be? If click level is strong enough to stimulate the contralateral ear, should the contralateral ear be masked? If masking is recommended, what kind of masking noise should be used, at what level, and how should the masking noise be quantified? Answers to these questions obviously are interrelated.

We rule out Sensation Level (SL), or a set number of decibels above the patient's threshold for the clicks, as a routine protocol for several reasons. (1) Except for patients with normal thresholds, level would not be consistent across patients, and not even for the same patient if the patient's threshold hearing level changes from examination to examination. (2) Inter-ear comparisons are based on equal physical levels at each ear, not equal psychophysical levels. (3) Inter-clinic comparisons would be difficult. (4) A set level, for example, 70 dB SL, may not be achievable in a patient with poor threshold sensitivity. (5) Click threshold has to be established before otoneurologic testing can begin. This may not be convenient with some patients and may be impossible with others unless thresholds were determined precisely by EPA.

Specifying click level in dB SPL may be the most practical approach. However, it is more common to specify level in dB nHL. If level is specified in dB nHL, what should the initial or protocol level be? It is not unusual to find clinical reports in which clicks as strong as 90 dB nHL have been used (Abramovich & Prasher, 1986; Stach & Delgado-Vilches, 1993). On the positive side, at these and stronger levels, waveforms with clearly distinguishable peaks usually can be elicited. On the negative side, these levels can be disturbingly uncomfortable to some patients, they require contralateral masking, they induce large artifacts into the response recording, and, remotely, could be damaging if the test procedure is long. Also, they may approach or be at the nonlinear portion of the operating range of the transducer. We are not dogmatic about any one starting level but do warn about the possible shortcomings of levels at or above 80 dB nHL.

A protocol click level of 70 dB nHL should be considered. Clicks this strong elicit clearly defined peaks from persons with normal ears and brains. Interaural attenuation for the clicks is about 70 dB when they are delivered by insert earphones. Therefore, contralateral masking may not be necessary. However, masking should be used to eliminate the possible confusing contribution of the non-test ear if there is uncertainty about the amount of interaural attenuation or if signals are delivered by circumaural earphones. If the protocol level does not elicit EPs whose peaks are not distinct enough for confident measures, then the test level can be increased in 5 dB steps until satisfactory EPs are recorded. The possible use of several levels requires establishing criteria for abnormality for a range of levels at and above 70 dB nHL.

The physical level for a 70 dB nHL click will be similar across clinics if the same criteria are used for selecting normal subjects on which to base 0 dB nHL and if the same psychophysical threshold procedures are used. Nevertheless, peak SPL for a 70 dB nHL click may differ by several dB from clinic to clinic, thus reducing the certainty of inter-clinic comparisons. Also, when periodic recalibration is done, new juries of normal listeners have to be put through the extensive psychophysical procedures. For these reasons, physical specification of the protocol level may be more desirable. According to Stapells, Picton, and Smith (1982), 106.4 dB peak SPL is the equivalent of 70 dB nHL.

If clinicians maintain a routine initial protocol for all patients, then contralateral masking should be used. White noise (equal energy per cycle) is the preferred masker because of the broad spectrum of the click. Pink noise (equal energy per octave) may be preferable for neonates and young infants. Even if the non-test ear has normal sensitivity, initial masking level need be no greater than 30 dB effective masking.

Click Rate

A compromise must be reached between data collection time and a long enough **intersignal interval (ISI)** to assure complete neuronal recovery and a well-defined AEP. An 11.1/s rate often suggested for threshold EPA also is a reasonable base rate for otoneurologic assessment. Schwartz and colleagues (1994) believe that rates between 17.1 and 21.1/s allow quick data collection without jeopardizing response definition. Test time can be saved by presenting fewer clicks per AEP. More will be said later about using increasingly faster rates as a diagnostic procedure after AEPs are obtained with an 11.1/s rate.

Sample Size and Replications

Sample Size (N per AEP)

When EPs were first studied, it was common to present as many as 4000 clicks for each AEP (N = 4000). With improved artifact-reject circuits and with clinical experience, clinicians lowered the N per AEP to 2000 and many, eventually, to 1000. Experience indicates that the signal-to-noise ratio (S/N) improves little after 500 samples. In fact, S/N can even deteriorate beyond 1000 samples if the patient becomes nervous and restless during data collection. A maximum of 800 samples—free of major artifact—per AEP should suffice for most patients.

Replications

It is common practice to obtain two AEPs for each test condition. We advocate at least three AEPs or replications for each test condition. The larger number the number of replications, the greater is the certainty about trace replicability. Also, composite AEPs made of the replications are more likely to have less interfering noise and to have better peak definition when they are made from three (or more) than from two replications.

Another practice is to make peak latency and amplitude measures from each AEP obtained for the same test condition and to report the average of the measures. We find little clinical value to this practice. One major virtue of EPs is their replicability. Differences from trace to trace reflect mainly differences in noise background, not physiologic differences in peak latency or amplitude. Measures can be made with greater certainty from the composite AEPs where the noise is less than in each of the constituent AEPs.

Silent Controls

Silent control AEPs should be obtained during clinical assessment despite the additional time they require and despite the certainty with which clinicians think that they can identify peaks in the signal-related AEPs. If composite control AEPs are relatively flat, they give the clinician greater confidence that the deflections in the signal-related AEPs really represent responses. If the control AEPs are bumpy, the clinician must judge the signal-related AEPs with more caution. Sometimes small, periodic artifacts that may be partially hidden by the response portion of the AEPs will be more apparent in the control AEPs.

A control AEP obtained before audible signals are presented alerts the audiologist to the kind and level of noise to be expected in the signal-related AEPs. However, the nature and amount of background noise can change during the test session. Therefore, another control AEP partway through the test procedure is in order.

Peak Measurements

Latency

Measures are made on waves I through V. The principal measures are the latencies of waves I, III, and V, and the I-III, III-V, and I-V intervals. The intervals often are called interwave or interpeak latencies. *Latency*, however, usually connotes the time between signal onset and the peak of interest. That is not what these intervals imply. Therefore, we prefer to call them interwave intervals (**IWI**) or interpeak intervals (**IPI**). Norms are established for each measure and bounds of normality are specified. All reported abnormalities are *longer* than normal.

Waves I, II, and III usually are single-peaked with only occasional bifid peaks that pose problems of peak identification and measurement. Wave IV, on the other hand, often merges with the positive upswing of wave V, especially in the ipsilateral response, and sometimes is identified only as an inflection in that upswing. At times, wave IV cannot be distinguished as a separate entity. Wave V often appears to be double-peaked. The most positive portion is followed within about 0.1 ms by a slight deflection sometimes described as a **shoulder**. Systematic changes in wave V with signal level or signal rate suggest that latency should be measured at the shoulder rather than at the preceding larger positivity. As mentioned earlier, identification of waves IV and V in the ipsilateral trace can be aided by reference to their location in the contralateral trace.

Amplitude

Amplitude customarily is measured from the positive peak to the following negative trough preceding the next positive peak. The negative trough following wave I and wave III usually can be identified with considerable confidence. Identifying the negative trough following wave V is more troublesome. The main problem is that often a positive inflection in the steep slope after wave V is followed by a further negative deflection. No strong recommendation can be made for choosing either the initial deflection or the later more negative deflection as the measuring point. We do advise, however, that each clinic establish guidelines for consistency of measurement within that clinic.

No norms have been established for absolute amplitude measures in microvolts against which patient values can be compared. Some clinicians use the relative value or the ratio of the amplitude of wave V to wave I. A V/I ratio less than 1.0 is suspect; a ratio of 0.5 or less is definitely abnormal.

Routine Protocol and Normative Values

A patient's threshold sensitivity is important in determining whether that patient's EPs are normal. Published norms for peak latencies and IPIs are based on panels of subjects with normal tone audiograms. These norms and their limits are discussed first. Corrections for norms when patients' thresholds are not normal will be discussed later.

For Patients with Normal Auditory Thresholds

The following test sequence is based on the recommended parametric conditions outlined in Figure 12-2. It assumes that the normality of the patient's threshold already has been established through voluntary behavioral response audiometry or, when necessary, by other procedures including EPA. Figure 12-3 outlines the steps. We now review the sequence.

Prepare the scalp for electrode placement, attach the electrodes, and check the inter-electrode impedances. If impedance(s) is(are) too high, determine the offending elec-

---

a. Prepare scalp and attach electrodes.

b. Check inter-electrode impedances and, if necessary, replace electrodes.

c. View ongoing EEG and, if necessary, eliminate sources of artifactual noise.

d. Obtain three silent-control traces to establish physiologic and instrumental noise baseline.

e. Obtain three EP traces for each ear for 70 dB nHL clicks at the standard signal rate of 11.1/s.

f. Repeat step (e) with clicks at 91.1/s.

g. If wave V shifts by more than the criterion limit at 91.1/s, obtain EPs for three additional intermediate rates, e.g., 31.1/s, 51.1/s, 71.1/s.

h. Obtain three more control EPs at the 11.1/s rate to confirm or to reestablish the noise baseline.

FIGURE 12-3   Recommended initial protocol sequence for otoneurologic assessment with EPs (ABR) as response index.

trode(s) and reattach (it) them after further cleansing or abrading of the attachment site. Place the acoustic transducer securely. View the ongoing EEG for artifacts that may introduce disturbing noise in the recording and, when necessary, correct the offending condition.

Establish a physiologic and instrumental noise baseline by means of silent-control EP traces. Set the signal level to no signal, or to –10 dB nHL if the test instrument does not have a no-signal setting. Do not try to get a no-signal condition by unplugging the earphones from the test instrument. Electric noise may be introduced by the transducer even without signal presentation. Unplugging the transducer will remove this noise. However, when the earphones are replugged and testing begins with audible signals, noise not present during the initial silent control condition will now enter the recording. Obtain at least three control traces.

Obtain at least three EP traces for each ear for 70 dB nHL clicks at the standard signal rate of 11.1/s. Then repeat the process for clicks at 91.1/s. If wave V shifts by more than the criterion limit at this fast rate, then obtain EPs for at least three additional intermediate rates, for example, 31.1/s, 51.1/s/, 71.1/s. At the completion of the rate study, obtain three more control EPs at the 11.1/s rate to confirm or to re-establish the noise baseline.

Testing need not stop here if further information is needed to assist in the diagnosis. However, proposing specific additional steps for all possible clinical contingencies that may arise is not feasible.

Norms and the Limits of Normality: Generalities

Replicability is a first consideration. Three (or more) traces obtained under identical recording and signal conditions are superimposed. Except for minor differences in noise background, the three superimposed traces should be alike. If they are, a composite AEP should be made and observations and measures, as described below, can be made. If the three traces differ markedly from each other, they and their composite should be compared with the control traces and their composite. If the signal-related traces exhibit larger activity than the control traces, the signal-related traces may be considered evidence of response. Their lack of replicability, therefore, may be pathognomonic of some ear or brain abnormality. This lack of replicability has diagnostic significance but no useful measures can be made of the peaks. However, before concluding that traces are not replicable, be certain that testing procedures and instrument performance are not faulty, and that patient tension or patient restlessness is not the basis for poor trace replicability.

Other conclusions have to be considered if signal-related traces might not be different from control traces. One obvious conclusion is that the test signals were below the patient's threshold or were insufficiently above threshold to elicit replicable activity. Another concern is that instrumental error or improper transducer placement resulted in no acoustic signal being delivered to the patient. If neither of these contingencies apply, then the absence of replicable, response-related peaks must be considered pathognomonic of some ear or brain abnormality. The diagnostic test should not be abandoned until testing is repeated with a longer analysis window (e.g., 20 ms) and with a lower high-pass filter setting (e.g., 10 Hz).

Assume now that replicable traces have been obtained with the recommended recording and signal parameters. With experience, a clinician learns to judge whether a patient's EPs look normal or abnormal. The impression often is based on whether all constituent peaks are present in the EP trace. Waves II and IV can be difficult to identify even in traces from subjects with normal ears and brains. Therefore, their absence in a patient's trace is insufficient basis for a judgment of abnormality. Sometimes even wave I is of questionable clarity. If the latencies of waves III and V are normal, it is usually safe to infer the normality of wave I. However, if either (or both) wave III or wave V is difficult to identify or is clearly absent, then abnormality of the trace is a reasonable conclusion.

Quantitative Measures

The eyeball approach to assessment of normality/abnormality is valuable. By itself, however, it seldom provides sufficient information for confident diagnosis. Eyeballing must be followed by measures of latency and of relative amplitudes.

Standard measures of EP peaks or waves are summarized in Figure 12-4, along with some characteristic values. The most effective measures are latencies of waves I, III, and V; I-III, III-V, and I-V IPIs; and differences for these measures for left and right ear stimulation at the same signal level. Two additional measures also are shown: increase in the latency of wave V with increase click rate, and the ratio of the amplitude of wave V to the amplitude of wave I. Less emphasis is placed on these measures because abnormalities in them seldom occur without concomitant abnormalities in peak latencies and IPIs. Figure 12-5 is an example of a worksheet that can be used to tabulate the measured values and to judge their normality/abnormality. The critical value (CV) represents the limit of normality for a particular clinic; values longer than the CV are considered abnormal. In this example, the CV is 2.5

---

a. Waveform replicability [qualitative]

b. General waveform configuration [qualitative]

c. Presence of waves I, III, and V in ipsilateral waveform [qualitative]

d. Absolute latency of principal waves (in ms)

      I: 1.7
     III: 3.8
      V: 5.7

e. Interwave intervals (in ms)

     I-III: 2.1
    III-V: 1.9
     I-V: 4.0

f. V/I amplitude ratio: 1.0 or greater

g. Difference of wave V latency between 11.1/s and 91.1/s signal rates: 0.4–0.8 ms

h. Inter-ear latency comparison (for normal threshold in both ears): within 0.2 ms

i. Comparison between sides of head for monotic stimulation [qualitative]

FIGURE 12-4   Observations and measures used to judge normality/abnormality of EPs to 70 dB nHL clicks. Latency values shown are representative of latencies reported in the literature, rounded to the closest 0.1 ms. Often, values are reported to the closest 0.01 ms. Each clinic must establish its own norms with its own filters, signal levels, signal rates, and so on.

	NORMS				PATIENT DATA		
Measure	Mean	Critical Value	Ear Difference	Critical Value	Left Ear	Right Ear	Difference
I	1.5	2.1	0.2	0.5	____	____	____
III	3.5	4.1	0.2	0.5	____	____	____
V	5.4	6.2	0.2	0.5	____	____	____
I-III	2.1	2.6	0.2	0.4	____	____	____
III-V	1.9	2.4	0.2	0.4	____	____	____
I-V	4.0	4.7	0.1	0.5	____	____	____

FIGURE 12-5   Sample worksheet for comparison of patient latency data illustrated with normative values for an 80 dB nHL click. All entries are rounded to the closest 0.1 ms. Values to the closest 0.01 ms can be used if latency measures are made with greater precision. Measurement differences greater (longer) than the Critical Values (+2.5 sd) are considered abnormal.

standard deviations longer than the normal average. Some clinics are more conservative and accept only values greater than 3.0 standard deviations as abnormal.

The normal values in Figure 12-5 are means across subjects of both genders between the ages of 18 and 25. It was noted in Chapter 5 that both gender and age affect peak latencies and IPIs. Head size also may affect latency measures. Insufficient data are available currently to present with confidence separate normal values according to age, gender, or head size.

For Patients with Hearing Loss

Many patients for whom otoneurologic assessment is requested have hearing losses. These hearing losses may affect the clarity of the EP peaks and also lead to peak latency prolongation. When peak latencies for a 70 dB nHL click are prolonged, the prolongation can be interpreted as an indicator of some abnormality of the auditory nerve or of portions of the brainstem or of both. Therefore, corrections for latency based on hearing loss have been proposed. The several correction formulae proposed focus primarily on high-frequency hearing losses, and especially on the loss at 4000 Hz. Correction formulae are not invoked until the hearing level at 4000 Hz is at least 40 dB.

No one of the proposed correction formulae has gained popular acceptance, probably because of the several factors that confound the certainty of any proposal. Most statements about correction formulae derive from studies of patients with sensorineural hearing losses, probably of cochlear origin. Do the same formulae apply if the losses are conductive or if they are neural? Most formulae are based on sloping audiograms. Do they apply if the audiogram is flat? Most formulae are based on a negative slope to the audiogram, that is, poorer hearing with increasing frequency. Are corrections to be made if the slope is positive, that is, if low-frequency threshold is distinctly poorer than high-frequency threshold? If slope is a consideration, does the steepness of the slope have to be taken into account as in one of the examples in the previous paragraph? Does the slope have to be monotonic, that is, continuously falling without any improvement in sensitivity at higher frequencies? For example, for many noise-induced hearing losses, the threshold at 8000 Hz is better than it is at 4000 Hz. Does this invalidate the use of a correction formula? Finally, if clicks are presented at equal sensation levels across patients, as recommended by some clinicians, should any correction be considered?

Given all the possible glitches in any correction formula, no one formula is endorsed here. If one is to be used, we suggest a conservative one proposed by Selters and Brackmann (1977), that is, subtract 0.1 ms from the measured latency of wave V for every 10 dB of hearing loss greater than 50 dB at 4000 Hz.

Correction for hearing loss also is important when a patient's ears have significantly different thresholds. Without correction for the effect of cochlear or more peripheral impairment, ear differences in peak latencies could be misinterpreted as evidence of some neural or brain disease. Unfortunately, there are no unequivocal guidelines for correction in cases of distinctly asymmetric hearing losses. Durrant and Fowler (1996) discuss various options and limitations of their validity. Among strategies to be considered are presentation of clicks to each ear well above a 70 dB nHL protocol level, use of brief tone bursts instead of clicks at frequencies where the poorer ear is most sensitive, and the correction factor for high-frequency loss discussed above. Clinicians have debated whether hearing loss also can alter IPIs to the point of their being interpreted as indicators of abnormality beyond the cochlea. That debate has not been resolved but the weight of evidence favors no clinically crucial changes in IPIs as a function of hearing loss (Fowler & Durrant, 1994).

Throughout, we have stressed corrections only for wave V because that is the most identifiable deflection in EPs. Also, if the latency of wave V (raw or corrected measure) is normal, the earlier waves cannot have been delayed to any pathologic extent.

Otoneurologic Applications of EPs

Diagnostic Goals

As stated several times, clinicians use AEP indices to establish the nature of the offending lesion as well as its site and size or extent. Sometimes the nature of the lesion, as revealed by AEPs, provides insight into its locus and extent. Conversely, the locus and extent of a lesion sometimes suggest the nature of the lesion. The focus of this section is on the site of the lesion.

Lesions either of the peripheral or of the central auditory nervous system are not necessarily discrete. For example, the pathologic process that produces a lesion of the middle ear also may produce a lesion of the inner ear. A lesion of the auditory nerve, part of the periphery, may accompany a lesion of the brainstem, part of the central nervous system. A lesion affecting lower parts of the brain may extend to more rostral regions of the brain. These examples illustrate the complex challenges to EPA when it is used for purposes of appraising otoneurologic damage.

It is beyond the scope of this book to provide examples of all possible combinations of lesions that a clinician may encounter in diagnostic applications of EPA. Instead, we restrict the following few examples to lesions that affect exclusively or primarily one limited area or one functional system within the periphery or within the brain. Patients who provide the examples of different pathologic conditions had their conditions defined by non-EPA procedures. We present the well-defined cases to give readers insight into the diagnostic implications of EPA results on patients whose undefined condition necessitates further study by EPA.

Peripheral Lesions

Middle Ear

The mechanical block imposed by whatever caused a conductive hearing impairment acts as a passive attenuator of the click. Rarely does the block attenuate all frequencies by the same amount. Therefore, the spectrum of a click at the cochlea must differ from the spectrum of the click at the tympanic membrane. One should, then, expect a patient's EP waveform to differ to some extent from what it might have been without the conductive block. Despite this expectation, patients with conductive hearing impairment as a group yield EPs that resemble EPs elicited from groups of normal-hearing listeners for clicks of equivalent Sensation Levels.

For the patient described in Figure 12-6, clicks at what is designated as 70 dB nSL (which in this instance is equivalent to 70 dB nHL) elicited EPs with peak latencies about

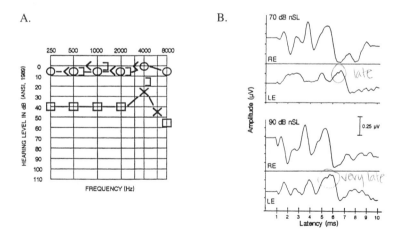

FIGURE 12-6   (A) Audiogram and (B) EPs to clicks from a 22-year-old woman with a conductive hearing loss. The stronger signals elicited EP configuration with left-ear stimulation similar to that elicited by right-ear stimulation but with longer peak latencies and smaller amplitudes.

[Reprinted with permission from Fowler & Durrant, "The effects of hearing loss on the auditory brainstem response," in J. T. Jacobson (Ed.), *Principles and applications in auditory evoked potentials.* ©Allyn & Bacon, 1994.]

equal to those elicited at about 40 dB nHL from a person with normal ears and brain. Latency-magnitude functions, as we pointed out in Chapter 10, usually do not provide sufficient additional diagnostic data to warrant the time to acquire them. However, if one can generate a function with at least three levels, the function should parallel a normal function. It will be displaced along the abscissa from the normal function by the amount of the conductive impairment (see Figure 12-7).

Cochlea

The patient described in Figure 12-8 had a high-frequency hearing loss of cochlear origin. At 50 dB nSL, the patient's wave V was barely discernible. As in Figure 12-7, nSL is equivalent to nHL. It resembles the kind of trace one obtains at 0 dB nHL for subjects with normal ears and brains. At 60 dB SL the latency of this patient's wave V was distinctly outside the range of values for normal subjects. With stronger signal levels, however, the latency of wave V closely approached normal values. Some clinicians consider the 60 dB/70 dB difference in this patient to be pathognomonic of a cochlear lesion and possibly an electrophysiologic equivalent of loudness recruitment.

The patient referred to in Figure 12-9 also had a cochlear impairment. It led to a threshold of about 60 dB SL for clicks. The patient's latency-magnitude function was barely distinguishable from similar functions obtained from normal subjects at those levels. In this instance, neither the EP traces nor the latency-magnitude function provided information to distinguish a cochlear from a middle-ear impairment.

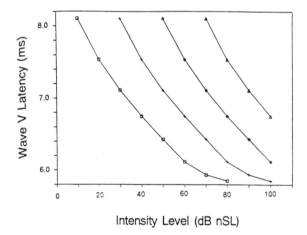

Intensity Level (dB nSL)

FIGURE 12-7   Hypothetic magnitude-latency functions for click-elicited wave V in conductive hearing losses (from left to right) of 0, 20, 40, and 60 dB.

[Reprinted with permission from Fowler & Durrant, "The effects of hearing loss on the auditory brainstem response," in J. T. Jacobson (Ed.), *Principles and applications in auditory evoked potentials*. ©Allyn & Bacon, 1994.]

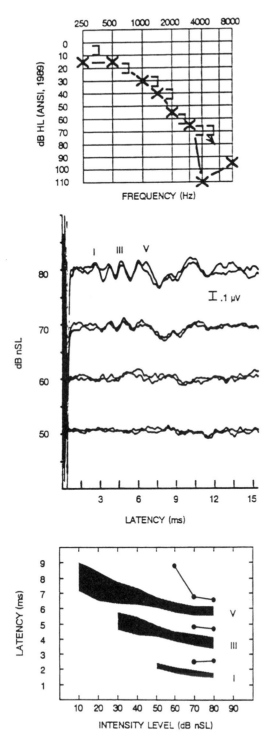

FIGURE 12-8   Audiogram, EP waveforms, and latency-magnitude functions for a patient with a high-frequency cochlear hearing loss.

[Reprinted with permission from Fowler & Durrant, "The effects of hearing loss on the auditory brainstem response," in J. T. Jacobson (Ed.), *Principles and applications in auditory evoked potentials.* ©Allyn & Bacon, 1994.]

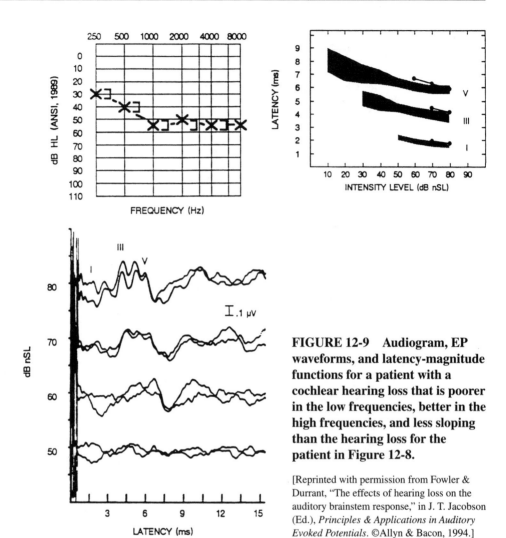

FIGURE 12-9   Audiogram, EP waveforms, and latency-magnitude functions for a patient with a cochlear hearing loss that is poorer in the low frequencies, better in the high frequencies, and less sloping than the hearing loss for the patient in Figure 12-8.

[Reprinted with permission from Fowler & Durrant, "The effects of hearing loss on the auditory brainstem response," in J. T. Jacobson (Ed.), *Principles & Applications in Auditory Evoked Potentials.* ©Allyn & Bacon, 1994.]

Comparison of these cases shows that obtaining EPs at more than one level *may* yield useful diagnostic information. As discussed in Chapter 10, some investigators believe that obtaining a latency-magnitude function also may indicate whether a patient has a steep high-frequency sensorineural hearing loss. On the other hand, as pointed out previously, often it is difficult to obtain a valid latency-magnitude function especially on those patients for whom such information may be the most needed.

VIII Nerve
Figure 12-10 illustrates distinct changes that can occur with a vestibular schwannoma. In this instance, the three major waves are present with stimulation of the affected (left) ear. Wave III, however, is smaller than it is in the non-affected ear, and the III-V interval is pro-

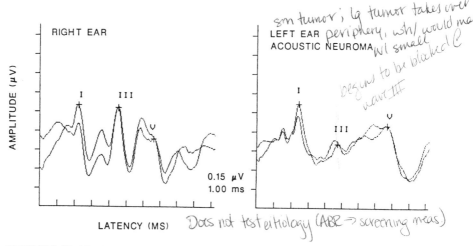

FIGURE 12-10   **Early potentials (EPs) from a 34-year-old woman with a 1.2 cm tumor arising from the superior branch of the vestibular nerve.**

[Reprinted with permission from Jacobson, Jacobson, Ramadan, & Hyde, "Auditory brainstem response measures in acoustic nerve and brainstem disease," in J. T. Jacobson (Ed.), *Principles and applications in auditory evoked potentials.* ©Allyn & Bacon, 1994.]

longed because of the abnormally long latency of wave V. The patient represented in Figure 12-11 had a large vestibular schwannoma which, for practical purposes, wiped out all five EP waves.

Central Lesions

Tumors

Intra-axial tumors, that is, lying wholly within the CNS, also may involve the periphery through pressure on the auditory nerve. Effects of these tumors are complex in that they usually are not discretely located only on one side of the brain and they may affect function below or above their locus. The example shown in Figure 12-12 seems to have had little effect on the periphery although wave I may be disproportionately large relative to wave III.

No deflections beyond wave III appear to be signal-related. This suggests that the tumor, a glioma, is low enough in the brainstem to interfere with the generators of wave IV and V, and large enough to interfere with the input from both ears.

Demyelinating Diseases

Demyelinating diseases, such as multiple sclerosis (MS), unlike tumors, which have a relatively discrete locus, usually are broadly, though not uniformly, disseminated throughout the brain. Therefore, their EPs ordinarily are not characterized by the absence or distortion of two or three successive waves. More characteristic are (1) replicability of traces obtained under identical conditions *poorer* than seen with more discrete peripheral or central lesions, (2) longer interpeak intervals (IPI) between most or all successive waves; the I-V interval

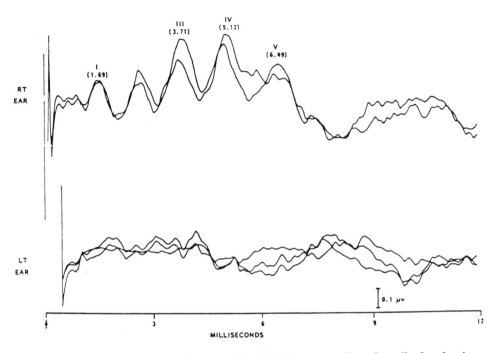

FIGURE 12-11   Ipsilateral early potentials (EPs) from a patient described as having a large left acoustic neuroma. All waves are clearly identifiable with right-ear stimulation but the III-V interval is slightly prolonged. No waves can be identified with confidence with left-ear stimulation.

[Reprinted with permission from Markand, "Brainstem auditory evoked potentials." *Journal of Clinical Neurophysiology, 11*:319–342, 1994.]

usually falls outside of clinical norms, and (3) abnormally large extensions of wave V latency with rapid signal presentations. Figure 12-13 provides an example of poor reproducibility of EPs. Figure 12-14 illustrates abnormal latency prolongations in traces that are reproducible.

Use of Other AEPs in Otoneurologic Diagnosis

SRPs

MPs

As defined earlier in this book, MPs are those signal-related deflections occurring between 10 and 50 ms in the AEP traces. Otoneurologic diagnostic applications of MPs were sidetracked by the myogenic-neurogenic controversy initiated by Bickford and colleagues. As a result, the clinical literature provides none of the secure quantitative guidelines that it offers for EPs and only a few observational generalities that an audiologist can apply with

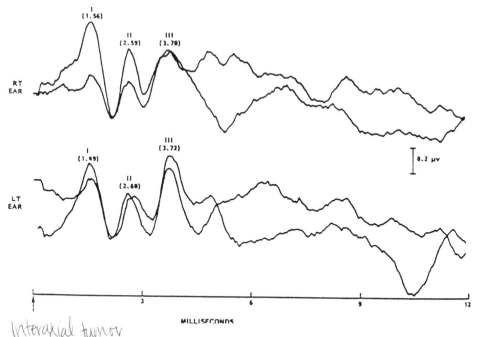

Interaxial tumor

FIGURE 12-12 **Ipsilateral early potentials (EPs) from a 15-year-old girl with a brainstem glioma. Waves I, II, and III are well-defined and occur at normal latencies. Waves IV and V cannot be defined with stimulation of either ear.**

[Reprinted with permission from Markand, "Brainstem auditory evoked potentials." *Journal of Clinical Neurophysiology, 11*:319–342, 1994.]

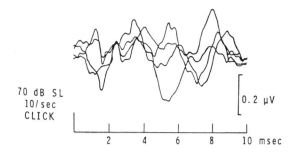

FIGURE 12-13   Early potentials (EPs) from patient with multiple sclerosis. Clicks of alternating polarity at 70 dB SL presented monotically at 10/s. The four traces were recorded consecutively. Note the poor replicability.

[Reprinted with permission from Keith & Jacobson, "Evoked potentials in multiple sclerosis and other demyelinating diseases," in J. T. Jacobson (Ed.), *Principles and applications in auditory evoked potentials.* ©Allyn & Bacon, 1994.]

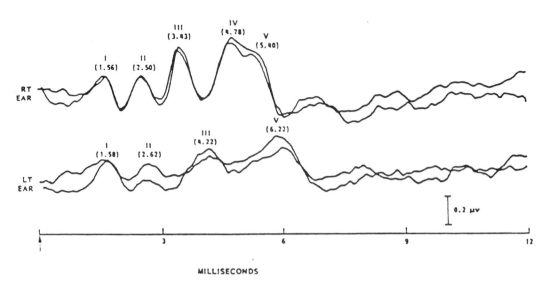

FIGURE 12-14 **Replicable ipsilateral early potentials (EPs) from a patient with multiple sclerosis. Right monotic stimulation elicits normal appearing peaks with normal latencies. Left monotic stimulation elicits smaller peaks with prolonged latencies and interpeak intervals.**

[Reprinted with permission from Markand, "Brainstem auditory evoked potentials." *Journal of Clinical Neurophysiology,* *11*:319–342, 1994.]

some confidence. Some of the information comes from studies on EPs in which the analysis window was extended beyond 10 ms to include portions of the MP time zone.

As a reminder, the designations EP, MP, and LP refer only to defined time periods within the analysis window for the AEP. They do not refer to specific generators within the brain even though speculations about generators are made by some authors.

Figure 12-15 shows examples of kinds of MP traces that may be obtained from patients whose communication impairment resulted from cortical lesions. One of the distinctly abnormal traces shows a gross distortion of what might be Pa and another shows nothing in the 10–50 ms time zone that can be interpreted as a signal-related response.

LPs

When the myogenic-neurogenic controversy diverted attention from the first 50 ms of the AEP, clinical investigators concentrated on activity beyond 50 ms, that is, LPs. We have already discussed LPs in terms of assessing threshold sensitivity and were able to identify some of their advantages and disadvantages for this purpose. In terms of assessing CNS disorders, however, descriptions are not nearly so discrete. The problem is that the plethora of LP clinical data is difficult to digest and to adapt clinically because of the wide range of clinical problems explored, the wide variety of signal and recording conditions, and the inherent variability of LPs. We have not been able to find clear enough cross-study commonalities to present as guidelines for analysis of CNS dysfunction. The only general

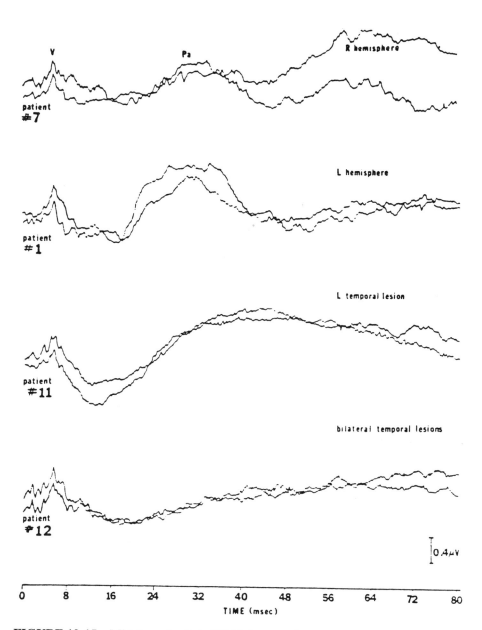

60dB HL

FIGURE 12-15   Middle potentials (MPs) from patients with cortical lesions.

Reprinted from Kraus, Özdamar, Hier, & Stein, "Auditory middle latency responses (MLRs) in patients with cortical lesions." *Electroencephalography and Clinical Neurophysiology, 54*:275–287, 1982. With kind permission from Elsevier Science Ireland Ltd., Bay 15K, Shannon Industrial Estate, Co. Clare, Ireland.]

guideline that we are able offer is to establish clinical norms for LPs to suprathreshold clicks under fixed signal and recording conditions and to determine normal ranges. Then, compare a patient's LPs under identical conditions.

If the patient's LPs lie outside the norm, then some CNS dysfunction may be inferred. The nature of the dysfunction cannot be ascertained, however, unless clearly defined abnormalities have been determined under identical conditions for a wide variety of possible CNS dysfunctions. Patients used for this determination must have had their dysfunctions qualified and quantified by clinical procedures that do not involve the use of EPs.

ERPs

In Chapters 1 and 8 we described ERPs mainly in terms of their application to assessing communication dysfunction. Just as with SRPs, ERPs also can be used to assess the nature, site, and extent of offending brain lesions. Application of ERPs for this purpose is more complex than that of SRPs because ERPs reflect the larger and more complex processing and storage portions of the brain as compared to the smaller and simpler transduction and transmission portions of the ear and brain. Some clinically relevant findings are emerging from ERP studies on patients with brain dysfunction. Abnormalities of both early and late ERPs have been reported but so far not enough commonalities have emerged to allow confident prediction of nature, site, or extent of brain lesions from the abnormalities noted in the ERPs.

C h a p t e r 13

Electrocochleography

This chapter focuses on the use of signal-related potentials from the cochlea and auditory nerve as indices for otologic diagnosis. We have already discussed auditory nerve potentials as waves I and II of early potentials (EPs). Now, we add cochlear microphonics (CM) and summating potentials (SP) to the list of peripheral potentials used in **electrocochleography (ECochG)**. Sometimes ECoG or other initials are used as initials for electrocochleography.

Figure 13-1 shows electrocochleographic responses elicited by distinctly suprathreshold clicks. Also, it shows how measures are made of CM, AP, and SP and characteristic normal values for those measures. Figure 13-2 shows CM and SP to tone bursts with measurement guidelines and characteristic normal values. SP is seen as a shift in the baseline on which CM is riding. With increasingly higher frequencies, that baseline shift becomes more negative.

Both CM and SP arise from the hair cells of the organ of Corti. When recorded with extratympanic electrodes, that is, distal to the tympanic membrane, CM and SP ordinarily are too small to be useful for threshold audiometry. Even in normal-hearing subjects, the recording noise usually obscures these potentials unless the eliciting signal is greater than 30 dB HL. This is especially true if the main electrode of the pair is outside the external auditory meatus, for example, on the earlobe. CM and SP are detectable near threshold when one recording electrode is placed through the tympanic membrane and against the promontory of the middle ear. These **transtympanic electrodes** must be placed by a physician with local or general anesthesia. That constraint on transtympanic electrodes precludes their routine use for either threshold audiometry or otologic diagnosis.

Historic Background

Wever and Bray (1930) and Davis, Derbyshire, and Saul (1933) in the United States, and Adrian (1931) in England did pioneer work on CM and AP from animals. They and other researchers and clinicians hoped to extrapolate animal findings to otologic diagnosis in human patients. With experimental animals, it was possible to place recording electrodes on

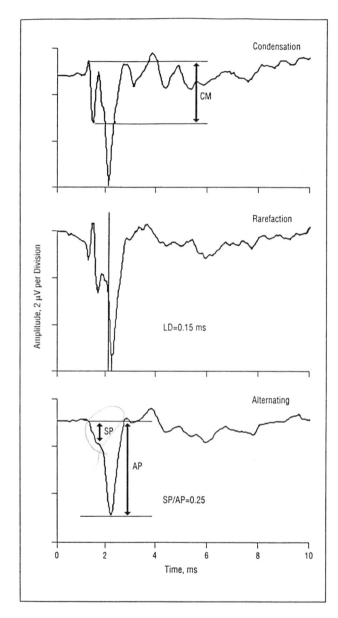

FIGURE 13-1   Click-evoked ECochG responses from a normal subject to condensation, rarefaction, and alternating suprathreshold clicks. Amplitude calculation criteria: action potential (AP)—from baseline to most negative peak; cochlear microphonic (CM)—peak-to-peak oscillation that precedes AP; summating potential (SP)— from baseline to inflection or knee that occurs on the leading edge of the AP. SP/AP ratio calculated from their respective measures. Latency of the largest negative peak used in determining AP latency difference (LD) between condensation and rarefaction clicks. Note the opposite polarity for CM in responses to the condensation and rarefaction clicks.

[Reprinted with permission from Margolis, Rieks, Fournier, & Levine, "Tympanic electro-cochleography for diagnosis of Meniere's disease." *Archives of Otolaryngology—Head and Neck Surgery, 121*:44–55, 1995. ©1995, American Medical Association.]

the round window membrane or directly into the cochlea. This allowed CM and AP to be visualized and measured oscilloscopically because they were much larger than the background physiologic and instrumental noise. Unfortunately, such near-field electrode placements were not feasible clinically for most patients. CM and AP picked up by far-field electrodes were small compared with the background noise. Electronic instruments and techniques of the 1930s were not able to extract the small CM and AP from the large background noise. Round-window recordings were obtained from some patients with tympanic

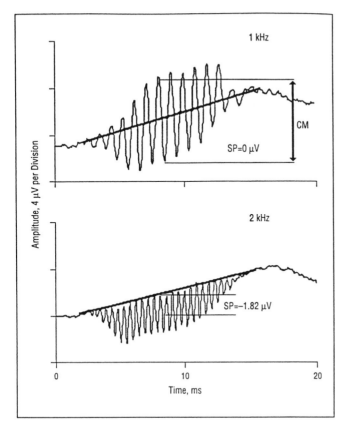

FIGURE 13-2 **ECochG responses from a normal subject to 1000 Hz and 2000 Hz suprathreshold tone bursts (5 ms rise/fall, 5 ms plateau). Peak-to-peak amplitude of cochlear microphonic (CM) measured at midpoint of response. For amplitude of summating potential (SP), a "moving" baseline (the ramp line in each of the figures) is determined by connecting the prestimulus baseline to the poststimulus baseline. The difference, a midpoint of the peak-to-peak waveform and the moving baseline, is taken as the SP. For this subject at 1000 Hz the moving baseline bisects the CM, thus making the SP 0 μV. At 2000 Hz, the midpoint of the CM is below the moving baseline resulting in an SP of −1.82 μV.**

[Reprinted with permission from Margolis, Rieks, Fournier, & Levine, "Tympanic electrocochleography for diagnosis of Meniere's disease." *Archives of Otolaryngology—Head and Neck Surgery, 121*:44–55, 1995. ©1995, American Medical Association.]

perforations and from some patients whose middle ear was exposed during exploratory or corrective surgery (Bordley, Ruben, & Lieberman, 1964; Fromm, Nylen, & Zotterman, 1935). The success of these recordings was not sufficient to encourage common use of CM and AP for clinical purposes.

In 1950, Davis, Fernández, and McAuliffe (1950) identified another signal-related cochlear potential in guinea pigs, the summating potential or SP. Others (Dallos & Cheatham, 1976) confirmed Davis' speculation that SP arises from the hair cells of the organ of Corti. CM, SP, and AP were not recorded from humans except during surgical procedures to eradicate disease or to improve hearing. Little clinical attention was given to any of the peripheral potentials until the advent of signal averaging. Even then, practical application of the peripheral potentials was not pursued vigorously until it became clear that at least AP could be recorded with far-field electrodes as waves I and II of the EPs.

At first, a transtympanic electrode was used with the exposed end of the penetrating electrode resting against the middle-ear promontory. As mentioned earlier, physician participation was essential not only to penetrate the tympanic membrane but also to anesthetize the skin of the external auditory meatus, and sometimes to anesthetize the patient. This constraint limited both research on and clinical application of ECochG. With improvement of extratympanic electrodes, and thus less discomfort and risk to the patient, research and clinical application of ECochG accelerated.

Despite the increased study of ECochG, that procedure still did not achieve clinical popularity. Nevertheless, several clinical needs helped to maintain interest in it . One of these was the need to determine the latency of wave I of the EPs for measures of I-III and I-V interwave intervals. As mentioned in the previous chapter, some patients do not yield a clearly identifiable wave I, especially if they have high-frequency sensorineural hearing losses. Obtaining the equivalent of wave I to clicks in ECochG recordings with extratympanic electrodes within the external auditory meatus is possible in many of these patients. A related need was to obtain an index for intra-operative monitoring that might be more sensitive than early brain potentials in detecting possibly harmful manipulation of the VIIIth nerve or of the vascular supply to the cochlea. The most propelling need, however, was for electrocochleographic evidence that a patient was suffering from Ménière's disease rather than from some other pathologic condition that could produce similar symptoms.

Clinicians have not used CM, SP, and AP as extensively as they have used potentials generated by the brain. Therefore, definitive clinical information about the peripheral potentials is not as extensive as information about electroencephalic potentials. We summarize the parameters and procedures as they have been presented by others (Ferraro, 1992, 1993) and offer only tentative conclusions about clinical implications. Also, we only discuss extratympanic electrodes, and just those extratympanic electrodes that can be applied without need for either local or general anesthesia.

Recording and Signal Parameters for Otoneurologic Assessment

Recording Parameters

Electrodes and Electrode Montages

The noninverting electrode is inserted in the ear canal. The inverting electrode, to be discussed later, and a ground or common-mode electrode are placed elsewhere on the head.

Insertion and placement may not be simple. Some ear canals are narrow. In such cases, visualization is difficult. Some patients have tortuous canals that also interfere with visualization and with inserting the electrode past the twists. Electrodes placed against the tympanic membrane generally require a microscope for proper visualization and placement (Levine, Margolis, Fournier, & Winzenburg, 1992). When the skin of the ear canal provides the electrode contact area, the skin has to be cleansed and sometimes abraded at the point where the active part of the electrode is to make contact. Narrow and tortuous canals make cleansing difficult. For any patient, the cleansing process usually is unpleasant and, at times, is uncomfortable enough to be disturbing. Despite all these difficulties, proper electrode insertion is not a major obstacle.

One type of ear-canal electrode, developed by Coats (1974), often is referred to as an "eartrode." It is a spring in the form of two small metal leaves hinged at one end. The exposed end of a silver recording wire terminates in a glob of silver on the outside of one leaf. The two leaves of the spring are pinched together with a forceps and inserted into the canal. When the forceps is withdrawn, the leaves separate and press against opposite sides of the canal. The metallic glob thus becomes the recording contact point. Spring tension holds the leaves in place against the skin of the canal. However, inadvertent tension on the recording wire can accidentally pull the metallic leaves from the canal. Therefore, the insulated portion of the recording wire is taped or otherwise secured to skin outside the canal.

Insertion of the spring leaves is relatively easy for skilled hands. Nevertheless, prior cleansing of the canal skin can be uncomfortable and is a negative feature of electrodes like the spring leaves. Another negative feature is that the spring pressure can cause the patient some discomfort if the spring has to remain in the ear for an extended period. Finally, electrode impedance usually is high.

Other kinds of electrodes include a disposable one that has soft porous material saturated with an electrolyte that contacts the skin of the meatus (Ruth, Lambert, & Ferraro, 1988). A metallic recording wire is attached to the porous material. A similar one has an opening in the porous material for passage of the stimulating sound. It, too, is disposable.

A rayon wick electrode also can be placed directly on the tympanic membrane, but it requires a microscope to insure the correct placement (Levine et al., 1992). When an insert-type transducer is used to deliver the sound, that insert holds the recording wire securely in place. An advantage of a wick electrode on the tympanic membrane is that it is closer to the CM, SP, and AP generators than are more distally placed electrodes. The larger potentials resulting from that placement produce a better signal-to-noise ratio than can be achieved by other extratympanic electrodes. On the down side, electrode impedance usually is several magnitudes higher than what usually is recommended. Nevertheless, proponents of this electrode (Margolis, Rieks, Fournier, & Levine, 1995) contend that high impedances *per se* do not cause any unusual recording problems. What is not clear is how the wick against the tympanic membrane affects the transmission of the acoustic signal delivered to the cochlea.

The most common site reported for the second, or inverting, electrode of the recording pair is the contralateral mastoid or earlobe. Some other sites reported are the vertex (Cz) and the high forehead (Fpz). The forehead or the nasion is the most frequently used placement for the ground or common-mode electrode.

Analysis Window

Strong clicks are the most commonly used eliciting signals. The crucial portions of the CM, SP, and AP in response to these clicks are complete by 5 ms. Therefore, if one wishes to obtain finely defined cochlear and VIIIth nerve potentials, a 5 ms window is desirable. However, 10 ms is a more commonly reported analysis window for ECochG. One reason for this is that 10 ms is the shortest epoch available on some commercial evoked potential units. A second reason is that clinicians and researchers often wish to record brainstem potentials simultaneously with the peripheral potentials. Another reason for using a 10 ms (or longer window) is to observe CM, SP, and sometimes AP to short tone bursts; a 5 ms window compromises full definition of the elicited peripheral potentials. Narrow-spectrum tone bursts have extended durations and require windows longer than 10 ms as in Figure 13-2.

Filter Passband

The time course of the CM, SP, and AP components in response to clicks indicates that their spectrum contains primarily high-frequency energy. Therefore, the 100–3000 Hz filter passband commonly used for recording EPs ordinarily is satisfactory for ECochG with clicks.

However, when tone bursts are used as eliciting signals, the resulting SP usually contains some defining energy in the frequency range below 100 Hz. Consequently, the high-pass end of the passband should be dropped to 50 Hz or lower. Margolis and colleagues (1995) used a 3–3000 Hz passband even for responses to clicks.

Signal Parameters

Spectrum

Clicks are the most commonly used signals in ECochG. Their spectrum, as described in previous chapters, is broad and parallels the frequency response curve of the transducer when operated below distortion levels. Tone bursts used as the eliciting signals have the major part of their energy at the fundamental frequency of the burst. As pointed out in Chapter 3, the extent of lower and higher harmonics depends mostly on the rise/fall and plateau durations.

Level

Levels ranging from 85 dB nHL to 100 dB nHL are commonly used. At these strong levels, traces usually have a good signal-to-noise ratio and the three separate peripheral potentials can be distinguished. Stronger levels have been used. However, patient discomfort and possible induced hearing loss increase with increasing signal level.

Polarity

Either rarefaction or condensation clicks can serve as signals. In the study by Margolis and colleagues (1995), rarefaction clicks elicited larger AP amplitudes from normal-hearing subjects at the strongest signal levels. Latencies did not differ significantly as a function of polarity. Alternating rarefaction/condensation clicks also can be used but should be avoided if a patient shows distinctly different traces with each polarity. Figure 13-1 illustrates how varying polarity can enhance the response components or, conversely, can reduce or eliminate one or the other. Figure 13-3 shows polarity manipulation more explicitly.

Rate

The 11.1/s rate used to elicit EPs also is satisfactory for ECochG. Routine use of rates slower and faster also has been reported. The latency of AP increases and amplitude decreases with increased signal rate, especially beyond 30/s. No particular diagnostic significance has been attributed to abnormal changes in AP with increasing signal rate.

Masking

One special virtue of ECochG is that contralateral masking usually is unnecessary. Activity picked up by the noninverting electrode ipsilateral to the stimulated ear comes almost entirely, or perhaps entirely, from the stimulated ear. In addition, if the acoustic transducer is the insert type, interaural attenuation will be about 70 dB. Sound reaching the contralateral ear ordinarily will be too weak to elicit large enough peripheral activity to contaminate or otherwise confuse the interpretation of the ipsilateral response. If there is some uncertainty about the possible contribution from the contralateral ear, that ear can be masked with white noise at no more than 30 dB effective masking.

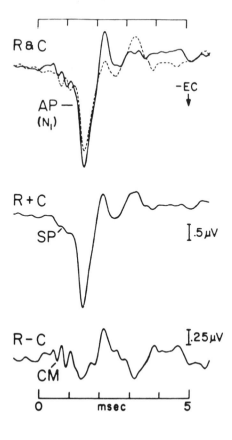

FIGURE 13-3   ECochG components to rarefaction (R) and condensation (C) clicks recorded from an ear-canal (EC) electrode: N₁ component of the whole nerve action potential (AP), summating potential (SP), cochlear microphonic (CM). Negativity of the non-inverting EC electrode relative to an inverting electrode indicated by a downward deflection. SP selectively enhanced by adding the R and C responses; CM enhanced by subtracting the C response from the R response.

[Reprinted with permission from Audiologic Evaluation Working Group on Auditory Evoked Potential Measurements, "Short Latency Auditory Evoked Potentials." *ASHA Desk Reference (Vol. 2, Audiology)*. Rockville MD: American Speech-Language-Hearing Association, 1995.]

Identification and Measurement of Peripheral Potentials

CM

CM mirrors the acoustic time course of the eliciting signal. This imaging includes polarity, that is, as the polarity of the eliciting signal reverses, CM polarity reverses correspondingly. CM has no measurable latency. It occurs simultaneously with the arrival of acoustic energy in the cochlea. The simultaneity sometimes makes it difficult to distinguish the biologic CM from the electric artifact associated with the transducer. Low inter-electrode impedances and careful shielding and grounding reduce the electric contamination. Also, presenting signals from remote transducers (either loudspeakers or smaller transducers attached to connecting tubing) separates electric artifact in time as well as space from the CM. Amplitude of CM is measured peak-to-peak at its maximum point.

SP

SP, like the CM, is present throughout the duration of the eliciting signal. It is seen as a unidirectional biasing or displacing of the baseline for the CM. In response to clicks, SP is

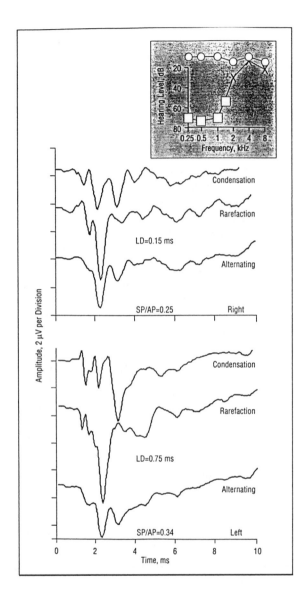

FIGURE 13-4   Responses to clicks from a 30-year-old woman with reversible endolymphatic hydrops. Inset shows air-conduction audiogram at time of ECochG. Right-ear responses are normal. With left-ear stimulation, the AP latency difference for condensation vs rarefaction clicks is abnormally large. Although the SP/AP ratio is larger with left-ear stimulation, that ratio (0.34) still is within normal limits.

[Reprinted with permission from Margolis, Rieks, Fournier, & Levine, "Tympanic electrocochleography for diagnosis of Meniere's disease." *Archives of Otolaryngology—Head and Neck Surgery, 121*:44–55. 1995, ©1995, American Medical Association.]

measured from an actual or estimated baseline to its maximum deflection, which appears as if it were an inflection in the large negative whole nerve action potential that follows it. Amplitude of SP in response to tone bursts is explained better through illustration (see Figure 13-2) than through verbal description.

AP

AP to clicks appears as a large negative spike—large, that is, in comparison to CM and SP amplitude. Its amplitude is measured from an actual or estimated baseline to the most negative deflection of the spike. Although it is possible to elicit identifiable AP to some tone bursts, clinically AP is studied primarily in response to clicks.

Example of Pathologic Responses

The pathologic condition that has received the most attention in ECochG studies is Ménière's disease or endolymphatic hydrops. Claims have been made that the ratio of the amplitude of SP to AP is abnormally large in patients with Ménière's disease. Levine and colleagues (1992) report a normal SP/AP of 0.31 with anything greater than 0.42 being abnormal. In their procedure, SP is best seen with alternating click polarity, which eliminates most of the CM contamination. An abnormally large SP is not evident in the traces shown in Figure 13-4 for a patient with Ménière's disease but what is noted for the affected ear is a larger than normal AP latency difference for condensation and rarefaction clicks. A larger than normal SP is seen, however, in the same patient's response to tone-bursts (Figure 13-5).

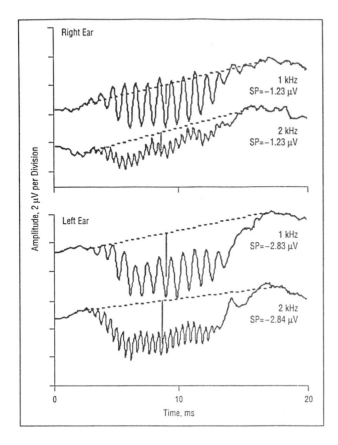

FIGURE 13-5 Responses to tone bursts from patient whose responses to clicks are shown in Figure 13-4. SPs for right-ear (better) stimulation are within the normal range; SPs for left-ear (poorer) stimulation are abnormally large.

[Reprinted with permission from Margolis, Rieks, Fournier, & Levine, "Tympanic electrocochleography for diagnosis of Meniere's disease." *Archives of Otolaryngology—Head and Neck Surgery, 121*:44-55, 1995. ©1995, American Medical Association.]

Chapter *14*

Visual and Somatosensory Averaged Evoked Potentials

Vision and somatosensation are not primary senses for audiologists to study. Nevertheless, some audiologists do record visual and somatosensory AEPs clinically for one of two purposes. First, audiologists may be the main electrophysiologic consultants in a clinical setting that concerns itself with a wide range of sensory and other neurologic problems. In this capacity, they may be asked to use visual and somatosensory AEPs to evaluate end-organ as well as central nervous system (CNS) integrity. Second, some patients whom audiologists assess for auditory dysfunction yield no signal-related auditory AEPs to signals of any frequency at any level. Is lack of response reflecting total deafness or is the brain incapable organizing recognizable auditory AEPs? If the patient does yield well-defined visual or somatosensory AEPs, the absence of definable auditory AEPs is strong presumptive evidence for total deafness or anacusis. On the other hand, the patient may be equally unresponsive electroencephalically to strong visual or somatosensory signals in the presence of behavioral evidence of responsivity in these modalities. If this is the case, then the lack of auditory AEPs is more indicative of brain than ear dysfunction.

Visual averaged evoked potentials are more commonly referred to simply as **visual evoked potentials** and the corresponding initials **VEP**. Similarly, **somatosensory averaged evoked potentials** are more commonly called **somatosensory evoked potentials** with corresponding initials **SSEP** or **SEP**. We elect to use the longer "visual averaged evoked potentials" and **VAEP**, and "somatosensory averaged evoked potentials" and **SAEP** (a) to maintain consistency with "auditory averaged evoked potentials" and (b) to avoid confusion with the practice by some to designate the auditory 40 Hz phenomenon with the initials SSEP. In most chapters we use the designation "auditory AEP" or drop the "auditory" entirely and use just AEP when the chapter deals solely with auditory phenomena. Because this chapter encompasses two different phenomena, we use VAEP and SAEP throughout.

In other chapters, for most figures, positivity of the noninverting electrode relative to the inverting electrode is shown by an upward deflection. Unfortunately, clinical electrophysiologists use an opposite convention, that is, they plot negativity as an upward deflection in VAEPs and SAEPs. We reproduce their VAEPs and SAEPs as they usually appear in the literature. Polarity convention has no interpretive significance. Readers who follow mostly clinical auditory literature in which figures show negativity as a downward deflection must be aware that most VAEPs and SAEPs are plotted according to a negative-up convention.

Historic Background

Historic landmarks in the evolution of visual and somatosensory AEPs as clinical indices parallel those already described for auditory evoked potentials. We do not elaborate further on historic aspects because the emphasis of this book is on auditory AEPs.

Visual Averaged Evoked Potentials

Differences between auditory and visual AEPs obviously arise from differences in effective signals and in ways in which those signals are transduced by the end-organs. Other differences arise from structural and organizational differences within the CNS. We emphasize those facets of VAEPs as they are used in neurologic assessment of the pre-chiasmal pathways. Assessment of vision *per se* will not be discussed.

The following recording, signal, and measurement parameters for visual averaged evoked potentials (VAEP) and for somatosensory averaged evoked potentials (SAEP) are based largely upon the guidelines promulgated by the American EEG Society (1994a), now the American Clinical Neurophysiology Society. Aminoff and Goodin (1994) provide an additional helpful overview of visual AEPs and their clinical applications.

Recording Parameters

Analysis Window
The analysis window should be 250 ms to have sufficient definition of the trace deflections most crucial for assessment of visual pathway integrity. Under some clinical circumstances, the analysis window may have to be extended beyond 250 ms for full definition of pathologically delayed peaks.

Filter Settings
A bandpass of 1–100 Hz encompasses most of the electroencephalic energy necessary to define VAEPs. The American EEG guidelines recommend that the slope for the low-frequency rolloff not exceed 12 dB/octave but that the high-frequency rolloff be 24 dB/octave.

Recording Sites

Recommended positions for the recording electrodes are: midoccipital region 5 cm above the inion (MO), lateral occipital region 5 cm to the left of MO (LO), lateral occipital region 5 cm to the right of MO (RO), and midline 12 cm above the nasion (MF). The ground electrode should be on the vertex. The electrode montage should be: LO-MF (channel 1), MO-MF (channel 2), RO-MF (channel 3), with MF being the common reference and noninverting input.

Signal Parameters

In early VAEP studies, common signals were light flashes created by a stroboscopic-type generator. Flash-evoked VAEPs then were supplanted by VAEPs evoked by reversals of a high-contrast, black-and-white checkerboard pattern (Figure 14-1). Pattern-reversal VAEPs proved to be more stable and predictable than flash-evoked VAEPs, thus making them more

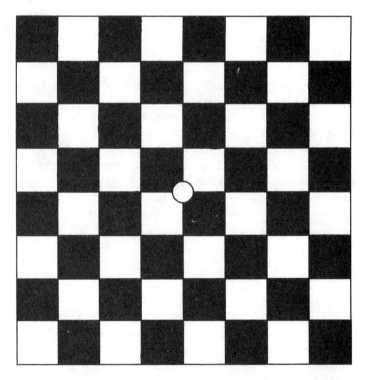

FIGURE 14-1   Black-and-white checkerboard pattern that is reversed two (or more) times per second to elicit visual averaged evoked potentials (VAEP). The patient fixates on a lighted spot in the center of the pattern. The reversing pattern is displayed on a TV screen or other oscilloscope, or by a system with light-emitting diodes.

reliable indices of normality or abnormality. Flashes still may have to be used for patients who cannot maintain the visual fixation required for the pattern-reversal procedure.

A common reversal rate is 2/s. The data sweep is synchronized to the instant of reversal. Each eye is stimulated separately. Patients are directed to fix their vision at the center of the checkerboard screen that should be at least 70 cm removed from the head. Different size checks are used for different diagnostic purposes. Check size is measured in minutes of arc subtended at the eye. The sizes commonly used are 15′, 30′, and 60′.

One hundred samples, free of large artifacts, usually suffice for each VAEP but as many as 200 samples may be necessary in some instances. As with auditory AEPs, the initial routine VAEP test should have the same number (e.g., 100) for each trace. The set protocol can then be modified if desirable or necessary when the traces obtained with the set protocol are equivocal. Likewise, the number of VAEPs obtained for each test condition should be the same, preferably three, even though two traces may seem sufficient for many patients.

Measures of VAEPs

Figure 14-2 illustrates the kinds of traces expected from persons with normal eyes and normal brains. Latencies of the peaks labeled N75 and P100 are important measures, both in

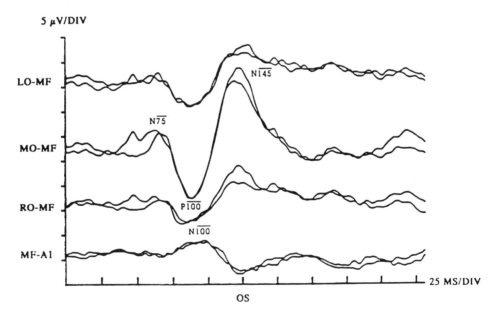

FIGURE 14-2   Normal visual averaged evoked potentials (VAEP) to a reversing checkerboard (1.88/s). Filter passband: 1-250 Hz; N per AEP: 400. LO (left occipital), MO (midoccipital), RO (right occipital), MF (Midfrontal), A1 (left earlobe).

[Reprinted with permission from "Guideline nine: Guidelines on evoked potentials." *Journal of Clinical Neurophysiology, 11*:40–73, 1994. ©American Electroencephalographic Society.]

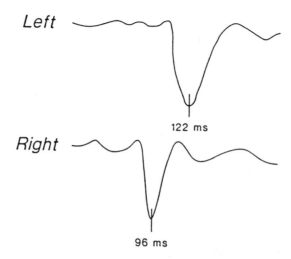

**FIGURE 14-3   Abnormal visual averaged
evoked potential (VAEP) to a reversing
checkerboard pattern from a patient with left
optic neuritis recorded with a Cz -Oz montage.
Negativity of the vertex electrode relative to
the occipital electrode indicated by an upward
deflection. Limit of normality for the reporting
laboratory for the large positive deflection is
117 ms.**

[Reprinted with permission from Misulis, *Essentials of clinical neurophysiology* (2nd ed.). Newton MA: Butterworth-Heinemann, 1997.]

terms of their absolute latencies and latency differences between the two eyes for each of the peaks. Amplitude measures (baseline-to-peak or peak-to-peak) also provide useful information, as do amplitude ratios for corresponding measures in each eye. Normal ranges for these measures in a given laboratory have to be established on populations equivalent to the spectrum of patients seen in that clinical laboratory, and for the signal and recording parameters routinely used in that laboratory.

Figure 14-3 provides an example of an abnormal VAEP. Traces are shown for only one recording channel (Cz-Oz). The patient whose responses are displayed had left optic neuritis.

Somatosensory Averaged Evoked Potentials

When an electric field of sufficient strength is introduced into the tissue surrounding a nerve, the axons depolarize. This results in a volley of action potentials that travels along sensory fibers toward the spinal cord and the brain. When electric activity from peripheral and CNS neurons to a succession of identical electric signals elicit are added and averaged, the resultant activity is a somatosensory averaged evoked potential or SAEP. Again, much of the material to follow is based on guidelines promulgated by the American EEG Society (1994a). Some additional examples of normal and pathologic SAEPs can be found in Tinazzi and Mauguière (1995) and Treede and Kunde (1995).

The eye and visual pathways all are contained in the head. By contrast, somatosensory end-organs are over the entire body, and afferent pathways are both peripheral and central. Furthermore, central pathways are in the spinal cord as well as the brain. In SAEP studies, the end-organs of major interest are primarily in the joints. Figure 14-4 shows schematically central pathways for proprioception or joint position sense that yield the somatosensory AEPs described. In practice, most attention is given to stimulating the arm and leg (Figure 14-5). Distribution of receptors and pathways add complexities beyond those encountered in eliciting and recording VAEPs. On the other hand, dispersion of receptors and pathways permit more precise location and assessment of somatosensory dysfunction.

Recording Parameters

Analysis Window

A 50 ms analysis window or recording epoch usually suffices to define SAEPs from the brain for upper extremity stimulation. However, the window should extend to 100 ms for recording brain AEPs resulting from lower extremity stimulation.

Filter Settings

A filter passband of 10 to 3000 Hz is wide enough to accommodate the high-frequency spectrum of the early somatosensory AEPs as well as the lower-frequency spectrum of the later components. Filter skirts of 12 dB/octave are recommended, but slope seldom is under the control of the clinician because slope values usually are designed into the instrument.

Recording Sites

Recording site depends on the particular nerve stimulated. Figure 14-6 shows some typical recording sites for upper extremity and for lower extremity stimulation.

Electrode Montage

The EEG Society guidelines recommend 4-channel recording for both upper and lower extremity studies. Not all laboratories, however, adhere to this recommendation. There are several popular alternative systems of electrode location and of channel arrangements. The inverting electrode is placed on the skin at the places indicated by the black dots in Figure 14-6. The noninverting electrode is placed on the forehead as a common reference. With this montage, the inverting electrode can be considered an active electrode because it is close to the generator. As a reminder, most clinicians record somatosensory AEPs traces with negativity of the active electrode with respect to the reference electrode by an upward deflection.

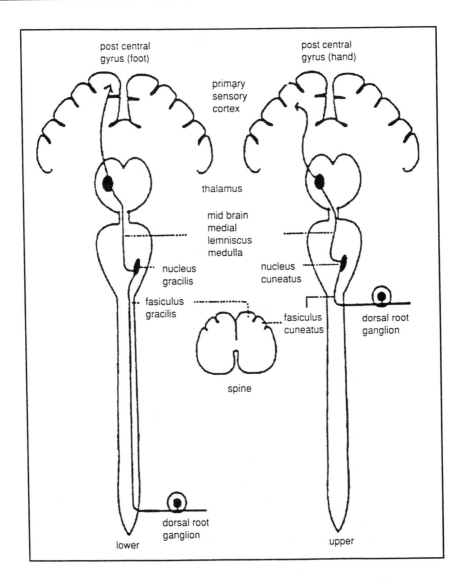

FIGURE 14-4   Neural pathway for proprioception or joint position sense responsible for somatosensory averaged evoked potentials (SAEP).

[Reprinted from Aldrich, "Clinical application of the somatosensory evoked potential." Cadwell, 1994. Courtesy of Cadwell Laboratories, Inc. Cadwell is a registered trademark of Cadwell Laboratories, Inc.]

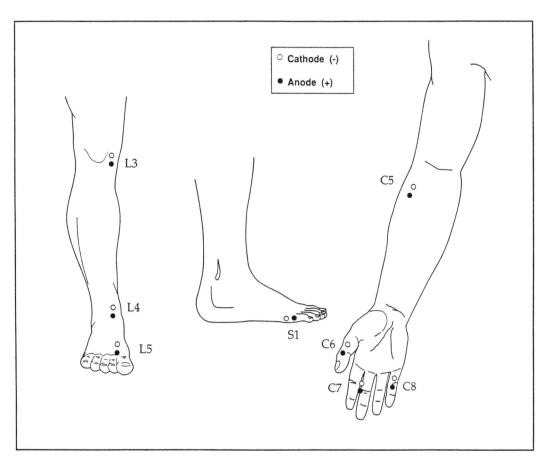

FIGURE 14-5   Common sites of stimulation for eliciting somatosensory averaged evoked potentials (SAEP) used for cervical levels C5 through C8 and lumbrosacral levels L3 to S1.

[Reprinted from Aldrich, "Clinical application of the somatosensory evoked potential." Cadwell, 1994. Courtesy of Cadwell Laboratories, Inc. Cadwell is a registered trademark of Cadwell Laboratories, Inc.]

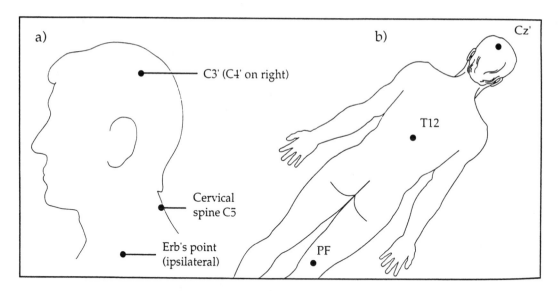

FIGURE 14-6   Common recording sites for somatosensory averaged evoked potentials (SAEP) for upper extremity (a, median nerve) and lower extremity (b, posterior tibial nerve) stimulation.

[Reprinted from Aldrich, "Clinical application of the somatosensory evoked potential." Cadwell, 1994. Courtesy of Cadwell Laboratories, Inc. Cadwell is a registered trademark of Cadwell Laboratories, Inc.]

Signal Parameters

Nature
A common signal is a direct current (DC) 0.2 ms pulse applied to the skin over a nerve. Electricity is delivered by a constant current or by a constant voltage source. Effective level is determined by observing the twitch of a muscle innervated by the motor fibers. Signal rates should vary between 2.7 and 3.3 pulses per second but should not be 3.0 per second.

Signal Number and Replications
Because of the good signal-to-noise ratio for most recordings, well-defined SAEPs usually can be obtained with 250 to 500 shocks. The number of replications of a signal condition depends largely on the degree of patient cooperation. In keeping with our recommendations for auditory and visual AEPs, we encourage a minimum of three replications of all signal conditions.

Measures of Somatosensory AEPs

Figures 14-7 and 14-8 show normal somatosensory AEPs resulting from stimulation of the median nerve of the wrist and of the tibial nerve at the ankle, respectively. The most

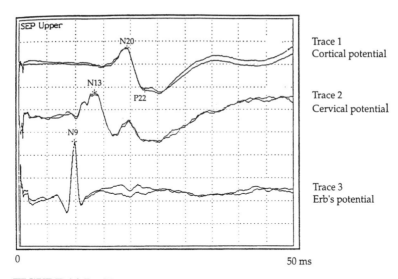

FIGURE 14-7   Normal somatosensory averaged evoked potentials (SAEP) from stimulation of the median nerve at the wrist for evaluation of the upper extremity.

[Reprinted from Aldrich, "Clinical application of the somatosensory evoked potential." Cadwell, 1994. Courtesy of Cadwell Laboratories, Inc. Cadwell is a registered trademark of Cadwell Laboratories, Inc.]

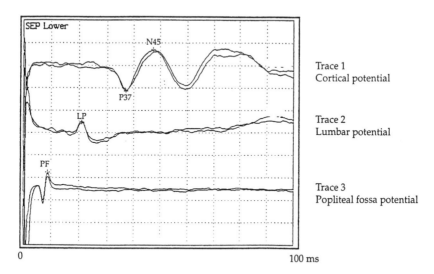

FIGURE 14-8   Normal somatosensory averaged evoked potentials (SAEP) from stimulation of the tibial nerve at the ankle for evaluation of the lower extremity. Note that the recording epoch is twice as long as that shown in Figure 14-7 to allow for longer travel time from the leg.

[Reprinted from Aldrich, "Clinical application of the somatosensory evoked potential." Cadwell, 1994. Courtesy of Cadwell Laboratories, Inc. Cadwell is a registered trademark of Cadwell Laboratories, Inc.]

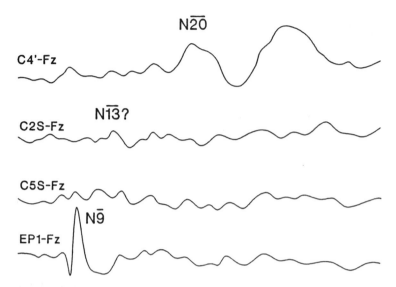

FIGURE 14-9   **Somatosensory averaged evoked potentials (SAEP) to left median nerve stimulation from a 31-year-old man with multiple sclerosis. Recording at the clavicular level (bottom trace) shows peaks in normal latency range. Traces at the C5 and C2 levels (middle 2 traces) show no definite peaks in the normal latency range. Scalp recording (top trace) shows an abnormally delayed N20 indicating a defect above the level of the brachial plexus.**

[Reprinted with permission from Misulis, *Evoked potential primer*. Newton, MA: Butterworth-Heinemann, revised edition, 1994.]

common abnormality encountered in patients is absence of identifiable responses. Sometimes responses that may be present cannot be analyzed because they are accompanied by excessive noise.

Figure 14-9 provides an example of abnormal SAEPs. The traces are from a 31-year-old man with multiple sclerosis but without clinically detectable sensory involvement.

Part V

Additional Topics

Chapter 15

Pragmatic Considerations

Early chapters stressed fundamentals of electroencephalic phenomena and their elicitation and recording. Later chapters described clinical applications of AEPs. In those descriptions, we mentioned some practical problems that can affect the feasibility of each application. Those problems are consolidated and expanded here in four sections: clinical decision making, equipment selection, patient management, and clinical reports. Although not completely independent, the sections are treated separately for convenience of highlighting salient points or issues.

Some discussion is in the form of questions, many of which are intentionally unanswered. Clinical situations are too varied to permit universally applicable answers. Also, the answers today may not be applicable tomorrow. However, the questions themselves change little over the years. Furthermore, they are kinds of questions that probably should be asked of any diagnostic audiologic procedure, not just EPA.

Clinical Decision Making

What Is the Question?

Primary Diagnostic Service
Audiology clinics seldom provide just primary diagnostic service or just management service or just consultative services on a referral basis. Most clinics do some of everything but an individual clinic may emphasize either primary service or secondary consultative or laboratory service. In this subsection we stress primary diagnostic responsibility, whether the patient was seen first in the clinic or was referred from another clinic for more definitive evaluation.

Before audiologists even consider turning on the power of the EPA system, they must ask several questions: "What information do I need for diagnosis or for recommendations for therapeutic management?" "What information do I already have from physical examinations, case history, and from previous tests?" "What additional information do I need for confident diagnosis and therapeutic recommendations?" "Which tests will give me the additional information that I need and which of these are the most practical to administer?" Only then should EPA be considered.

Estimating how often EPA will be necessary is not possible because each clinic differs in the kinds of patients it sees for diagnosis. The only safe generality is that EPA would be done less often in those clinics where it is a common procedure if the appropriate questions had been asked first. This may seem like heresy from authors who promote EPA as a desirable and useful procedure. Nevertheless, the wisest, kindest, and most economic step may be *not* to do EPA when its use is of questionable value.

We move now to the assumption that EPA *is* the most appropriate next procedure for a particular patient. Additional preliminary questions need to be asked. "What *unique* information do I need from EPA?" and "How can I best structure the EPA procedure to give me that unique information?"

Consultative or Referral Diagnostic Service

Audiologists in these clinics usually do not have the luxury of asking the initial questions just discussed. Most commonly, they are asked (or ordered) to do EPA on a referred patient. Nevertheless, if circumstances permit, they should contact the referring physician or other source about the information that the referrer wishes to have. They should ask as diplomatically as possible whether they have the privilege of obtaining the needed information in the way that they (the audiologists) deem best.

Even if audiologists have no decision about whether to do EPA on a referred patient, they can still ask themselves the questions about the best way to structure the EPA to give the requested information. Sometimes, however, the referring source requests a specified fixed EPA procedure. In these cases, audiologists cannot exercise their discretion. Nevertheless, they can still protect their professional integrity by how they interpret and report their data.

One-Size-Fits-All

Some EPA procedures are so commonly accepted that audiologists and other clinicians run them routinely whether or not they provide the answers to the questions discussed above. Even a name has become routinized. The usual request is "Do that brainstem test." It makes no difference whether the response they elicit comes from the brainstem, the cerebral cortex, muscles of the head and neck, or from any other part of the body. Almost everything done auditorily with the EPA equipment is labeled "brainstem" done with a "brainstem machine."

Some routinization is desirable. However, good clinical practice dictates asking pertinent guideline questions before deciding *which* routine procedure to use first. The routine "brainstem" procedure may result in identifiable AEPs but those AEPs may not necessarily be the ones required to provide the best diagnostic information. On the other hand, failure to obtain replicable AEPs with routine "brainstems" on a patient does not necessarily mean that the whole EPA session is a failure. It may just imply that the routine "brainstem" procedure was not the best one to use or not the only one to use to obtain valuable diagnostic data.

Routinization is acceptable if it works for the patient's benefit. However, if a one-size-fits-all procedure is done primarily for the benefit of the clinician's convenience or wallet, then it is poor clinical practice. ,

Establish Routines for Comparative Purposes

Some routinization of diagnostic procedures, EPA or otherwise, is desirable. It permits meaningful comparison across patients and even for the same patient from visit to visit. Routine does not imply the one-size-fits-all concept just discussed. For example, the routine for threshold EPA on an adult should be different from the routine for otoneurologic assessment on the same adult. Also, the routine for threshold EPA on a 3-month-old infant probably should be different from the routine threshold EPA on a 30-year-old adult.

EPA routinization usually is not compatible with the common practice of on-line eyeball judgments of AEP traces and immediate choices of subsequent signal or recording parameters. Examples of pretest routinization are given in earlier chapters and will not be repeated here. We do repeat, however, that discretionary changes *after* a routine procedure are acceptable. They are even desirable if the initial routine EPA has not yielded enough data to answer the clinical question(s) posed before the procedure was begun.

Equipment Selection

Clinic Setup or Organization

Most clinicians work in settings in which a variety of audiologic services are offered, including EPA. It is wise, therefore, to consider criteria for EPA equipment selection in the context of the setting in which the equipment will be used. Does the clinic have a primary medical orientation or a primary rehabilitation and educational emphasis, or are both facets equally stressed? Is there a major medico-legal or forensic component to the service? Is there an otoneurologic emphasis requiring electronystagmography and facial nerve conduction studies? Is there a large neurologic component to the service requiring assessment of somatosensory and visual function along with auditory function?

Do all services take place within a totally self-contained clinic or does the clinic also participate in intra-operative monitoring in a hospital's surgical unit, do neonatal hearing screening in a hospital's nursery, provide evoked potential services for satellite clinics or contract clinics, and so on? Does the clinic serve patients of all ages and conditions or does it limit itself to patients whose behavioral cooperation is not a problem? Answers to all these questions, and others soon to be discussed, are important determinants to consider along with the intrinsic properties of available equipment before purchasing EPA equipment.

Operational and Service Personnel

Will the EPA equipment be operated by an audiologist experienced with EPA or by a technician with occasional supervision by an experienced audiologist? Is there a staff electronics technician capable of routine maintenance, trouble-shooting, making repairs, and modifying equipment or computer programs to accommodate an audiologist's requests? How available is the equipment vendor for in-service training and for rapidly needed repairs? How long is the warranty period or service contract?

Systems Decisions

Modular versus Integrated

Should the EPA system be amassed from separate modules (signal generator, amplifiers, signal averager, etc.) or should it be a commercial stand-alone unit with all components integrated at the factory? Modular systems generally have greater flexibility and versatility than integrated systems and can be adapted to new clinical procedures with relative ease. It is easier to identify and fix modular problems and breakdowns than problems occurring in integrated systems. Although not always so, the initial cost of a modular system generally is cheaper than a commercial, integrated system. Long-term costs also may be less because modules can be adapted rather than replaced. A less flexible commercial unit may have to be replaced in 5 to 8 years if it cannot be used for some of the rapidly evolving test procedures. Unfortunately, some clinicians continue to use less-than-effective procedures because they cannot afford to replace their limited commercial unit.

On the down side, modular systems may be larger than integrated systems and less portable or mobile. Modular systems also require operator knowledge of modular interconnections or else the service of an in-house electronics technician. Modular systems usually are more susceptible to difficult-to-trace ground loops and 60 Hz interference. Most integrated commercial systems have carefully wired circuits that minimize 60 Hz and other electric artifacts. Finally, patient safety in terms of current leakage usually is well controlled in contemporary commercial units. Assistance from someone skilled in patient safety regulations and procedures is essential before a modular system can be used clinically or experimentally.

Single Purpose versus Multipurpose Integrated EPA System

Because of the cost of commercial integrated EPA systems, users understandably want units that serve many purposes (e.g., neonatal hearing screening, threshold EPA, otoneurologic assessment in the three major sensory modalities, generate clinical reports). Having a multipurpose EPA system also means that the user has to learn and become facile with only one system. Different systems for different uses, even if made by the same manufacturer, limit the ease with which the clinician can shift from one procedure to another. If the different systems are from different companies, shifting mental gears is even more difficult.

On the down side, a multipurpose unit usually is larger and heavier than a special purpose unit. Some multipurpose units are truly portable but with all of their necessary peripheral accoutrements, they can be heavy and clumsy to carry. Another unfavorable aspect of a multipurpose unit is that it can be in only one place at a time. If EPA is not a large portion of one's clinical practice despite a wide range of applications, simultaneous need for the equipment is not a problem. However, if EPA is a major part of the practice and if it has to be done in several settings (e.g., office, neonatal ICU, operating room), economic scheduling of a multipurpose unit can be a problem.

Incorporation of Integrated EPA System with Multipurpose
Audiometric System

Several manufacturers have developed integrated EPA systems as part of larger systems that serve a variety of audiologic purposes: voluntary behavioral response audiometry, acoustic-immittance measures, otoacoustic emissions measures, hearing aid selection, and so on. Although the initial cost of a multipurpose audiometric unit is high, the cost per procedure is not. One component of the unit (e.g., sound delivery portion) serves several purposes and does not have to be duplicated for each purpose. Such units are large, but the total space they occupy usually is smaller than the space occupied by individual pieces of equipment that serve the same purposes.

The multipurpose audiometric units that incorporate EPA also have their shortcomings.

1. Initial cost is higher than for any one of the separate portions if they were purchased as separate portions. Although the overall cost for the larger unit may be smaller than the sum of the costs of the individual portions, the initial outlay may be prohibitive for some clinics.
2. The net space for the larger unit may be less than the sum of the space for the other units. However, it may be difficult to find a sufficiently large space adjacent to the test booth.
3. Portability for a large unit is out of the question, and even mobility is difficult to accomplish.
4. Despite its versatility, the multipurpose audiometric unit can be used for only one purpose at a time. A clinic, therefore, has to be able to afford successive rather than simultaneous use of its key equipment.
5. A breakdown in one component of the large unit may shut down all operations of the system.
6. Because all sub-units are closely interwoven, altering just the EPA portion when the need for procedural modification arises may not be possible.

Manufacturer or Vendor

An EPA unit or system may satisfy a clinician based on answers to questions or concerns already discussed. However, it may not be the instrument or system of choice if the quality of its construction and the backing of the manufacturer or vendor is not certain. A trade name alone is not sufficient assurance. In the corporate world, companies swallow each other. A manufacturer of impeccable integrity and quality may not be able to sustain either if new corporate managers find these admirable traits incompatible with profit. It is impossible for a prospective buyer to assess with confidence the insides of a packaged unit or the insides of the sustaining natures of the humans who market the unit. Nevertheless, a prospective purchaser can seek answers to some helpful questions either of the manufacturer or the vendor. Following are some questions that a prospective buyer should consider.

How many years has the manufacturer been in business? What is its financial solvency? Will it stay in business long enough to service its products? If it is a new company, how qualified are its design and technical personnel? What kind of free warranty does the manufacturer offer and what is the record of honoring warranties? What is the company's record of equipment breakdowns, recalls, and retrofitting? Does the company field test its equipment thoroughly and work out the bugs before placing a product on the market? Does the product live up to its promotional build-up? Does the equipment live up to the technical specifications published in its promotional brochures?

Patient Management

Patient Safety

Patient management begins before any patient is scheduled for EPA. As mentioned, equipment must be checked for harmful levels of current leakage that could pass from the equipment, through the electrodes, and then through the patient. Most commercial integrated EPA systems have been tested carefully for excessive current leakage. In addition, they come equipped with a special male safety plug for the power cord that is plugged into the 60 Hz power receptacle. If one has constructed an EPA system from separate modules, one must be certain that it, too, has the appropriate safety power plug as well as all other leakage controls.

If a clinic plans to control difficult-to-manage patients with drugs, medical personnel should be available to administer or to supervise administration of drugs. Also, qualified medical personnel should be available to monitor the status of the patient after drugs have been administered and should be available for resuscitation if that is necessary. This caution also implies that monitoring and resuscitation equipment be immediately available.

We have not had a single unfortunate event in our long experience with patients for whom sedation or anesthesia was necessary. This is because of extraordinary precautions before, during, and after drug administration—and because of luck. Luck is not to be trusted. Many patients for whom EPA is necessary are those whose central nervous systems are not normal. The same CNS disorder that leads to auditory dysfunction also may lead to aberrant or unexpected reactions to drugs that are benign for most patients.

One uncommon but important syndrome deserves special safety attention, the Jervell and Lange-Nielsen syndrome (Gorlin & Sedano, 1970). Two conditions characterize this syndrome that is associated with genetic, and probably congenital, deafness: prolonged Q-T interval in the electrocardiogram (**ECG**) and unpredictable fainting spell or syncope. Sometimes there is no recovery from the syncope and the patient, usually a child, dies. There is no clear indication that sedation or anesthesia increases the likelihood of syncope or death. However, the emotional and legal consequences would be devastating if by chance alone such a child would die during EPA for which the child had been sedated or anesthetized. A pre-EPA ECG should be taken on any child for whom the cause of a probable hearing loss is totally uncertain. Pre-EPA ECGs on all children who are to be sedated or anesthetized is an even safer course of action despite its cost.

Preparation, Explanations, and Instructions for Patients and Patients' Families

We tried in the earlier chapters to take the mystery out of averaged evoked potentials and evoked potential audiometry. Nevertheless, despite our explanations and equivalent explanations by others, even many experienced audiologists see EPA as something entirely different from conventional behavioral response audiometry. They may even ascribe special attributes to it that are unwarranted. Patients and patients' families, who do not have clinical backgrounds, are even more awed by thoughts of electrodes and brain waves. Often, they expect miraculous results from EPA. As a result, they can be fearful for themselves or for their children before EPA is started, and they can be disappointed with the limited information in terms of test results when they receive a report of the test results.

Simply stated but accurate written information should be given to adult patients and to parents of young children after EPA has been scheduled. Statements should include something about why EPA is going to administered, the procedure itself, and what information can be expected after test results are analyzed. Different wording has to be used for adult patients than for parents of young children.

One instruction we always gave to parents was to wash their child's hair the day before or the morning before the EPA. The cleansing helps to remove oils, dirt, and dead skin that can interfere with electrode attachment and low inter-electrode impedance. Parents usually want their children to look their best when they go to a doctor or any place in public. Therefore, they sometimes put an oily dressing on their child's hair after they have washed it. We caution them against this because the hair dressing has to be removed before electrodes are attached.

Physical Management of Young, Difficult-to-Control Patients

Throughout this book we have stressed testing patients with behavioral response procedures first and resorting to EPA if other procedures cannot be accomplished or cannot provide sufficient information for proper diagnosis and remediation. The assumption in this subsection, therefore, is that other procedures have been attempted and that EPA is a desirable next step. One reason for resorting to EPA is that a patient, usually a child, cannot be restrained physically for the other procedures. A logical conclusion is that attempts at EPA also will be futile unless the child can be sedated or anesthetized.

Sedation or anesthesia carefully administered and monitored seldom has adverse biologic effects on a child. Nevertheless, some risks, known and unknown, accompany pharmacologic control. A natural question ensues: Should a child ever be sedated or anesthetized for EPA? The answer is "occasionally" because EPA rarely, if ever, is crucial for the child's survival or physical well being. Sometimes remedial measures cannot be initiated with sufficient confidence without the EPA results, and reliable EPA results cannot be obtained unless a child is subdued pharmacologically. More often, however, sedation and anesthesia are administered for the economic benefit of the clinician or the clinic. Waiting out a child, as will be described shortly, can be costly because of not being able to give time to other revenue-generating procedures.

Getting a young child to fall into natural sleep during EPA often can be accomplished by exhausting a child sufficiently before the procedure begins. Keeping a child awake one hour later than usual the evening before and waking the child one hour earlier than usual on the morning of the EPA promotes this exhaustion. Care has to be exercised not to let the child sleep in the car on the way to the clinic. If at all possible, the child should be brought to the clinic close to ordinary nap time.

Some clinicians wait until a child is asleep, naturally or induced, before applying electrodes. The child is easier to manage when asleep than when awake. However, electrode application time uses some of that sleep time, which, ordinarily, is brief. Also, a child's sleep often is disrupted during the manipulation necessary for applying electrodes and earphones. It may be wiser to apply electrodes as quickly as possible after the tired child is brought to the clinic. After the electrodes are attached, diapers should be changed if the child is an infant. (A supply of disposable diapers in the clinic may be as vital as a supply of electrodes.) Then the child should be fed. By that time, the child usually is so tired that natural deep sleep will follow. A favorite doll, toy, or blanket sometimes is helpful in calming a child before or during a test. Earphones should be placed as soon as the child is asleep. Testing can then begin.

If a child is compliant but not asleep, begin the test anyway. Testing will be satisfactory because there are no movement artifacts to introduce disrupting noise into the recordings. The child sometimes relaxes when test signals are strong enough to be audible. Sometimes the monotonous sounds are soporific enough to induce sleep. Most adults and older children find it difficult to remain awake unless the tester focuses their attention on the test signals.

Management Immediately before, during, and after Test Procedure

Do not assume that satisfactory test conditions at the start of a test will persist throughout. Even when the patient is totally cooperative by being physically still, electrode paste may dry leading to increased inter-electrode impedance with consequent increase in recording noise. If the patient is a young child, that child most likely will move during the procedure, sometimes with considerable vigor. Movement not only introduces disrupting artifacts but may also loosen electrodes and dislodge earphones. An assistant should be alongside the child to monitor attachment of electrodes and secure placement of the earphones.

Presence of Parents, Guardians, Spouses during EPA

Having parents, guardians, or spouses present during EPA can be beneficial. Parents can assist in management of their children during electrode application and can comfort their children when necessary after the procedure has begun. An additional benefit of having families or caretakers present is that they witness the complexities of EPA and they have concrete references for some of the vocabulary in the written report that they will receive.

Family members and caretakers also can be hindrances. Most test areas are small and extra bodies get in the way. Another negative aspect is that parents get oversolicitous when their child cries during scalp preparation and electrode attachment. If one could communicate to the child the benign and generally comfortable nature of the entire procedure, EPA probably would not be necessary. The awake child who does not fuss or cry during electrode application is the exception. A third potential problem is that few procedures begin without a hitch. Artifacts have to be reduced, sometimes requiring replacement of electrodes. Also, earphones may have to be replaced. Any of these common preliminary adjustments can be interpreted by others as faulty procedure, reducing the observer's confidence in the eventual results.

Explaining Test Results

Some explanation has to be given to the patient or to the patient's parents or guardians after the procedure is finished. Patients or families would like definitive test results before leaving. Complying with that wish, however, is hazardous. If a set protocol (such as we have recommended) is used, immediate definitive results must wait for compositing and aligning of traces and careful measurement analysis. If initial eyeballing of the traces shows clear-cut replicability at one level (or one ear or one frequency) but not at a lower level, the clinician may wish to risk giving preliminary indications of test results. If the patient was evaluated for otoneurologic purposes and if no abnormality was evident in the traces, a preliminary indication of normality may be risked. Even in these cases, clinicians should stress the tentative nature of the conclusions, and that final results will be conveyed in writing after careful analysis of the traces obtained that day.

Those clinicians (the majority) who make immediate eyeball judgments of response versus no response or normality versus abnormality during the procedure may be more comfortable with giving results to patients or families at the conclusion of the EPA procedure. Even these clinicians should stress the tentative nature of their conclusions.

To give or not give EPA results immediately is a moot issue for those patients who are evaluated on consultative referral from a physician or other professional person. Test results should go to the referrer without even tentative information given to patient or family unless the audiologist or other clinician is given explicit permission to give tentative results first.

Management of Delayed Negative Reactions

As mentioned, adverse reactions from sedation or anesthesia are unlikely to occur during EPA if proper precautions are taken before and during EPA. Likewise, the probability of delayed reaction is small. Nevertheless, the possibility is there. A more likely scenario, especially for a young child, is that the child may have been incubating a bacterial or viral infection that did not manifest itself until hours or days after the EPA. Parents are apt to attribute the child's illness to the sedation or anesthesia. It is important, therefore, warn parents about the possibility, however minimal it may be, of delayed reactions and to urge them to contact the child's primary care physician at once if adverse reactions do occur.

Another post-EPA problem is an allergic reaction to the scalp cleanser, electrode paste, or electrode itself. Welts can occur on the scalp at the spot of electrode placement. Usually, these welts gradually disappear without treatment. Nevertheless, parents should be cautioned about the possibility of allergic reactions and should be urged to contact the child's primary care physician if allergic welts do occur.

Clinical Reports

The old saw "The job's not finished 'til the paper work's done" clearly applies to EPA. As much thought must be given to the written report as to all other phases of EPA. Report writing can be routinized in the interest of convenience and economy but reports must be tailored to some extent for each patient.

We cite "Guidelines for Writing Clinical Evoked Potential Reports" published by The American EEG Society (1994b) because, for the most part, their recommendations are consonant with our own practices. The introduction to the "Guidelines" states valuable generalities.

> The clinical evoked potential report should provide a basic minimal level of information allowing a knowledgeable reader to judge the adequacy and reliability of testing and the accuracy of interpretation. Further numerical data or descriptive information may be added to this basic minimum as desired. Numerical data allow a better evaluation by an informed reader than does a purely descriptive report.
>
> The clinical report should also provide a meaningful guide to the referring physician concerning relevance of the electrophysiologic findings to the clinical problem under investigation.
>
> The format of presentation should follow a logical and orderly sequence. As test reports often travel widely, local idiosyncratic terminology should be avoided for the sake of clarity.
>
> An evoked potential report should generally include: identification, clinical information, technical data, results, description, and interpretation (including impressions and clinical correlation). (p. 74)

The American EEG Society guidelines are intended for otoneurologic applications of EPA (as well as for visual and somatosensory testing). Nevertheless, the principles enunciated can be applied to threshold EPA as well. Some of our extensions of the American EEG Society guidelines may seem obvious and trivial. We know from experience, however, that these obvious and seemingly trivial points frequently are neglected, leading to needless and sometimes distressful confusion.

Reports can be on printed sheets with blanks for specific data on the particular patient on whom EPA was done. Reports also can be in narrative form on clinic letterhead. Most often, a brief letter accompanies a printed data form. Sometimes the accompanying letter is expanded to provide information or recommendations that cannot easily be written on the data form. The following discussion pertains only to data report forms.

Clinic and Operator Identification

Report forms should clearly identify the clinic and the parent institution if it is not a stand-alone clinic. Besides address and phone number, the form should include the name of the person responsible for the clinic's operation and the name of the person responsible for the particular EPA that is being reported. The form should indicate the date of the test as well as date of the report.

Patient Identification

Provide all pertinent information that you can without violating a patient's legal right of or personal desire for privacy. In addition to the patient's name, give the birthdate, gender, address, telephone number, and clinic file number. Include the patient's middle name or initial. Also include the maiden name for married women who have taken their husbands' last name. In other words, do everything possible to provide a unique identity for the patient and avoid confusing the patient with other patients with similar names.

Background Clinical Information

The most important fact to be given here is why the patient has been referred for EPA and what information is expected to be derived from the procedure. Provide some background on the patient's condition, results of other physical and laboratory examinations, results of previous audiologic assessments, and inconsistencies that need to be resolved or uncertainties that need to be clarified. Usually, only highlights can be given on a form. If it is vital to extend comments, do so in a covering letter.

Technical Details of EPA Procedure

We have stressed throughout this book that EPA results must be interpreted in the context of the restraints of test parameters and conditions. Despite several well-intentioned tries at test standardization, there is no one set procedure either for threshold EPA or for otoneurologic assessment. Just as one cannot give a speech discrimination score without specifying the test material, how it was administered, and so on, a clinician cannot report threshold levels or peak latencies without specifying the parameters or conditions under which those data were obtained. Intra-patient or inter-clinic comparisons are seriously compromised without these specifications.

Recording parameters include electrode placement, inter-electrode impedances, analysis window, and filters. Signal parameters include the acoustic transducer, nature of the acoustic signal(s), signal rates, and signal level(s). Also to be included is N per AEP and the number of replications per signal condition. Finally, patient state should be described. Was the patient awake or asleep? Was sedation or anesthesia used? If so, what kind and how much? Did changes in the patient's state affect acquisition or interpretation of the AEPs?

Results

Results should be presented as actual traces, tabulation of measures on the traces, and, when necessary, descriptions of those relevant features of the AEPs that are not obvious from inspection or mensuration. Individual superimposed AEPs for each replication of a signal condition as well as the corresponding composite AEP trace should accompany the report form and the cover letter. Time and amplitude axes should be labeled clearly. Polarity also should be clearly indicated, that is, which direction on the trace represents electric positivity. Polarity should not have to be shown; that is, a deflection above a baseline automatically should indicate positivity. Unfortunately, however, many neurologists with EEG experience still plot positivity below the baseline.

The stimulated ear should be identified along with each trace or set of traces: right, left, or binaural. If clicks of only one polarity (rarefaction or condensation) are the test signals, only one notation need be made on the form. However, if polarity is varied throughout the procedure, then rarefaction, condensation, or alternating should be shown for each trace or set of traces.

Tabulated measures are difficult to specify in advance because EPA done for different reasons requires different time, magnitude, or other measures. Some clinics automatically tabulate latencies of waves I through V for specified signal levels as well as the I-V, I-III, and III-V interpeak intervals. Avoid reporting latencies or other measures with more significant figures than the instrument's resolution allows.

Interpretation

This is a ticklish issue because some referring physicians and other professionals want to interpret on their own. In these cases, they use the EPA service as a laboratory to provide them with specifically requested data. Interpretation by the EPA clinician can be regarded as an intrusion, especially if the patient receives a copy of the information sent to the referrer. More often, the clinician is asked to interpret the EPA results, at least in terms of the initial question(s) posed and shown on the report form. Yes, sensitivity impairment can be a significant basis for the failure of this 3-year-old child to develop intelligible speech. No, EP peak latencies and interpeak intervals and changes of latency with signal rate are not compatible with a vestibular neurilemmoma. Further interpretation of EPA can be added in terms of the compatibility or correlation of the EPA results with the patient's history and with the results of other examinations.

Results of threshold EPA are self-explanatory because they are expressed in dB nHL. Normality or abnormality of latency measures for otoneurologic purposes is not always obvious. Therefore, they should be accompanied by a list of the range of normal values with limits of normality expressed in standard deviations. Interpretation entered on the report form should be concise and brief. Interpretive elaboration, if necessary, can be made part of the cover letter.

Recommendations

We restrict discussion here only to recommendations for further EPA evaluations. For example, threshold EPA was done on a 4-month-old child only with clicks at widely spaced signal levels of 10, 50, and 90 dB nHL. Replicable AEPs were obtained for each ear at 90 dB nHL but not at 50 or 10 dB nHL. If educational management depends upon more precise threshold levels, the audiologist might recommend another threshold EPA with clicks at levels of 60, 70, and 80 dB nHL, or with tone bursts of two different frequencies at those same narrower levels. As another example, an adult patient with an unclassified language communication disorder has had a typical otoneurologic evaluation with EPs to clicks as the response index. That EPA yielded no abnormality. The audiologist might recommend an additional EPA with MPs and LPS as response indices, or might suggest an EPA with early event-related potentials as the response index.

Often, well-meaning referrers have unrealistic expectations of EPA. A physician may ask the audiologist if surgery is indicated by the results of an otoneurologic EPA with early EPs as the response index. Another audiologist may ask whether monaural or binaural hearing aids should be placed on a child as the results of threshold EPA with MPs as the response index. If these, or similar questions, were the bases of the referral for EPA, the audiologist should clarify the limitations of the requested EPA procedure before the patient is accepted on referral.

Chapter *16*

AEP Generators and Brain Function

Audiologists and other clinicians need not know the exact anatomic contributors to the AEPs that they use clinically or the precise psychophysiologic significance of each deflection in those AEPs to make correct clinical decisions. They base their diagnoses mainly on reliable, empirically derived, correlations between AEP abnormalities and auditory or otoneurologic abnormalities. Nevertheless, knowledge of AEP generators and of the ear and brain functions they represent is of unquestioned value for providing (a) fuller understanding of each patient's dysfunction, (b) bases for refinement of current EPA procedures, and (c) bases for developing new approaches to assessing auditory and otoneurologic dysfunctions.

Earlier chapters include some segments on the AEP/brain relations. The goal of this chapter is to provide a general framework upon which those segments can be consolidated and expanded. Logically, this material should have been presented early in the book to strengthen the understanding of the AEPs obtained in various clinical contexts. However, as pointed out in the Preface, the reader may not have had sufficient experience with AEPs to integrate this background material with other portions of the book. Earlier chapters now can be reread from a different perspective after completion of this chapter.

The theoretic orientation in this chapter differs markedly from what we call the *traditional* or *classical* view or concept of the central auditory nervous system (CANS). In this chapter we restate in summary form that classical view of central auditory nervous system anatomy and function. We refer to our orientation simply as an *alternate* view or concept. Most of the alternate concept described in this chapter has been published earlier in different contexts (Goldstein, 1963, 1967, 1973, 1980, 1982). The present version does not differ fundamentally from earlier versions. However, it has been updated and it includes more clinical implications.

We define the **peripheral auditory system (PAS)** to include anything from the pinna to the termination of the fibers of the VIIIth or auditory nerve in the cochlear nuclei of the brainstem. The central auditory nervous system (CANS) includes any neural structure wholly contained within the brain that can be activated by auditory signals. The CANS begins with the cells in the cochlear nuclei on which the VIIIth nerve fibers terminate.

Classical or Traditional View of the CANS

Following is a general overview based on writings too vast to cite individually. What we present is, in our opinion, a consensus of the extant views of CANS anatomy and physiology. Exceptions may be found in the literature that contradict our general statements.

Anatomy

The essence of the CANS in this view is the **lemniscal system** or the **primary auditory projection system (PAPS)**. Refer back to Figure 2-1, which is a characteristic representation of the system. The PAPS consists of large fiber pathways (lemnisci) with interconnecting nuclei. The rostral termination of the PAPS, the **primary auditory reception area**, is **Heschl's gyrus** on the superior surface of the temporal lobe. This gyrus (or pair of gyri) is surrounded in the cerebral cortex by what are designated as **auditory association areas**. Also included in some versions of the traditional view is part of the central nervous system called the **reticular formation** that serves all sensory systems, not just audition.

Function

Finding clear statements relating specific auditory phenomena to specific portions of CANS anatomy for this traditional view is difficult. However, juxtaposition in the literature of figures, such as Figure 2-1, with descriptions of auditory phenomena lead to the impression that the PAPS alone is responsible for most auditory phenomena. Exceptions to this are roles assigned to the reticular formation: (a) participation in auditory reflexes and (b) arousing or alerting the cerebral cortex to incoming auditory signals.

The literature implies progressive processing of the auditory signal at each of the nuclear waystations as the message moves rostrally, and that it is the *processed* message that is conveyed to the next nuclear waystation or processing center. Conscious awareness of sound in the normal brain does not occur until the neural messages reach the cerebral cortex. However, some processing of auditory signals leading to auditory perceptions occurs at all levels of the brain. For example, the initial processing for localization occurs at the lowest level of the brain at which there are interconnections between the neural inputs from each ear.

Relation to AEPs

Each successive peak of the AEP, at least through about 30 ms, is attributed to activity of discrete nuclei and/or pathways of the PAPS. For example, wave III of the early AEP usually is attributed to the cochlear nuclei of the brainstem, wave IV to superior olivary complex, and wave V to the lateral lemniscus. Some later waves presumably arise from activity of higher level nuclei and pathways. Beyond 30 ms it is difficult to ascribe discrete waves to discrete nuclei or pathways. Some later waves presumably result from the overlap or superimposition of electric activity from two or more structures of the PAPS. Most of the later peaks are believed to arise mainly from cortical structures.

Strengths and Weaknesses of Traditional View

Several observations argue for the validity of the traditional view of CANS anatomy and function. First, what has been described as the PAPS, the main constituent of the traditional CANS, unquestionably relates to auditory function. Furthermore, the heavily myelinated lemniscal portions and their discrete one-to-one nuclear interconnections appear responsive only to auditory signals. Input from other modalities neither activates nor inhibits those portions nor modifies their functions. Also, given the usual signal and recording conditions used to obtain early signal-related potentials, individual peaks in the AEPs can probably be ascribed primarily to some discrete CANS nuclei and to their major lemniscal interconnections.

The weaknesses of the traditional system, however, outweigh its strengths. A few weaknesses are described as examples. If processing were occurring at each level of the PAPS and if only processed signals were transmitted rostrally to the next nuclear waystation, different kinds of electrophysiologic activity would be recorded in each of the large fiber pathways or in their discrete nuclear interconnections. No evidence supports this prediction. In fact, tonotopic studies suggest the maintenance of frequency mapping from caudal through the most rostral portions of the PAPS. Furthermore, tuning curves for individual neurons maintain their same general properties. Given the limited available evidence, it appears that the same *unprocessed* information is being transmitted rostrally along the entire large-fiber portion of the PAPS.

The traditional view cannot account for several key temporal psychoacoustic phenomena. Backward masking, in particular, poses a theoretic challenge, especially to the role of the PAPS in conscious awareness of auditory signals. Consider this situation. The skull of a person is opened and a recording electrode is placed on Heschl's gyrus. A sound is presented to the person and electric evidence of response is recorded within 15 to 20 ms after signal onset. A second sound is presented 20 ms after the onset of the first and electric evidence of response to the second signal occurs within 15 to 20 ms after its onset. Theoretically, the listener should hear two successive sounds that are equally loud. However, the first sound will be softer than when it is presented alone, or will be inaudible, that is, it will be backwardly masked by the second sound.

A clinical observation provides another challenge to the validity of the traditional view of CANS anatomy and function. If conscious perception of sound occurs only after auditory messages arrive at the cerebral cortex, then bilateral destruction of Heschl's gyrus should produce total, permanent deafness. The reality is that no case of permanent sensitivity impairment has ever been reported in which there was confirmed bilateral cortical damage in the Sylvian fissure along with confirmed integrity of the peripheral auditory system (PAS). However, there are reports of confirmed bilateral cortical damage and presumed normality of the PAS in which there was little or no clinically significant, permanent sensitivity impairment or hypacusis.

A fourth example of the inadequacy of the traditional view comes from EPA threshold estimates when early signal-related AEPs are used as the response index. Given the usual signal and recording conditions for threshold EPA, the peaks of the AEPs within the first 30 ms almost certainly are generated by the PAPS. If the PAPS is involved in the conscious perception of sound, then EPA thresholds should be distinctly different if the patient is asleep or awake; and if awake, measured thresholds should be different if the patient is in reverie or is attending carefully to the test sounds. The reality is, however, that reliable threshold estimates are indistinguishable clinically when early AEPs are used as the response index regardless of patient state.

Alternate View of the CANS

Just as with the traditional view of the CANS, literature pertaining to or supporting this alternate view is incomprehensibly vast. However, because the alternate view has not been generally promoted, several references that support specific points will be cited. Some writings have had a more general influence on the evolution of the alternate view. Although, they support specific points as well, they will not be cited at those points. The writings of the neurophysiologist George H. Bishop (1958, 1961), as well as personal interactions with him, had the most profound influence on the evolution of the alternate view. Some other early influences came from Mildred A. McGinnis (McGinnis, Kleffner, & Goldstein, 1956) and from the writings of E. Roy John and colleagues (John, Bartlett, Shimokochi, & Kleinman, 1973; Kleinman & John, 1975). In addition, clinical experience helped create and mold the alternate view.

Anatomy and Function

Function helps to define anatomy in the alternate view of the CANS. Therefore, anatomy and function will be interwoven in the following descriptions. Some details of this alternate view are given now to form the backdrop for the appreciation of AEPs as indices for assessing central auditory dysfunction.

The core of the entire **central nervous system (CNS)**, which serves all sensory and motor functions, is the unmyelinated (or thinly myelinated), multisynaptic, reticulate gray matter that surrounds the fluid-filled central canal of the spine and brain. The gray matter of the brain is the part of the CNS with which we feel, see, and hear. It is represented schematically in Figure 16-1 by the large ice-cream-cone-like structure.

Figure 16-1 is a functional representation of the CANS and bears no resemblance to its actual structure. When one does look at a real spinal cord and brain in cross section, one notes that in the spine and lower brainstem, large-fiber motor and sensory pathways neatly enclose the central gray matter. This neat arrangement is disturbed at upper brain levels by interspersal of motor and sensory pathways of the cranial nerves. Nevertheless, the gray matter still clusters closer to the central canal than to the lateral surfaces of the brain. At the top of the brain, no large-fiber pathways box in the gray matter; therefore, it overflows and covers the entire brain as the cerebral cortex.

Additional features characterize the central gray matter of the brain. We describe these

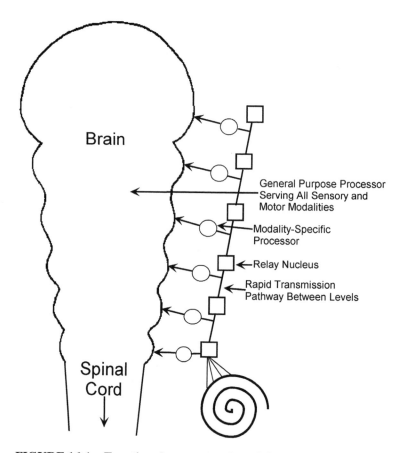

**FIGURE 16-1   Functional representation of the central auditory
nervous system (CANS) according to the alternate view of the
CANS described in the text. The large general purpose processor
comprises all the gray matter of the brain and serves all sensory
and motor modalities, not just audition.**

features in the context of the input aspect of audition. The gray matter does not function as
a single continuous entity. It is a series of brains that developed phylogenetically, hence the
indentations or bumps in Figure 16-1. The number of successive brains is uncertain. Whatever the number, each newer brain is larger and more complex than the one below it, and
has regulatory control over the lower brain(s) without replacing it(them). Part of the regulatory control takes place through connections within the central gray matter. Each brain or
brain level must receive the *same unprocessed message* from the periphery or the ear. Under
normal conditions, the unprocessed, all-or-none messages received at each brain level must
be processed in some way before the central gray matter can use them meaningfully.

    In summary, the CANS consists of: fast conducting pathways, which deliver the same
unprocessed neural messages from the periphery to all brain levels; associated processors,

which convert the original messages into some form that can be used meaningfully by the central gray matter; and the central gray matter, which is the core of the brain, processes the processed message even further and, if appropriate, brings it into consciousness.

The fast conducting pathways and their associated interconnecting nuclei are the same as the PAPS of the traditional view of the CANS. The central gray matter of the brain, other than the cerebral cortex, is the same as the reticular formation of the traditional view.

The PAPS conveys its messages rapidly and without distortion because of the secure one-to-one synaptic connections at each successive nuclear waystation. It is always open, that is, it always can be activated from the periphery whether the person is awake and attentive, awake and in reverie, drowsy, asleep and in any stage of sleep. Only the ear activates the PAPS. Stimuli in other modalities cannot affect the PAPS activity initiated by the ear.

At each nuclear waystation, along with the secure one-to-one connection, other sub-nuclei receive the same message as has been transmitted to the one-to-one connection. These sub-nuclei process or convert the all-or-none discharges to extract different aspects of the original message: spectrum, magnitude, time, and direction. They are local, dedicated processors.

The dual arrangement of nuclei just described is most clearly illustrated at the cochlear nucleus of the brainstem, the original auditory input to the brain (Figure 16-2). Each fiber of the auditory nerve bifurcates or splits into two branches. One branch (ascending) terminates usually just on one cell in the anteroventral cochlear nucleus. The most common pattern of nerve discharge through these interconnections is the so-called **primary discharge pattern** (see the **post-stimulus [PST] histograms** in Figure 16-3). The other branch (descending) terminates diffusely on a variety of cells mainly in the posteroventral and dorsal cochlear nucleus. These are the local dedicated processors at the lowest level of the CANS. Discharge patterns from these latter cells are varied (Figure 16-3) and they reflect the processing of information embedded in the all-or-none discharges of the auditory nerve. It is this processed information that is fed to the central gray matter for further processing and integration. This dual transmission-processing arrangement holds true for all the nuclear waystations up through Heschl's gyrus.

Determining which of the sub-nuclei at any of the nuclear waystations is part of the rapid transmission system and which serve as local dedicated processors is not easy. Distinction can be aided by (a) the synaptic wiring (secure one-to-one connections of the rapid transmission system versus diffuse multisynaptic connections of the processors) and (b) by the nature of the neural discharge patterns as defined by the PSTs (primary pattern for the rapid transmission system versus other patterns for the processing system).

Processors are not necessarily immediately adjacent to the main portion of the nuclear waystations. The medial superior olivary nucleus (MSO), for example, is anatomically disjointed from the cochlear nucleus complex (of which it may or may not be a part), and its specialized cells are activated by only one neuron from each side of the brain. The processed message delivered by the axon of each cell contains information about the relative timing of an acoustic signal delivered to each ear.

The same unprocessed acoustic message is delivered to each brain or brain level for initial processing at each level. From this, one can speculate that *all* auditory functions take place or are negotiated at each level. This speculation is borne out by observations of auditory behavior in patients with damage at various levels of the brain. The nature of brain damage rarely, if ever, is so discrete that only one portion of the CANS at one level is

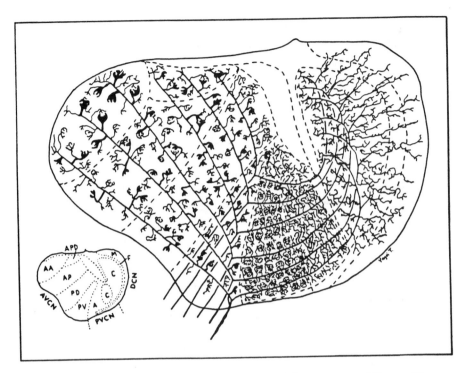

FIGURE 16-2   Diagrammatic representation of the entrance of the auditory (VIII) nerve into the cochlear nucleus of the cat. The nerve bifurcates with the ascending branch (left) terminating in the anteroventral cochlear nucleus (AVCN) and the descending branch (right) terminating in the posterventral and dorsal cochlear nucleus (PVCN and DCN).

[Reprinted with permission from Tsuchitani, "Lower auditory brain stem structures of the cat," in Naunton & Fernandez (Eds.), *Evoked electrical activity in the auditory nervous system*. New York: Academic Press, 1978.]

affected and all other portions of the CANS at that and other levels are spared. Nevertheless, clinical observations make it evident that speech communication through hearing is possible despite severe bilateral damage to Heschl's gyrus and the medial geniculate bodies (Landau, Goldstein, & Kleffner, 1960). Even an anencephalic infant showed cardiac orienting responses to various sounds, responses similar to those elicited from normal infants (Graham, Leavitt, Strock, & Brown, 1978).

Although the same auditory functions are carried out at each level, the sophistication of those functions increases at successively higher levels. Furthermore, each higher level exercises greater control over the functions that take place at the lower levels.

The principles of the alternate view of the CANS are not complex. However, the anatomic organization and wiring required to operate the CANS defy description at this time. The complicated description above of the alternate view of the CANS is a gross simplification to allow the principles to be illustrated or caricatured. Missing from the descrip-

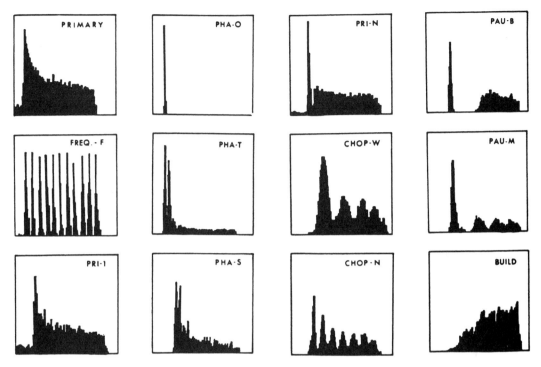

FIGURE 16-3 Examples of discharge patterns of auditory neurons in the form of poststimulus time (PST) histograms. The PST histograms represent the temporal distribution of neural spikes after signal (tone bursts) onset. Bin width is 0.2 ms; total analysis time is 40 ms. The primary-type PST histogram (upper left) comes mainly from neurons in the anteroventral cochlear nucleus (AVCN). Other forms of PSTs come mainly from neurons in the posteroventral or the dorsal cochlear nucleus (PVCN and DCN).

[Reprinted with permission from Tsuchitani, "Lower auditory brain stem structures of the cat," in Naunton & Fernandez (Eds.), *Evoked electrical activity in the auditory nervous system.* New York: Academic Press, 1978.]

tion are the complex interactions between levels within the central gray matter, interactions between the two sides of the brain, intermodality interactions, interactions with the autonomic nervous system, and sensorimotor interactions.

Another question to be dealt with is "What constitutes the CANS anatomically?" Is it just those structures that can be clearly delineated or do other, less well-defined portions of the brain participate in auditory functions? An old and common observation is that a novel auditory signal elicits distinct changes in the EEG recorded from nearly all parts of the brain, including the occipital lobe. After several repetitions of the same auditory signal, notable changes in the EEG no longer take place in the region of the occipital lobe. Now, each repetition of that auditory signal is paired with a visual signal. After several such conditioning trials, the auditory signal by itself elicits a distinct change in the EEG in the occipital region of the brain (Jasper & Shagass, 1941). Does this make the occipital lobe part of the CANS? The cerebellum ordinarily is not stressed or included in descriptions of the CANS despite unequivocal connections to and interactions with well-defined auditory portions of the brainstem (Marsh & Worden, 1964). Is the cerebellum part of the CANS? Obviously, these questions are difficult to answer. Just as obviously, the circumstances described challenge a simple anatomic description of the CANS.

Equally difficult to delineate is what constitutes an overall response of the brain to an auditory signal. In the description in the previous paragraph, the occipital region of the brain (as well as other nontemporal regions of the brain) ceases to react electrophysiologically to repetitions of the same sound. Most subcortical portions of the brain also cease to respond to repetitive auditory signals. This non-response conveys information to the central general processor of the brain. The brain now knows that it is dealing primarily with an auditory message; other sensory mechanisms can be excluded, at least from the initial processing.

We have implied that what others have called the reticular formation is part of what we regard as the central general integrative processor. Unfortunately, anatomists and physiologists have not clearly delineated anatomically what they believe to be the reticular formation. We include *all* of the central gray matter from the bottom of the spinal cord to the cerebral cortex in our circumscription of the central general processor.

The reticulate structure of the central general processor is not haphazardly diffuse and all parts of it are not functionally equivalent. Speaking now only of the input aspects, the portions of the central processor closest to the sensory input are devoted primarily to the modality of that input—olfaction, gustation, vision, somatosensation, or audition. However, unlike the rapid transmission portions of the nuclei, the processing portions devoted primarily to one modality can be affected by activity in other modalities. Their circuits may not be hard-wired but they are not diffusely wired, especially the portions closest to the input from the local dedicated processors attached to the fast relay nuclei. Those portions closest to the input probably are genetically programmed to deal in some meaningful way with the transformed properties of the all-or-none sensory message, the processed properties as reflected in the wide variety of discharge patterns other than the primary variety. Yes, the programs can be modified through learning, but they are not as plastic or malleable as portions of the process more remote from the input.

The concepts just expressed tie closely to the notion of centrality. Most audiologists and other clinicians have been taught that rostral implies centrality, that is, the higher a structure is in the brain, the more central are the functions it serves. This notion of centrality implies increasing sophistication from the more caudal to the more rostral portions of the brain.

There is another equally valid and equally useful notion of centrality—that is, integration. The closer a portion of the central processor is toward the central canal (and away from the input), the more general is the function of that portion. It works more to integrate input from all sensory modalities *and* from the motor modalities. Further, the more central the portion is anatomically, the more plastic or modifiable it is functionally.

How and where the central general processor uses its memory are relevant to applications of event-related potentials (ERPs) in assessing central auditory function or dysfunction. Short-term memory resides primarily in that portion closest to the local dedicated processors. Those diffuse portions of that central computer closest to the central canal are most responsible for long-term memory.

Finally, there are three magic numbers or time constants important for understanding central auditory functions and their AEP counterparts. These numbers are 1.5–2.0 ms, 15–20 ms, and 150–200 ms. For convenience, we continue only with the larger number of the pairs. Here are sample illustrations of these time constants.

1. Two successive signals (e.g., clicks) must be separated by at least 2 ms before they can be perceived as separate signals. This time constant seems to be determined mainly by the periphery.

2. 20 ms must elapse between two different successive signals (e.g., 1000 Hz and 2000 Hz tone bursts) before the listener can be certain which of the pair occurred first. This time constant appears to be determined mainly by the local dedicated processors and immediately surrounding portions of the central general processor. Backward masking occurs if the local processing of the first signal is interrupted by the action of the second signal.

3. A signal (e.g., 1000 Hz tone) must be presented for at least 200 ms for full temporal integration to occur, i.e., for the lowest (weakest) signal to be effective as a threshold signal. This time constant appears to be determined mainly, if not solely, by reticulate gray matter of the central general processor. These magic numbers appear to be key to psychoacoustic and electrophysiologic phenomena.

Relation to AEPs

Figure 16-4 is a summary depiction of the statements that follow. Three kinds of electric activity occur at each brain or brain level. They reflect three categories of physiologic processes in response to a single signal input:

1. Reception of untransformed input messages and subsequent relaying of the untransformed message to the next level.

2. Initial processing of the input message at each level to extract its temporal, tonal, magnitude, and spatial implications.

3. Reception of the transformed or processed messages by the gray matter at that level and further integrative processing of the message. The last stage also includes transmission of the integratively transformed message up *and* down *within* the central gray reticulate system or computer.

The first of the three waves at each level is drawn to be smallest. Primary, untransformed messages are carried by fewer neurons than are necessary for negotiating subsequent transformation processes. The time course of the initial wave also implies a higher frequency spectrum than for the two later waves. Untransformed messages are carried by groups of neurons that discharge nearly synchronously in time. Therefore, the distribution of discharge energy is more compact in time than is energy representing later transformation processes. Dedicated processors at each level use a larger pool of neurons and their activity is more broadly distributed in time. These conditions lead to a larger second wave with more low-frequency composition. Also, the processing requires input from the untransformed signals, which means it must begin its activity at some finite later time. The

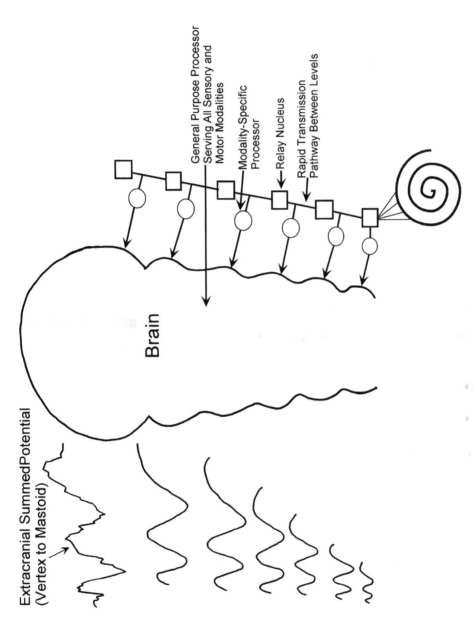

FIGURE 16-4 Three phases of electroencephalic activity at each brain level in the alternate view of the central auditory nervous system (CANS). Activation is by brief acoustic signals. The first phase or wave represents activity of the fast conducting pathway; the second wave, activity of the modality-specific processor; the third wave, activity of the general purpose processor. Each of the six traces was hand-drawn. The extracranial tracing at the top is an actual summing of the six traces below. See text for further details.

central general processor uses even a larger neuron pool with its activity distributed more widely in time. Thus, its electric manifestation is still larger and more dominantly low frequency.

Although Figure 16-4 shows the three waves as successive, they overlap partially in time. The second wave representing activity of the local dedicated processors begins before the residual activity of the fast transmission pathways has completely ended. Likewise, activity begins within the central general processor before the electric activity within the local dedicated processors ceases entirely.

Figure 16-4 shows a finite transmission time between brain levels, that is, the activity at each brain begins a few milliseconds later than the activity of the lower level. This transmission delay, along with the time overlap at each brain mentioned above, leads to an overall temporal smearing of electroencephalic activity. When customary extracranial electrodes record activity across the billions of neurons in between, they record this temporal smearing or blur along with the inevitable spatial blur. The net activity depicted on the top of Figure 16-4 reflects the combined temporal-spatial blur. The net summed potential at the top of the figure is an actual algebraic addition of the three artificially constructed waves at each of the brain levels below. The little wiggles superimposed on the larger deflections are not instrumental or physiologic noise. If the constituent waves below represent physiologic activity in response to a sound, then each of the large and small deflections has some physiologic significance. In an actual electroencephalic recording, the complex AEP picked up with extracranial electrodes also will include physiologic and instrumental noise. One sobering conclusion based on the total complexity is that it is difficult and risky to draw firm diagnostic inferences from individual waves of AEPs as they ordinarily are recorded. *When an abnormality appears in a net trace is not always a safe indication of where in the brain that the pathologic process has occurred or of what the pathologic condition is.*

In Chapters 5 through 8, we described ways (e.g., analysis window size, filter passbands, signal rates, etc.) by which certain signal- and event-related portions of the AEP could be sufficiently isolated from other portions to be used for specific clinical purposes (e.g., threshold audiometry, location of site of lesion) with reasonable certainty. In concluding this chapter, we stress only capitalizing on origins of AEPs, as detailed earlier, to assess the three major systems of the CANS and of the brain as a whole.

Use of AEPs for Systems Analysis

What follows is a restatement in modified form of portions of previous chapters in which we discussed diagnostic strategy. Start with some broad clinical questions that must be asked first before AEP indices and procedures are selected. "Is the purpose of the test to determine the site, nature and extent of a lesion; or is the purpose to determine the basis for the patient's auditory disorder?" "If it is the latter, is the patient's auditory communication problem peripherally or centrally based, or both?" "If the disorder is centrally based, is it caused by disruption of the system for transmission of unprocessed messages, by the failure of the local dedicated processors to perform the initial transformation of the message, or by the failure of the central integrative system to accept or to appropriately interpret the transformed message?" "Is the patient's auditory problem modality-specific or is it a manifestation of a more pervasive problem encompassing other sensory modalities?"

Signal-related AEPs are sufficient to determine the integrity of the periphery for most clinical purposes. Clinicians can establish, at least as a first approximation, whether the ear is delivering normal, predictable signals to the CANS. Early and middle signal-related AEPs (EPs and MPs) provide indices of normality or abnormality of the rapid transmission of unprocessed messages in the brain. Patterns of late AEPs (LPs) provide gross indication of normality/abnormality of the initial and subsequent transformation processing of the messages received by the brain from the periphery.

Transformation processing by the CANS is best assessed by event-related potentials or ERPs: early ERPs to appraise the integrity of the local dedicated processors and late ERPs to appraise the integrity of the central integrative processor.

It is wise to sweep diagnostically from the periphery through the successive stages of central transmission, early central transformation processing, and later integrative processing. What appears to be a high-level dysfunction may only be a later inevitable consequence of an earlier, more primitive dysfunction.

Finally, a diagnostician must make certain that the auditory dysfunction under scrutiny is just that and not part of a broader problem involving other sensory modalities. Therefore, the same diagnostic sweep applied to audition may have to be applied to other modalities as well to complete the assessment of the auditory dysfunction.

References

ABRAMOVICH, S., & PRASHER, D. K. (1986). Electro-cochleography and brain-stem potentials in Ramsay Hunt syndrome. *Archives of Otolaryngology, 112,* 925–928.

ADAMS, J. C., & BENSON, D. A. (1973). Task-contingent enhancement of the auditory evoked response. *Electroencephalography and Clinical Neurophysiology, 35,* 249–257.

ADES, H. W., & BROOKHART, J. M. (1950). The central auditory pathway. *Journal of Neurophysiology, 11,* 189–206.

ADRIAN, E. D. (1931). The microphonic action of the cochlea: An interpretation of Wever and Bray's experiments. *Journal of Physiology, 71,* 28P–29P.

AINSLIE, P. J., & BOSTON, J. R. (1980). Comparison of brain stem auditory evoked potentials for monaural and binaural stimuli. *Electroencephalography and Clinical Neurophysiology, 49,* 291–302.

ALDRICH, W. M. (1994). *Clinical application of the somatosensory evoked potential.* Kennewick, WA: Cadwell Laboratories.

ALEXANDER, B., BINNIE, C. D., & MARGERISON, J. H. (1971). CNVs for the simple minded. *American Journal of EEG Technology, 11,* 161–164.

ALHO, K., SAMS, M., PAAVILAINEN, P., & NÄÄTÄNEN, R. (1986). Small pitch separation and the selective-attention effects on the ERP. *Psychophysiology, 23,* 189–197.

ALHO, K., TÖTTÖLÄ, K., REINIKAINEN, K., SAMS, M., & NÄÄTÄNEN, R. (1987). Brain mechanism of selective listening reflected by event-related potentials. *Electroencephalography and Clinical Neurophysiology, 68,* 458–470.

ALLISON, T., HUME, A. L., WOOD, C. C., & GOFF, W. R. (1984). Developmental and aging changes in so-matosensory, auditory, and visual evoked potentials. *Electroencephalography and Clinical Neurophysiology, 58,* 14–24.

American EEG Society. (1994a). Guideline nine: Guidelines on evoked potentials. *Journal of Clinical Neurophysiology, 11,* 40–73.

American EEG Society. (1994b). Guideline ten: Guidelines for writing clinical evoked potential reports. *Journal of Clinical Neurophysiology, 11,* 74–76.

American National Standards Institute. (1989). *Specifications for audiometers, ANSI S3.6-1989.* New York: ANSI.

American Speech and Hearing Association. (1978). Guidelines for manual pure-tone audiometry. *Asha, 20,* 297–301.

AMINOFF, M. J., & GOODIN, D. S. (1994). Visual evoked potentials. *Journal of Clinical Neurophysiology, 11,* 493–499.

ANTHONY, P. F., DURRETT, R., PULEC, J. L., & HARTSTONE, J. L. (1979). A new parameter in brain stem evoked response: Component wave areas. *Laryngoscope, 89,* 1569–1578.

ARAVABHUMI, S., IZZO, K. L., & BAKST, B. L. (1987). Brainstem auditory evoked potentials: Intraoperative monitoring technique in surgery of posterior fossa tumors. *Archives of Physical Medicine and Rehabilitation, 68,* 142–146.

ASHA Audiologic Evaluation Working Group on Auditory Evoked Potential Measurements. (1988). *The short latency auditory evoked potentials.* Rockville, MD: American Speech-Language-Hearing Association.

BALLACHANDA, B. B., RUPERT, A., & MOUSHEGIAN, G. (1994). Asymmetric frequency-following responses. *Journal of the American Academy of Audiology, 5,* 133–137.

BARAN, J. A., LONG, R. R., MUSIEK, F. E., & OMMAYA, A. (1988). Topographic mapping of brain electrical activity in the assessment of central auditory nervous system pathology. *American Journal of Otology, 9(Supplement),* 72–76.

BARNET, A. B., & LODGE, A. (1967). Click evoked EEG responses in normal and developmentally retarded infants. *Nature, 214,* 252–255.

BARNET, A. B., OHLRICH, E. S., WEISS, I. P., & SHANKS, B. (1975). Auditory evoked potentials during sleep in normal children from ten days to three years of age. *Electroencephalography and Clinical Neurophysiology, 39,* 29–41.

BARRETT, K. A. (1992). *The effect of small variations in signal intensity on early event-related potentials.* Doctoral dissertation, University of Wisconsin-Madison.

BARSKY-FIRKSER, L., & SUN, S. (1997). Universal newborn hearing screenings: A three-year experience. *Pediatrics, 99,* E41–E45.

BAUCH, C. D., OLSEN, W. O., & POOL, A. F. (1996). ABR indices: Sensitivity, specificity, and tumor size. *American Journal of Audiology, 5(1),* 97–104.

BAUCH, C. D., ROSE, D. E., & HARNER, S. G. (1980). Brainstem responses to tone pip and click stimuli. *Ear and Hearing, 1,* 181–184.

BEADLE, K. R., & CROWELL, D. H. (1962). Neonatal electrocardiographic responses to sound: Methodology. *Journal of Speech and Hearing Research, 5,* 112–123.

BEAGLEY, H. A. (1970). Characteristic of the auditory evoked response in a group of aphasic children. *Sound, 4,* 62–64.

BEATTIE, R. C., GARCIA, E., & JOHNSON, A. (1996). Frequency-specific auditory brainstem responses in adults with sensorineural hearing loss. *Audiology, 35,* 194–203.

BEATTIE, R. C., & KENNEDY, K. M. (1992). Auditory brainstem response to tone bursts in quiet, notch noise, highpass noise, and broadband noise. *Journal of the American Academy of Audiology, 3,* 349–360.

BECKER, D. E., & SHAPIRO, D. (1981). Physiological responses to clicks during Zen, Yoga, and TM meditation. *Psychophysiology, 18,* 694–699.

BENTIN, S., MCCARTHY, G., & WOOD, C. C. (1985). Event-related potentials, lexical decision and semantic priming. *Electroencephalography and Clinical Neurophysiology, 60,* 343–355.

BERTOLINI, M., & DUBINI, S. (1969). Contributo allo studio del potenziale evocato acustico durante il sonno in pazienti psicotici. *Revista di Neurologia, 39,* 492–503.

BICKFORD, R. G., JACOBSON, J. L., & CODY, T. R. (1964). Nature of average evoked potentials to sound and other stimuli in man. *Annals of the New York Academy of Sciences, 112,* 204–223.

BISHOP, G. H. (1958). The place of cortex in a reticular system. In *Reticular formation of the brain* (pp. 413–421). Boston: Little, Brown and Company.

BISHOP, G. H. (1961). The organization of the cortex with respect to its afferent supply. *Annals of the New York Academy of Sciences, 94,* 559–569.

BLOCK, E. P. (1984). *Tonal bone-conduction thresholds by electroencephalic audiometry.* Master's thesis, University of Wisconsin-Madison.

BOGACZ, J., VANZULLI, A., & GARCIA-AUSTT, E. (1962). Evoked responses in man. IV. Effects of habituation, distraction and conditioning upon auditory evoked responses. *Acta Neurologica Latino Americano, 8,* 244–252.

BORDLEY, J. E., & HARDY, W. G. (1949). A study in objective audiometry with the use of a psychogalvanic response. *Annals of Otology, Rhinology and Laryngology, 58,* 751–760.

BORDLEY, J. E., RUBEN, R. J., & LIEBERMAN, A. T. (1964). Human cochlear potentials. *Laryngoscope, 74,* 463–479.

BORG, E., & LÖFQVIST, L. (1981). Brainstem response (ABR) to rarefaction and condensation clicks in normal hearing and steep high-frequency hearing loss. *Scandinavian Audiology, 13,* 99–101.

BORSANYI, S. J. (1964). Some aspects of auditory potentials in man. *Annals of Otology, Rhinology and Laryngology, 73,* 61–71.

BUCHSBAUM, M. S., HENKIN, R. I., & CHRISTIANSEN, R. L. (1974). Age and sex differences in averaged evoked responses in a normal population, with observations on patients with gonadal dysgenesis. *Electroencephalography and Clinical Neurophysiology, 37,* 137–144.

BURKARD, R., & HECOX, K. (1983). The effect of broadband noise on the human brainstem auditory evoked response. II. Frequency specificity. *Journal of the Acoustical Society of America, 74,* 1214–1223.

BURKARD, R., SHI, Y., & HECOX, K. E. (1990). Brainstem auditory-evoked responses elicited by maximum length sequences: Effect of simultaneous masking noise. *Journal of the Acoustical Society of America, 87,* 1665–1672.

CALLAWAY, E. (1966). Averaged evoked responses in psychiatry. *Journal of Nervous and Mental Disease, 143,* 80–94.

CHEOUR-LUHTANEN, M., ALHO, K., KUJALA, T., SAINIO, K., REINIKAINEN, K., RENLUND, M., AALTONEN, O., EEROLA, O., & NÄÄTÄNEN, R. (1995). Mismatch negativity indicates vowel discrimination in newborns. *Hearing Research, 82,* 53–58.

CHERTOFF, M. E., GOLDSTEIN, R., & MEASE, M. R. (1988). Early event-related potentials with passive subject participation. *Journal of Speech and Hearing Research, 31,* 460–465.

CHUEDEN, H. (1972). The masking noise and its effect upon the human cortical evoked potential. *Audiology, 11,* 90–96.

CLARK, J. L., MOUSHEGIAN, G., & RUPERT, A. L. (1997). Interaural time effects on the frequency-following response. *Journal of the American Academy of Audiology, 8,* 308–313.

CLEMIS, J. D., & MITCHELL, C. (1977). Electrocochleogrphy and brain stem responses used in the diagnosis of acoustic tumors. *Journal of Otolaryngology, 6,* 447–459.

COATS, A. C. (1974). On electrocochleographic electrode design. *Journal of the Acoustical Society of America, 56,* 708–711.

COATS, A. C. (1983). Instrumentation. In E. J. Moore (Ed.), *Bases of auditory brain-stem evoked responses* (pp. 197–220). New York: Grune and Stratton.

COATS, A. C., & MARTIN, J. L. (1977). Human auditory nerve action potentials and brain stem evoked responses. *Archives of Otolaryngology, 103,* 605–622.

COBURN, K. L., CAMPBELL, K. C. M., KUHN, M. J., & MORENO, M. A. (1996). Electrophysiological and structural abnormalities in a long-term survivor of trisomy 13 (Patau's syndrome). *American Journal of Audiology, 5,* 35–43.

COHEN, J., & POLICH, J. (1997). On the number of trials needed for P300. *International Journal of Psychophysiology, 25,* 249–255.

COLLET, L., CHANAL, J. M., HELLAL, H., GARTNER, M., & MORGAN, A. (1989). Validity of bone conduction stimulated ABR, MLR and otoacoustic emissions. *Scandinavian Audiology, 18,* 43–46.

CONE-WESSON, B. (1995). Bone-conduction ABR tests. *American Journal of Audiology, 4,* 14–19.

CONE-WESSON, B., MA, E., & FOWLER, C. G. (1997). Effect of stimulus level and frequency on ABR and MLR binaural interaction in human neonates. *Hearing Research, 106,* 163–178.

CONE-WESSON, B., & RAMIREZ, G. M. (1997). Hearing sensitivity in newborns estimated from ABRs to bone-conducted sound. *Journal of the American Academy of Audiology, 8,* 299–307.

COOK, E. W. III, & MILLER, G. A. (1992). Digital filtering: Background and tutorial for psychophysiologists. *Psychophysiology, 29,* 350–367.

DALLOS, P., & CHEATHAM, M. A. (1976). Production of cochlear potentials by inner and outer hair cells. *Journal of the Acoustical Society of America, 60,* 510–512.

DALLOS, P. J., & OLSEN, W. O. (1964). Integration of energy at threshold with gradual rise-fall tone pips. *Journal of the Acoustical Society of America, 36,* 743–757.

DAUMAN, R., SZYFTER, W., CHARLET DE SAUVAGE, R., & CAZALS, Y. (1984). Low frequency thresholds assessed with 40 Hz MLR in adults with impaired hearing. *Archives of Oto-Rhino-Laryngology, 240,* 85–89.

DAVIS, H. (1936). Some aspects of the electrical activity of the cerebral cortex. *Cold Spring Harbor Symposia on Quantitative Biology, 4,* 285–291.

DAVIS, H. (1964). Enhancement of evoked cortical potentials in humans related to a task requiring a decision. *Science, 145,* 182–183.

DAVIS, H. (1965). Slow cortical responses evoked by acoustic stimuli. *Acta Oto-Laryngologica, 59,* 179–185.

DAVIS, H. (1976). Principles of electric response audiometry. *Annals of Otology, Rhinology and Larygology, 85[supplement],* 1–96.

DAVIS, H., BOWERS, C., & HIRSH, S. K. (1968). Relations of the human vertex potential to acoustic input: Loudness and masking. *Journal of the Acoustical Society of America, 43,* 431–438.

DAVIS, H., DAVIS, P. A., LOOMIS, A. L., HARVEY, E. N., & HOBART, G. (1939). Electrical reactions of the human brain to auditory stimulation during sleep. *Journal of Neurophysiology, 2,* 500–514.

DAVIS, H., & DERBYSHIRE, A. J. (1972). Reminiscences of the pioneer days of electroencephalography and electroencephalic audiometry. Videotape of a program sponsored by the Department of Communicative Disorders, University of Wisconsin-Madison.

DAVIS, H., DERBYSHIRE, A. J., & SAUL, L. J. (1933). Further analysis of the electrical phenomena of the auditory mechanism. *American Journal of Physiology, 105,* 27–28.

DAVIS, H., ENGEBRETSON, M., LOWELL, E. L., MAST, T., SATTERFIELD, J., & YOSHIE, Y. (1964). Evoked responses to clicks recorded from the human scalp. *Annals of the New York Academy of Sciences, 112,* 224–225.

DAVIS, H., FERNÁNDEZ, C., & MCAULIFFE, D. R. (1950). The excitatory process in the cochlea. *Proceedings of the National Academy of Sciences, 36,* 580–587.

DAVIS, H., & HIRSH, S. K. (1979). A slow brain stem response for low-frequency audiometry. *Audiology, 18,* 445–461.

DAVIS, H., HIRSH, S. K., SHELNUTT, J., & BOWERS, C. (1967). Further validation of evoked response audiometry (ERA). *Journal of Speech and Hearing Research, 10,* 717–732.

DAVIS, H., HIRSH, S. K., TURPIN, L. L., & PEACOCK, M. E. (1985). Threshold sensitivity and frequency specifity in auditory brainstem response audiometry. *Audiology, 24,* 54–70.

DAVIS, H., MAST, T., YOSHIE, H., & ZERLIN, S. (1966). The slow response of the human cortex to auditory stimuli. *Electroencephalography and Clinical Neurophysiology, 21,* 105–113.

DAVIS, H., SILVERMAN, S. R., & MCAULIFFE, D. R. (1951). Some observations on pitch and frequency. *Journal of the Acoustical Society of America, 23,* 40–42.

DAVIS, H., & ZERLIN (1966). Acoustic relations of the human vertex potential. *Journal of the Acoustical Society of America, 39,* 109–116.

DEMPSEY, J. J., CENSOPRANO, E., & MAZOR, M. (1986). Relationship between head size and latency of the auditory brainstem response. *Audiology, 25,* 258–262.

DERBYSHIRE, A. J., & FARLEY, J. C. (1959). Sampling auditory responses at the cortical level. *Annals of Otology, Rhinology and Laryngology, 69,* 675–697.

DERBYSHIRE, A. J., FRASER, A. A., MCDERMOTT, M., & BRIDGE, A. (1956). Audiometric measurements by electroencephalography. *Electroencephalography and Clinical Neurophysiology, 8,* 467–478.

DINIZ, J. JR., MANGABEIRA-ALBERNAZ, P. L., MUNHOZ, M. S. L., & FUKUDA, Y. (1997). Cognitive potentials in children with learning disabilities. *Acta Oto-Laryngologica, 117,* 211–213.

DIRCKX, J. J. J., DAEMERS, K., SOMERS, T., OFFECIERS, F. E., & GOVAERTS, P. J. (1996). Numerical assessment of TOAE screening results: Currently used criteria and their effect on TOAE prevalence figures. *Acta Oto-Laryngologica, 116,* 672–679.

DOBIE, R. A., & NORTON, S. J. (1980). Binaural interaction in human auditory evoked potentials. *Electroencephalography and Clinical Neurophysiology, 49,* 303–313.

DOHERTY, K. A., BARRETT, K. A., & GOLDSTEIN, R. (1991). Effect of sample size on early event-related potentials [Abstract]. *Asha, 33,* 152.

DON, M., EGGERMONT, J. J., & BRACKMANN, D. E. (1979). Reconstruction of the audiogram using brain stem responses and high-pass noise masking. *Annals of Otology, Rhinology, and Laryngology, 57 [supplement],* 1–20.

DON, M., & ELBERLING, C. (1994). Evaluating residual background noise in human auditory brain-stem responses. *Journal of the Acoustical Society of America, 96,* 2746–2757.

DON, M., & ELBERLING, C. (1996). Use of quantitative measures of auditory brainstem response peak amplitude and residual background noise in the decision to stop averaging. *Journal of the Acoustical Society of America, 99,* 491–499.

DONCHIN, E., & MCCARTHY, G. (1979). Event-related brain potentials in the study of cognitive processes. In C. L. Ludlow & M. E. Doran-Quine (Eds.), *The neurological bases of language disorders in children: Methods and directions for research* (pp. 109–128). Bethesda, MD: U.S. Department of Health, Education, and Welfare.

DOWNS, M. P., & STERRITT, G. M. (1964). Identification audiometry for neonates: A preliminary report. *Journal of Auditory Research, 4,* 69–80.

DOWNS, M. P., & STERRITT, G. M. (1967). A guide to newborn and infant hearing screening programs. *Archives of Otolaryngology, 85,* 37–44.

DOYLE, D. J., & HYDE, M. L. (1981). Analogue and digital filtering of auditory brainstem responses. *Scandinavian Audiology, 10,* 81–89.

DUNCAN-JOHNSON, C. C., & DONCHIN, E. (1977). On quantifying surprise: The variations in event-related potentials with subjective probability. *Psychophysiology, 14,* 455–467.

DURRANT, J. D. (1983). Fundamentals of sound generation. In E. J. Moore (Ed.), *Bases of auditory brainstem evoked responses* (pp. 15–49). New York: Grune and Stratton.

DURRANT, J. D., BOSTON, J. R., & MARTIN, W. H. (1990). Correlation study of two-channel recordings of the brain stem auditory evoked potential. *Ear and Hearing, 11,* 215–221.

DURRANT, J. D., & FOWLER, C. G. (1996). ABR protocols for dealing with asymmetric hearing loss. *American Journal of Audiology, 5(3),* 5–6.

DURRANT, J. D., NOZZA, R. J., HYRE, R. J., & SABO, D. L. (1989). Masking level difference at relatively high masker levels: Preliminary report. *Audiology, 28,* 221–229.

DURRANT, J. D., SABO, D. L., & HYRE, R., J. (1990). Gender, head size, and ABRs examined in large clinical sample. *Ear and Hearing, 11,* 210–214.

EBENBICHLER, G., UHL, F., LANG, W., LINDINGER, G., EGKHER, A., & DEECKE, L. (1997). Cortical DC potential shifts accompanying central processing of visually presented analogue and digital time displays. *Neuropsychologia, 35,* 349–357.

EISENBERG, R. B. (1966). Electroencephalography in the study of developmental disorders of communication. *Journal of Speech and Hearing Disorders, 31,* 183–186.

EISENBERG, R. B. (1970). The organization of auditory behavior. *Journal of Speech and Hearing Research, 13,* 453–471.

ELBERLING, C., & DON, M. (1984). Quality estimation of averaged auditory brainstem responses. *Scandinavian Audiology, 13,* 187–197.

ELBERLING, C., & DON, M. (1987). Detection functions for the human auditory brainstem response. *Scandinavian Audiology, 16,* 89–92.

ELBERLING, C., & PARBO, J. (1987). Reference data for ABRs in retrocochlear diagnosis. *Scandinavian Audiology, 16,* 49–55.

EYSHOLDT, U., & SCHREINER, C. (1982). Maximum length sequences—a fast method for measuring brainstem auditory evoked responses. *Audiology, 21,* 242–250.

FERRARO, J. A. (1992). Electrocochleography: How - part I. *Audiology Today, 4(6),* 26–28.

FERRARO, J. A. (1993). Electrocochleography: How - part II. *Audiology Today, 5(3),* 31–33.

FINITZO-HIEBER, T., FREEMAN, F. J., GERLING, I. J., DOBSON, L., & SCHAEFER, S. D. (1982). Auditory brainstem response abnormalities in adductor spasmodic dysphonia. *American Journal of Otolaryngology, 3,* 26–30.

FISHER, R. S., RAUDZENS, P., & NUNEMACHER, M. (1995). Efficacy of intraoperative neurophysiologic monitoring. *Journal of Clinical Neurophysiology, 12,* 97–109.

FOLSOM, R. C. (1985). Auditory brain stem responses from human infants: Pure-tone masking profiles for clicks and filtered clicks. *Journal of the Acoustical Society of America, 78,* 555–562.

FOLSOM, R. C., & WYNNE, M. K. (1986). Auditory brain stem responses from human adults and infants: Restriction of frequency contribution by notched-noise masking. *Journal of the Acoustical Society of America, 80,* 1057–1064.

FORD, J. M., ROTH, W. T., DIRKS, S. J., & KOPELL, B. S. (1973). Evoked potential correlates of signal recognition between and within modalities. *Science, 181,* 465–466.

FOWLER, C. G., & DURRANT, J. D. (1994). The effects of peripheral hearing loss on the auditory brainstem response. In J. T. Jacobson (Ed.), *Principles and applications in auditory evoked potentials* (pp. 237–250). Boston: Allyn and Bacon.

FOWLER, C. G., & MIKAMI, C. M. (1992). Effects of cochlear hearing loss on the ABR latencies to clicks and 1000 Hz tone pips. *Journal of the American Academy of Audiology, 3,* 324–330.

FOWLER, C. G., & NOFFSINGER, D. (1983). Effects of stimulus repetition rate and frequency on the auditory brainstem response in normal, cochlear-impaired, and VIII nerve/brainstem-impaired subjects. *Journal of Speech and Hearing Research, 26,* 560–567.

FOWLER, C. G., & SWANSON, M. R. (1989). The 40-Hz potential and SN_{10} as measures of low-frequency thresholds. *Scandinavian Audiology, 18,* 27–33.

FRANKLIN, B. (1983). Newborn screening: Are common auditory stimulus frequencies too high? *Hearing Journal, 36,* 19–21.

FROMM, B., NYLEN, C. O., & ZOTTERMAN, Y. (1935). Studies in the mechanism of the Wever and Bray effect. *Acta Oto-Laryngologica, 22,* 477–486.

FRYE-OSIER, H. A. (1983). *Simultaneous early and middle components of the averaged electroencephalic response elicited from neonates by narrow-spectrum signals.* Doctoral dissertation, University of Wisconsin-Madison.

GAILLARD, A. W. K. (1977). The late CNV wave: Preparation versus expectancy. *Psychophysiology, 1977, 14,* 563–568.

GALAMBOS, R., & HECOX, K. E. (1978). Clinical applications of the auditory brain stem response. *Otolaryngologic Clinics of North America, 11,* 709–722.

GALAMBOS, R., MAKEIG, S., & TALMACHOFF, P. J. (1981). A 40-Hz auditory potential recorded from the human scalp. *Proceedings of the National Academy of Sciences, 78,* 2643–2647.

GALAMBOS, R., & WILSON, M. (1994). Newborn hearing thresholds measured by both insert and earphone methods. *Journal of the American Academy of Audiology, 5,* 141–145.

GEISLER, C. D., FRISHKOPF, L. S., & ROSENBLITH, W. A. (1958). Extracranial responses to acoustic clicks in man. *Science, 128,* 1210–1211.

GEISLER, C. D., & ROSENBLITH, W. A. (1962). Average responses to clicks recorded from the human scalp. *Journal of the Acoustical Society of America, 34,* 125–127.

GERLING, I. J., & FINITZO-HIEBER, T. (1983). Auditory brainstem response with high stimulus rates in normal and patient populations. *Annals of Otology, Rhinology and Laryngology, 92,* 119–123.

GOLDSTEIN, R. (1956). Effectiveness of conditioned electrodermal responses (EDR) in measuring puretone thresholds in cases of non-organic hearing loss. *Laryngoscope, 66,* 119–130.

GOLDSTEIN, R. (1963). Electrophysiologic audiometry. In J. Jerger (Ed.), *Modern developments in audiology* (pp. 167–192). New York: Academic Press.

GOLDSTEIN, R. (1967). Electroencephalic audiometry, In A. B. Graham (Ed.), *Sensorineural hearing processes and disorders* (pp. 301–312). Boston: Little, Brown and Company.

GOLDSTEIN, R. (1973). Electroencephalic audiometry. In J. Jerger (Ed.), *Modern developments in audiology* (2nd ed.)(pp. 407–435). New York: Academic Press.

GOLDSTEIN, R. (1980). Components of the extracranial AER: Convenience vs concept. *Revue de Laryngologie, Otologie, Rhinologie (Bordeaux), 101,* 209–227.

GOLDSTEIN, R. (1982). Neurophysiology of hearing. In N. J. Lass, L. V. McReynolds, J. L. Northern, & D. E. Yoder (Eds.), *Speech, language and hearing* (pp. 180–192). Philadelphia: W. B. Saunders.

GOLDSTEIN, R., & FRYE-OSIER, H. A. (1984). Simultaneous recording of early- and middle-latency averaged electroencephalic responses for neonatal hearing screening or evaluation. In R. H. Nodar & C. Barber (Eds.), *Evoked potentials II* (pp. 543–547). Boston: Butterworth.

GOLDSTEIN, R., KARLOVICH, R. S., TWEED, T. S., & KILE, J. E. (1983). Psychoacoustic tuning curves and averaged electroencephalic responses in a patient with low-frequency sensory-neural hearing loss. *Journal of Speech and Hearing Disorders, 48,* 70–75.

GOLDSTEIN, R., KENDALL, D. C., & ARICK, B. E. (1963). Electroencephalic audiometry in young children. *Journal of Speech and Hearing Disorders, 28,* 331–354.

GOLDSTEIN, R., & McRANDLE, C. C. (1976). Middle components of the averaged electroencephalic response to clicks in neonates. In S. K. Hirsh, D. H. Eldredge, I. J. Hirsh, & S. R. Silverman (Eds.), *Hearing and Davis: Essays honoring Hallowell Davis* (pp. 445–456). St. Louis: Washington University Press.

GOLDSTEIN, R., & RODMAN, L. B. (1967). Early components of averaged evoked responses to rapidly repeated auditory stimuli. *Journal of Speech and Hearing Research, 10,* 697–705.

GOLDSTEIN, R., & TAIT, C. (1971). Critique of neonatal hearing evaluation. *Journal of Speech and Hearing Disorders, 36,* 1–18.

GORGA, M. P., BEAUCHAINE, K. L., KAMINSKI, J. R., & BERGMAN, B. M. (1992). Use of tone bursts in ABR evaluation. *American Journal of Audiology, 1,* 11–12.

GORGA, M. P., & NEELY, S. T. (1994). Stimulus calibration in auditory evoked potential measurements. In J. T. Jacobson (Ed.), *Principles and applications in auditory evoked potentials* (pp. 85–97). Boston: Allyn and Bacon.

GORGA, M. P., REILAND, J. K., & BEAUCHAINE, K. A. (1985). Auditory brainstem responses in a case of high-frequency conductive hearing loss. *Journal of Speech and Hearing Disorders, 50,* 346–350.

GORGA, M. P., & THORNTON, A. R. (1989). The choice of stimuli for ABR measurements. *Ear and Hearing, 10,* 217–230.

GORLIN, R. J., & SEDANO, H. (1970). Profound childhood deafness with ECG abnormalities, fainting spells, and sudden death. (Jervell and Lange-Nielsen's syndrome, cardio-auditory syndrome, surdo-cardiac syndrome). *Modern Medicine, 38,* 138–139.

GOTO, H., ADACHI, T., UTSUNOMIYA, T., NAKANO, H., & CHIN, K. (1978). EEG evoked response, P300 and CNV during processing of sentence information: Clinical application. *T.-I.-T. Journal of Life Sciences, 8,* 55–58.

GRAHAM, F. K., LEAVITT, L. A., STROCK, B. D., & BROWN, J. W. (1978). Precocious cardiac orienting in a human anencephalic infant. *Science, 199,* 322–324.

GRASS, E. R., & JOHNSON, E. (1980). *An introduction to evoked response signal averaging.* Quincy, MA: Grass Instrument Company.

GUTNICK, H. G., & GOLDSTEIN, R. (1978). Effect of contralateral noise on the middle components of the averaged electroencephalic response. *Journal of Speech and Hearing Research, 21,* 613–624.

HAGOORT, P., BROWN, C. M., & SWAAB, T. Y. (1996). Lexical-semantic event-related potential effects in patients with left hemisphere lesions and aphasia, and patients with right hemisphere lesions without aphasia. *Brain, 119,* 627–649.

HALL, J. W. III. (1992). *Handbook of auditory evoked responses.* Boston: Allyn and Bacon.

HALL, J. W., III., BULL, J. M., & CRONAU, L. H. (1988). Hypo- and hyperthermia in clinical auditory brain stem response measurement: Two case reports. *Ear and Hearing, 9,* 137–143.

HALL, J. W., III., MORGAN, S. H., MACKEY-HAGARDINE, J., AGUILAR, E. A., III, & JAHRSDOERFER, R. A. (1984). Neuro-otologic applications of simultaneous multi-channel auditory evoked response recordings. *Laryngoscope, 94,* 883–889.

HARDY, W. G., & PAULS, M. D. (1952). The test situation in PGSR audiometry. *Journal of Speech and Hearing Disorders, 17,* 13–24.

HARKER, L. A., HOSICK, E., VOOTS, R. J., & MENDEL, M. I. (1977). Influence of succinylcholine on middle component auditory evoked potentials. *Archives of Otolaryngology, 103,* 133–137.

HECOX, K., & GALAMBOS, R. (1974). Brainstem auditory evoked responses in human infants and adults. *Archives of Otolaryngology, 99,* 30–33.

HERRMANN, B. S. (1994). Perspectives and implications of early identification of hearing loss. *Current Opinion in Otolaryngology & Head and Neck Surgery, 2,* 449–454.

HERRMANN, B. S., THORNTON, A. R., & JOSEPH, J. M. (1995). Automated infant hearing screening using the ABR: Development and validation. *American Journal of Audiology, 4(2),* 6–14.

HILLYARD, S. A. (1985). Electrophysiology of human selective attention. *Trends in NeuroSciences, 8,* 400–405.

HOOD, L. J., & BERLIN, C. I. (1986). *Auditory evoked potentials.* Austin TX: Pro-Ed.

HORWITZ, S. F., LARSON, S. J., & SANCES, A. J. JR. (1966). Evoked potentials as an adjunct to the auditory evaluation of patients. *Proceedings of the Symposium on Biomedical Engineering, 1,* 49–53.

HOTH, S. (1986). Reliability of latency and amplitude values of auditory-evoked potentials. *Audiology, 25,* 248–257.

HUMES, L. E., & OCHS, M. G. (1982). Use of contralateral masking in the measurement of the auditory brainstem response. *Journal of Speech and Hearing Research, 25,* 528–535.

HYDE, M. L. (1994a). Signal processing and analysis. In J. T. Jacobson (Ed.), *Principles and applications in auditory evoked potentials* (pp. 47–83). Boston: Allyn and Bacon.

HYDE, M. L. (1994b). The slow vertex potential: Properties and clinical applications. In J. T. Jacobson (Ed.), *Principles and applications in auditory evoked potentials* (pp. 179–218). Boston: Allyn and Bacon.

IVEY, R. G. (1986). Survey of school age children referred for central auditory assessment. *Human Communication Canada, 10,* 5–10.

JACOBSON, G. P., CALDER, J. A., NEWMAN, C. W., PETERSON, E. L., WHARTON, J. A., & AHMAD, B. K. (1996). Electrophysiological indices of selective auditory attention in subjects with and without tinnitus. *Hearing Research, 97,* 66–74.

JACOBSON, G. P., JACOBSON, J. T., RAMADAN, N., & HYDE, M. (1994). Auditory brainstem response measures in acoustic nerve and brainstem disease. In J. T. Jacobson (Ed.), *Principles and applications in auditory evoked potentials* (pp. 387–426). Boston: Allyn and Bacon.

JACOBSON, J. T., JACOBSON, C. A., & SPAHR, R. C. (1990). Automated and conventional ABR screening techniques in high risk infants. *Journal of the Academy of Audiology, 1,* 187–195.

JASPER, H. H., & SHAGASS, C. (1941). Conditioning occipital alpha rhythm in man. *Journal of Experimental Psychology, 28,* 373–388.

JERGER, J., CHMIEL, R., FROST, J. D. JR., & COKER, N. (1986). Effect of sleep on the auditory steady state evoked potential. *Ear and Hearing, 7,* 240–245.

JERGER, J., CHMIEL, R., GLAZE, D., & FROST, J. D. JR. (1987). Rate and filter dependence of the middle-latency response in infants. *Audiology, 26,* 269–283.

JEWETT, D. L. (1970). Volume-conducted potentials in response to auditory stimuli as detected by averaging in the cat. *Electroencephalography and Clinical Neurophysiology, 28,* 609–618.

JEWETT, D. L., ROMANO, M. N., & WILLISTON, J. S. (1970). Human auditory evoked potentials: Possible brain stem components detected on the scalp. *Science, 167,* 1517–1518.

JEWETT, D. L., & WILLISTON, J. S. (1971). Auditory-evoked far fields averaged from the scalp of humans. *Brain, 94,* 681–696.

JOHN, E. R., BARTLETT, F., SHIMOKOCHI, M., & KLEINMAN, D. (1973). Neural readout from memory. *Journal of Neurophysiology, 36,* 893–924.

JOHN, E. R., CHABOT, R. J., PRICHEP, L. S., RANSOHOFF, J., EPSTEIN, F., & BERENSTEIN, A. (1989). Real-time intraoperative monitoring during neurosurgical and neuroradiological procedures. *Journal of Clinical Neurophysiology, 6,* 125–158.

KAMPMEIER, O. F., COOPER, A. R., & JONES, T. S. (1957). *A frontal section anatomy of the head and neck.* Urbana, IL: University of Illinois Press.

KATBAMMA, B., METZ, D. A., BENNETT, S. L., & DOKLER, P. A. (1996). Effects of electrode montage on the spectral composition of the infant auditory brainstem response. *Journal of the American Academy of Audiology, 7,* 269–273.

KATZ, J., CHERTOFF, M., & SAWUSCH, J. R. (1984). Dichotic training. *Journal of Auditory Research, 24,* 251–264.

KEITH, R. W., & JACOBSON, J. T. (1994). Evoked potentials in multiple sclerosis and other demyelinating diseases. In J. T. Jacobson (Ed.). *Principles and applications in auditory evoked potentials* (pp. 427–445). Boston: Allyn and Bacon.

KJÆR, M. (1979). Differences of latencies and amplitudes of brainstem evoked potentials in subgroups of normal material. *Acta Neurologica Scandinavica, 59,* 72–79.

KLEINMAN, D., & JOHN, E. R. (1975). Contradiction of auditory and visual information by brain stimulation. *Science, 187,* 271–273.

KNAPP, P. H. (1948). Emotional aspects of hearing loss. *Psychosomatic Medicine, 10,* 203–222.

KÖHLER, W., & WEGENER, J. (1955). Currents of the human auditory cortex. *Journal of Cellular and Comparative Physiology, 45 (supplement),* 25–54.

KRAUS, N., MCGEE, T., & COMPERATORE, C. (1989). MLRs in children are consistently present during wakefulness, stage 1, and REM sleep. *Ear and Hearing, 10,* 339–345.

KRAUS, N., MCGEE, T., FERRE, J., HOEPPNER, J., CARRELL, T., SHARMA, A., & NICOL, T. (1993). Mismatch negativity in the neurophysiologic/behavioral evaluation of auditory processing deficits: a case study. *Ear and Hearing, 14,* 223–234.

KRAUS, N., MCGEE, T, & STEIN, L. (1994). The auditory middle latency response. In J. T. Jacobson (Ed.), *Principles and applications in auditory evoked potentials* (pp. 155–178). Boston: Allyn and Bacon.

KUPPERMAN, G. L., & MENDEL, M. I. (1974). Threshold of the early components of the averaged electroencephalic response determined with tone pips and clicks during drug-induced sleep. *Audiology, 13,* 379–390.

LANDAU, W. M., GOLDSTEIN, R., & KLEFFNER, F. R. (1960). Congenital aphasia: A clinicopathologic study. *Neurology, 10,* 915–921,

LEVINE, R. A. (1981). Binaural interaction in brainstem potentials of human subjects. *Annals of Neurology, 9,* 384–393.

LEVINE, S. C., MARGOLIS, R. H., FOURNIER, E. M., & WINZENBURG, S. M. (1992). Tympanic electrocochleography for evaluation of endolymphatic hydrops. *Laryngoscope, 102,* 614–622.

LINS, O. G., PICTON, T. W., BOUCHER, B. L., DURIEUX-SMITH, A., CHAMPAGNE, S. C., MORAN, L. M., PEREZ-ABALO, M. C., MARTIN, V., & SAVIO, G. (1996). Frequency-specific audiometry using steady-state responses. *Ear and Hearing, 17,* 81–96.

LOWELL, E. L., TROFFER, C. L., WARBURTON, E. L., & RUSHFORD, G. M. (1960). Temporal evannation: A new approach in diagnostic audiology. *Journal of Speech and Hearing Disorders, 25,* 342–345.

LOWELL, E. L., WILLIAMS, C. T., BALLINGER, R. M., & ALVIG, D. P. (1961). Measurement of auditory threshold with a special purpose analog computer. *Journal of Speech and Hearing Research, 4,* 105–112.

MACKENZIE, M. A., VINGERHOETS, D. M., COLON, E. J., PINCKERS, A. L. J. G., & NOTERMANS, S. L. H. (1995). Effect of steady hypothermia and normothermia on multimodality evoked potentials in human poikilothermia. *Archives of Neurology, 52,* 52–58.

MAEDA, H., MORITA, K., KAWAMURA, K., & NAKAZAWA, Y. (1996). Amplitude and area of the auditory P300 recorded with eyes open reflect remission of schizophrenia. *Biological Psychiatry, 39,* 743–746.

MARCUS, R. E. (1951). Hearing and speech problems in children. *Archives of Otolaryngology, 53,* 134–146.

MARCUS, R. E., GIBBS, E. L., & GIBBS, F. A. (1949). Electroencephalography in the diagnosis of hearing loss in the very young child. *Diseases of the Nervous System, 10,* 170–173.

MARGOLIS, R. H., RIEKS, D., FOURNIER, E. M., & LEVINE, S. E. (1995). Tympanic electrocochleography for diagnosis of Meniere's disease. *Archives of Otolaryngology-Head and Neck Surgery, 121,* 44–55.

MARKAND, O. N. (1994). Brainstem auditory evoked potentials. *Journal of Clinical Neurophysiology, 11,* 319–342.

MARSH, J. T., MCCARTHY, D. A., SHEATZ, G., & GALAMBOS, R. (1961). Amplitude changes in evoked auditory potentials during habituation and conditioning. *Electroencephalography and Clinical Neurophysiology, 13,* 224–234.

MARSH, J. T., & WORDEN, F. G. (1964). Auditory potentials during acoustic habituation: Cochlear nucleus, cerebellum and auditory cortex. *Electroencephalography and Clinical Neurophysiology, 17,* 685–692.

MARSH, J. T., WORDEN, F. G., & SMITH, J. C. (1970). Auditory frequency-following response: Neural or artifact? *Science, 169,* 1222–1223.

MARSH, R. R. (1988). Digital filtering of auditory evoked potentials. *Ear and Hearing, 9,* 101–107.

MARSH, R. R. (1991). The auditory brainstem response recorded with 60 Hz notch filters. *Ear and Hearing, 12,* 155–158.

MARTIN, B. A., SIGAL, A., KURTZBERG, D., & STAPELLS, D. R. (1997). The effects of decreased audibility produced by high-pass noise masking on cortical event-related potentials to speech sounds /ba/ and /da/. *Journal of the Acoustical Society of America, 101,* 1585–1599.

MARTIN, L., BARAJAS, J. J., FERNANDEZ, R., & TORRES, E. (1988). Auditory event-related potentials in well-characterized groups of children. *Electroencephalography and Clinical Neurophysiology, 71,* 375–381.

MASON, S. M., & MELLOR, D. H. (1984). Brain-stem, middle latency and late cortical evoked potentials in children with speech and language disorders. *Electroencephalography and Clinical Neurophysiology, 59,* 297–309.

MAURIZI, G., PALUDETTI, G., OTTAVIANI, F., & ROSIGNOLI, M. (1984). Auditory brainstem responses to middle- and low-frequency tone pips. *Audiology, 23,* 75–84.

MCCANDLESS, G. A., & ROSE, D. E. (1970). Evoked cortical responses to stimulus change. *Journal of Speech and Hearing Research, 13,* 624–634.

MCFARLAND, W. H., VIVION, M. C., & GOLDSTEIN, R. (1977). Middle components of the AER to tone-pips in normal-hearing and hearing-impaired subjects. *Journal of Speech and Hearing Research, 20,* 781–798.

MCFARLAND, W. H., VIVION, M. C., WOLF, K. E., & GOLDSTEIN, R. (1975). Reexamination of effects of stimulus rate and number on the middle components of the averaged electroencephalic response. *Audiology, 14,* 456–465.

MCGEE, T., KRAUS, N., & MANFREDI, C. (1988). Toward a strategy for analyzing the auditory middle-latency response waveform. *Audiology, 27,* 119–130.

MCGINNIS, M. A., KLEFFNER, F. R., & GOLDSTEIN, R. (1958). Teaching aphasic children. *Volta Review, 58,* 239–244.

MCRANDLE, C., & GOLDSTEIN, R. (1973). Effect of alcohol on the early and late components of the averaged electroencephalic response to clicks. *Journal of Speech and Hearing Research, 16,* 353–359.

MCRANDLE, C. C., SMITH, M. A., & GOLDSTEIN, R. (1974). Early averaged electroencephalic response to clicks in neonates. *Annals of Otology, Rhinology and Otolaryngology, 83,* 695–702.

MENCHER, L., & MENCHER, G. T. (1993). Identification of infants born with hearing loss: A North American perspective. *Volta Review, 95,* 9–18.

MENDEL, M. I., & GOLDSTEIN, R. (1969). The effect of test conditions on the early components of the averaged electroencephalic response. *Journal of Speech and Hearing Research, 12,* 344–350.

MENDEL, M. I., & GOLDSTEIN, R. (1969). Stability of the early components of the averaged electroencephalic response. *Journal of Speech and Hearing Research, 12,* 351–361.

MENDEL, M. I., & KUPPERMAN, G. L. (1974). Early components of the averaged electroencephalic response to constant level clicks during rapid eye movement sleep. *Audiology, 13,* 23–32.

MICHALEWSKI, H. J., & WEINBERG, H. L. (1977). The contingent negative variation (CNV) and speech production: Slow potentials and the area of Broca. *Biological Psychology, 5,* 83–96.

MICHELS, M. W., & RANDT, C. T. (1947). Galvanic skin response in the differential diagnosis of deafness. *Archives of Otolaryngology, 45,* 302–311.

MILLER, C. L., MORSE, P. A., & DORMAN, M. F. (1977). Cardiac indices of infant speech perception: Orienting and burst discrimination. *Quarterly Journal of Experimental Psychology, 29,* 533–545.

MISULIS, K. E. (1989). Basic electronics for clinical neurophysiology. *Journal of Clinical Neurophysiology, 6,* 41–74.

MISULIS, K. E. (1994). *Evoked potential primer.* Revised edition. Newton, MA: Butterworth-Heinemann.

MISULIS, K. E. (1997). *Essentials of clinical neurophysiology* (2nd ed.). Newton, MA: Butterworth-Heinemann.

MITCHELL, C., KEMPTON, J. B., CREEDON, T., & TRUNE, D. (1996). Rapid acquisition of auditory brainstem responses with multiple frequency and intensity tone-bursts. *Hearing Research, 99,* 38–46.

MOKOTOFF, B., SCHULMAN-GALAMBOS, C., & GALAMBOS, R. (1977). Brain stem auditory evoked responses in children. *Archives of Otolaryngology, 103,* 38–43.

MØLLER, A, R. (1988). Use of zero-phase digital filters to enhance brainstem auditory evoked potentials (ABRs). *Electroencephalography and Clinical Neurophysiology, 71,* 226–232.

MØLLER, A. R. (1994a). Neural generators of auditory evoked potentials. In J. T. Jacobson (Ed.), *Principles and applications in auditory evoked potentials* (pp. 23–46). Boston: Allyn and Bacon.

MØLLER, A. R. (1994b). Auditory neurophysiology. *Journal of Clinical Neurophysiology, 13,* 284–308.

MORA, J. A., EXPÓSITO, M., SOLÍS, C., & BARAJAS, J. J. (1990). Filter effects and low stimulation rate on the middle-latency response in newborns. *Audiology, 29,* 329–335.

MORRONGIELLO, B. A., & CLIFTON, R. K. (1984). Effects of sound frequency on behavioral and cardiac orienting in newborn and five-month-old infants. *Journal of Experimental Child Psychology, 38,* 429–446.

MUSIEK, F. E., & BARAN, J. A. (1986). Neuroanatomy, neurophysiology, and central auditory assessment. Part I: Brain stem. *Ear and Hearing, 7,* 207–219.

MUSIEK, W. W., & LEE, W. W. (1997). Conventional and maximum length sequences middle latency response in patients with central nervous system lesions. *Journal of the American Academy of Audiology, 8,* 173–180.

NÄÄTÄNEN, R. (1982). Processing negativity: An evoked-potential reflection of selective attention. *Psychological Bulletin, 92,* 605–640.

NÄÄTÄNEN, R. (1990). The role of attention in auditory information processing as revealed by event-related potentials and other brain measures of cognitive function. *Behavioral and Brain Sciences, 13,* 201–288.

NÄÄTÄNEN, R. (1995). The mismatch negativity: A powerful tool for cognitive neuroscience. *Ear and Hearing, 16,* 6–18.

NÄÄTÄNEN, R., & MICHIE, P. T. (1979). Early selective attention effects on the evoked potential. A critical review and reinterpretation. *Biological Psychology, 8,* 81–136.

National Institutes of Health (NIH). (1993). Early identification of hearing impairment in infants and young children. *National Consensus Statement, 11,* 1–24.

OADES, R. D., DITTMAN-BALCAR, A., SCHEPKER, R., EGGERS, C., & ZERBIN, D. (1996). Auditory event-related potentials (ERPs) and mismatch negativity (MMN) in healthy children and those with attention-deficit or Tourette/tic symptoms. *Biological Psychology, 43,* 163–185.

OKEN, B. S., & SALINSKY, M. (1992). Alertness and attention: Basic science and electrophysiologic correlates. *Journal of Clinical Neurophysiology, 9,* 480–494.

OKU, T., & HASEGAWA, M. (1997). The influence of aging on auditory brainstem response and electrocochleography in the elderly. *ORL; Journal of Oto-Rhino-Laryngology and Its Related Specialties, 59,* 141–146.

OUDESLUYS-MURPHY, A. M., & HARLAAR, J. (1997). Neonatal hearing screening with an automated auditory brainstem response screener in the infant's home. *Acta Pædiatrica, 86,* 651–655.

ÖZDAMAR, Ö., DELGADO, R. E., EILERS, R. E., & URBANO, R. C. (1994). Automated electrophysiologic hearing testing using a threshold-seeking algorithm. *Journal of the American Academy of Audiology, 5,* 77–88.

PAMPIGLIONE, M. C. (1952). The phenomenon of adaptation in human E.E.G. *Revue Neurologique, 27,* 197–198.

PARKER, D. J. (1981). Dependence of the auditory brainstem response on electrode location. *Archives of Otolaryngology, 107,* 367–371.

PARVING, A., & SALOMON, G. (1996). The effect of neonatal universal hearing screening in a health surveillance perspective—a controlled study of two health authority districts. *Audiology, 35,* 158–168.

PEKKONEN, E., JOUSMÄKI, V., KÖNÖNEN, M., REINIKAINEN, K., & PARTANEN, J. (1994). Auditory sensory memory impairment in Alzheimer's disease: An event-related potential study. *NeuroReport, 5,* 2537–2540.

PICTON, T. W. (1992). The P300 wave of the human event-related potential. *Journal of Clinical Neurophysiology, 9,* 456–479.

PICTON, T. W., CHAMPAGNE, S. C., & KELLETT, A. J. C. (1992). Human auditory evoked potentials recorded using maximum length sequences. *Electroencephalography and Clinical Neurophysiology, 84,* 90–100.

PICTON, T. W., HILLYARD, S. A., KRAUSZ, H. I., & GALAMBOS, R. (1974). Human auditory evoked potentials. I: Evaluation of components. *Electroencephalography and Clinical Neurophysiology, 36,* 179–190.

PIHAN, H., ALTENMÜLLER, E., & ACKERMANN, H. (1997). The cortical processing of perceived emotion: A DC-potential study on affective speech prosody. *NeuroReport, 8,* 623–627.

PLOMP, R., & BOUMAN, M. A. (1959). Relation between hearing threshold and duration for pure tones. *Journal of the Acoustical Society of America, 31,* 749–758.

POLICH, J. (1990). P300, probability, and interstimulus interval. *Psychophysiology, 27,* 396–403.

POLICH, J., ALEXANDER, J. E., BAUER, L. O., KUPERMAN, S., MORZORATI, S, O'CONNOR, S. J., PORJESZ, B., ROHRBAUGH, J., & BEGLEITER, H. (1997). P300 topography of amplitude/latency correlations. *Brain Topography, 9,* 275–282.

POLICH, J., HOWARD, L., & STARR, A. (1985). Stimulus frequency and masking as determinants of P300 latency in event-related potentials from auditory stimuli. *Biological Psychology, 21,* 308–318.

POLICH, J., & KOK, A. (1995). Cognitive and biological determinants of P300: An integrative review. *Biological Psychology, 41,* 103–146.

POLICH, J., & LUCKRITZ, J. Y. (1995). Electrophysiological assessment of young, middle-age, and elderly adults. In M. Bergener, J. C. Brockelhurst, & S. I. Finkel (Eds.), *Aging, health, and healing* (pp. 153–170). New York: Springer Publishing Company.

POLICH, J. M., & STARR, A. (1983). Middle-, late-, and long-latency auditory evoked potentials. In E. J. Moore (Ed.), *Bases of auditory brain-stem evoked responses* (pp. 345–361). New York: Grune & Stratton.

PRICE, L. L., & GOLDSTEIN, R. (1966). Averaged evoked responses for measuring auditory sensitivity in children. *Journal of Speech and Hearing Disorders, 31,* 248–256.

PRICE, L. L., ROSENBLÜT, B., GOLDSTEIN, R., & SHEPHERD, D. C. (1966). The averaged evoked response to auditory stimulation. *Journal of Speech and Hearing Research, 9,* 361–370.

PSAROMMATIS, I. M., TSAKANIKOS, M. D., KONTORGIANNI, A. D., NTOUNIADAKIS, D. E., & APOSTOLOPOLOUS, N. K. (1997). Profound hearing loss and presence of click-evoked otoacoustic emissions in the neonate: A report of two cases. *International Journal of Pediatric Otorhinolaryngology, 39,* 237–243.

ROBIER, T, C., FABRY, D. A., LEEK, M. R., & VAN SUMMERS, W. (1992). Improving the frequency specificity of the auditory brain stem response. *Ear and Hearing, 13,* 223–227.

ROMANI, A., BERGAMASCHI, R., VERSINO, M., ZILIOLI, A., SARTORI, I., CALLIECO, R., MONTOMOLI, C., & COSI, V. (1996). Estimating reliability of evoked potential measures from residual scores: An example using tibial SSEPs. *Electroencephalography and Clinical Neurophysiology, 100,* 204–209.

ROSENHAMER, H., & HOLMKVIST, C. (1982). Bilaterally recorded auditory brainstem responses to monaural stimulation. *Scandinavian Audiology, 11,* 197–202.

RUBIN, S. S., NEWHOFF, M., PEACH, R. K., & SHAPIRO, L. P. (1996). Electrophysiological indices of lexical processing: The effects of verbal complexity and age. *Journal of Speech and Hearing Research, 39,* 1071–1080.

RUHM, H. B., & CARHART, R. (1958). Objective speech audiometry: A new method based on electrodermal response. *Journal of Speech and Hearing Research, 1,* 169–178.

RUHM, H., WALKER, E., & FLANIGIN, H. (1967). Acoustically evoked potentials in man: Mediation of early components. *Laryngoscope, 77,* 806–822.

RUTH, R. A., HILDEBRAND, D. L., & CANTRELL, R. W. (1982). A study of methods used to enhance wave I in the auditory brain stem response. *Otolaryngology—Head and Neck Surgery, 90,* 635–640.

RUTH, R. A., LAMBERT, P. R., & FERRARO, J. A. (1988). Electrocochleography: Methods and clinical applications. *American Journal of Otology, 9 [supplement],* 1–11.

SALAMY, A. (1984). Maturation of the auditory brainstem response from birth through early childhood. *Journal of Clinical Neurophysiology, 1,* 293–329.

SCHULMAN-GALAMBOS, C., & GALAMBOS, R. (1975). Brain stem auditory evoked responses in premature infants. *Journal of Speech and Hearing Research, 18,* 456–465.

SCHWARTZ, D. M., LARSON, V. D., & DECHICCHIS, A. R. (1985). Spectral characteristics of air and bone conduction transducers used to record the auditory brain stem response. *Ear and Hearing, 6,* 274–277.

SCHWARTZ, D. M., MORRIS, M. D., & JACOBSON, J. T. (1994). The normal auditory brainstem response and its variants. In J. T. Jacobson (Ed.), *Principles and applications in auditory evoked potentials* (pp. 123–153). Boston: Allyn and Bacon.

SELTERS, W. A., & BRACKMANN, D. E. (1977). Acoustic tumor detection with brain stem electric response audiometry. *Archives of Otolaryngology, 103,* 181–187.

SININGER, Y. S., ABDALA, C., & CONE-WESSON, B. (1997). Auditory threshold sensitivity of the human neonate as measured by the auditory brainstem response. *Hearing Research, 104,* 27–38.

SMITH, L. L., & GOLDSTEIN, R. (1973). Influence of background noise on the early components of the averaged electroencephalic response to clicks. *Journal of Speech and Hearing Research, 16,* 488–497.

SOHMER, H., & FEINMESSER, M. (1967). Cochlear action potentials recorded from the external ear in man. *Annals of Otology, Rhinology and Laryngology, 76,* 427–436.

SOHMER, H. & FEINMESSER, M. (1970). Cochlear and cortical audiometry conveniently recorded in the same subject. *Israel Journal of Medical Sciences, 6,* 219–223.

SQUIRES, N., AINE, C., BUCHWALD, J., NORMAN, R., AND GALBRAITH, G. (1980). Auditory brainstem response abnormalities in severely and profoundly retarded adults. *Electroencephalography and Clinical Neurophysiology, 50,* 172–185.

STACH, B. A., & DELGADO-VILCHES, G. (1993). Sudden hearing loss in multiple sclerosis: Case report. *Journal of the American Academy of Audiology, 4,* 370–375.

STAPELLS, D. R. (1994). Low-frequency hearing and the auditory brainstem response. *American Journal of Audiology, 3(2),* 11–13.

STAPELLS, D. R., PICTON, T. W., & DURIEUX-SMITH, A. (1994). Electrophysiologic measures of frequency-specific auditory function. In J. T. Jacobson (Ed.). *Principles and applications in auditory evoked potentials* (pp. 251–283). Boston: Allyn and Bacon.

STAPELLS, D. R., PICTON, T. W., PÉREZ-ABALO, M., READ, D., & SMITH, A. (1985). In J. T. Jacobson (Ed.). *The auditory brainstem response* (pp. 147–177). San Diego: College Hill Press.

STAPELLS, D. R., PICTON, T. W., & SMITH, A. D. (1982). Normal hearing thresholds for clicks. *Journal of the Acoustical Society of America, 72,* 74–79.

STARR, A., & ACHOR, L. J. (1975). Auditory brain stem responses in neurological disease. *Archives of Neurology, 32,* 761–768.

STARR, A., & SQUIRES, K. (1982). Distribution of auditory brain stem potentials over the scalp and nasopharynx in humans. *Annals of the New York Academy of Sciences, 388,* 427–442.

STEVENS, S. S. (1935). The relation of pitch to intensity. *Journal of the Acoustical Society of America, 8,* 150–154.

STUART, A., YANG, E. Y., & GREEN, W. B. (1994). Neonatal auditory brainstem response to air- and bone-conducted clicks: 0 to 96 hours postpartum. *Journal of the American Academy of Audiology, 5,* 163–172.

STUDENT, M., & SOHMER, H. (1978). Evidence from auditory nerve and brainstem evoked responses for an organic brain lesion in children with autistic traits. *Journal of Autism and Childhood Schizophrenia, 8,* 13–20.

SUTTON, S., BRAREN, M., ZUBIN, J., & JOHN, E. R. (1965). Evoked-potential correlates of stimulus uncertainty. *Science, 150,* 1187–1188

SUTTON, S., TUETING, P., ZUBIN, J., & JOHN, E. R. (1967). Information delivery and the sensory evoked potential. *Science, 155,* 1436–1439.

SUZUKI, T., KOBAYASHI, K., AOKI, K., & UMEGAKI, Y. (1992). Effect of sleep on binaural interaction in auditory brainstem response and middle latency response. *Audiology, 31,* 25–30.

SUZUKI, T., KOBAYASHI, K., & UMEGAKI, Y. (1994). Effect of natural sleep on auditory steady state responses in adult subjects with normal hearing. *Audiology, 33,* 274–279.

THARPE, A. M., & CLAYTON, E. W. (1997). Newborn hearing screening: Issues in legal liability and quality assurance. *American Journal of Audiology, 6(2),* 5–12.

THORNTON, A. R., MENDEL, M. I., & ANDERSON, C. (1977). Effect of stimulus frequency and intensity on the middle components of the averaged electroencephalic response. *Journal of Speech and Hearing Research, 20,* 81–94.

TINAZZI, M., & MAUGUIÈRE, F. (1995). Assessment of intraspinal and intracranial conduction by P30 and P39 tibial nerve somatosensory evoked potentials in cervical cord, brainstem, and hemispheric lesions. *Journal of Clinical Neurophysiology, 12,* 237–253.

TREEDE, R. D., & KUNDE, V. (1995). Middle-latency somatosensory evoked potentials after stimulation of the radial and median nerves: Component structure and scalp topography. *Journal of Clinical Neurophysiology, 12,* 291–301.

TSUCHITANI, C. (1978). Lower auditory brain stem structures in the cat. In R. F. Naunton & C. Fernández (Eds.), *Evoked electrical activity in the auditory nervous system* (pp. 373–401). New York: Academic Press.

VAN DER DRIFT, J. F. C., BROCAAR, M. P., & VAN ZANTEN, G. A. (1988). Brainstem response audiometry. I. Its use in distinguishing between conductive and cochlear hearing loss. *Audiology, 27,* 260–270.

VAN OLPHEN, A. F., RODENBURG, M., & VERWEY, C. (1978). Distribution of brain stem responses to acoustic stimuli over the human scalp. *Audiology, 17,* 511–518.

VIVION, M. C., HIRSCH, J. E., FRYE-OSIER, J. L., & GOLDSTEIN, R. (1980). Effects of stimulus rise-fall time and equivalent duration on middle components of the AER. *Scandinavian Audiology, 9,* 223–232.

WALTER, W. G., COOPER, R., ALDRIDGE, V. J., MCCALLUM, W. C., & WINTER, A. L. (1964). Contingent negative variation: An electric sign of sensori-motor association and expectancy in the human brain. *Nature, 203,* 380–384.

WATKIN, P. M. (1996). Outcomes of neonatal screening for hearing loss by otoacoustic emission. *Archives of Disease in Childhood—Fetal and Neonatal Edition, 75,* F158–F168.

WATSON, C. S., & GENGEL, R. W. (1969). Signal duration and signal frequency in relation to auditory sensitivity. *Journal of the Acoustical Society of America, 46,* 989–997.

WATSON, D. R. (1996). The effects of cochlear hearing loss, age and sex on the auditory brainstem response. *Audiology, 35,* 246–258.

WEBER, B. A. (1992). Patient-specific normative values for auditory brain stem response audiometry. *American Journal of Audiology, 1,* 24–26.

WEBER, B. A., & ROUSH, P. A. (1995). Use of maximum length sequence analysis in newborn hearing testing. *Journal of the American Academy of Audiology, 6,* 187–190.

WELCH, D., GREVILLE, K. A., THORNE, P. R., & PURDY, S. C. (1996). Influence of acquisition parameters on the measurement of click evoked otoacoustic emissions in neonates in a hospital environment. *Audiology, 35,* 143–157.

WEVER, E. G., & BRAY, C. W. (1930). Action currents in the auditory nerve in response to acoustical stimulation. *Proceedings of the National Academy of Sciences, 16,* 344–350.

WILLIAMS, H. L., TEPAS, D. I., & MORLOCK, H. C. (1962). Evoked responses to clicks and electroencephalographic stages of sleep in man. *Science, 138,* 685–686.

WILSON, M. J., KELLY-BALLWEBER, S., & DOBIE, R. A. (1985). Binaural interaction in auditory brain stem responses: Parametric studies. *Ear and Hearing, 6,* 80–88.

WITHROW, F. B., & GOLDSTEIN, R. (1958). An electrophysiologic procedure for determination of auditory threshold in children. *Laryngoscope, 68,* 1676–1999.

WOLF, K. E., & GOLDSTEIN, R. (1978). Middle component averaged electroencephalic responses to tonal stimuli from normal neonates: Initial report. *Archives of Otolaryngology, 104,* 508–513.

WOLF, K. E., & GOLDSTEIN, R. (1980). Middle component AERs from neonates to low-level tonal stimuli. *Journal of Speech and Hearing Research, 23,* 185–201.

Wu, C., & Stapells, D. R. (1994). Pure-tone masking profiles for human auditory and middle latency responses to 500-Hz tones. *Hearing Research, 78,* 169–174.

Yang, E. Y., Stuart, A., Stenstrom, R., & Green, W. B. (1987). Test-retest reliability of the auditory brainstem response to bone-conducted clicks in newborn infants. *Audiology, 32,* 89–94.

Yardanova, J. Y., & Kolev, V. N. (1996). Developmental changes in the alpha response system. *Electroencephalography and Clinical Neurophysiology, 99,* 527–538.

Zerlin, S., & Naunton, R. F. (1974). Early and late averaged electroencephalic responses at low sensation levels. *Audiology, 13,* 366–378.

Glossary

These are words or terms highlighted in the text the first time that they are used. They occur again at least two more times in the text. The only words or terms highlighted are those peculiar to evoked potential audiometry (EPA) or to concepts relevant to the main topics in the book.

40 Hz phenomenon Enhancement of middle-latency potentials (middle potentials) by superimposing them in the same 50–100 millisecond analysis window when the eliciting signals are presented at 40 per second.

addresses Memory storage locations in a computer, equally spaced in time in the analysis window or recording epoch, at which the EEG is digitized, quantified, and stored; used synonymously with "stations" in this book.

aliasing If the sampling rate or temporal resolution of a computer is not fine enough, some high frequencies in the EEG will be reproduced as lower frequencies in the averaged evoked potential.

alpha rhythm Periodic brain activity, as recorded in the electroencephalogram, occurring about 10 times per second.

amplification Instrumental increase in the magnitude of an electric signal; usually expressed as a ratio of the voltage output of an amplifier to the initial or input signal. Often used synonymously with gain.

amplifier Instrument for increasing the magnitude of an electric signal.

amplitude A measure of the absolute magnitude of a physical event. In the context of evoked potential audiometry, amplitude refers to the size (in microvolts) of a selected peak or wave in an averaged evoked potential (AEP), usually measured from its most positive point to the following negative trough; or from a baseline to the most positive or negative point of interest.

amplitude resolution Smallest amplitude change that can be measured by the computer. The fineness or coarseness of the resolution will determine whether a peak in one averaged evoked potential can be considered larger or smaller than a corresponding peak in another averaged evoked potential.

analog Implies a continuous representation over time of a signal or response; averaged evoked potential traces as ordinarily displayed are in analog form.

analog-to-digital conversion Process by which selected points in the continuously varying EEG are assigned discrete numeric values that are stored in and manipulated by a computer.

analysis window Selected time period, usually in milliseconds, after (or before) signal onset during which the EEG is digitized, quantified, and stored; used synonymously with "recording epoch" in this book.

area-under-the-curve Area between the baseline and the beginning and end of a peak. Expressed as microvolts x milliseconds, or milliseconds $\times$ microvolts (μV-ms or ms-μV).

artifact reject circuit Electronic buffer system that examines the digital values of the EEG in a sweep and then adds that sweep to the ongoing averaging if all voltages are within a preset limit; or discards that sweep if the voltage at any address exceeds the preset limit.

audiometry Measurement of hearing.

auditory association area Portion of the cerebral cortex adjacent to Heschl's gyrus or the primary auditory reception area.

auditory brainstem response Series of peaks of the auditory averaged evoked potential generated by the auditory nerve and auditory-related nuclei and pathways in the brainstem. Peak latencies of the auditory brainstem response (ABR) are usually less than 10 milliseconds (ms).

averaged evoked potential Sum or addition of segments of the EEG following a number of repetitions of the identical test signals divided by the number of repetitions or segments that contributed to the sum.

averaged response computer Instrument that digitally sums and averages changes in EEG in response to repetitions of identical test signals. It enhances desired portion of the EEG and reduces the unwanted background noise.

bandpass filter Instrument that allows energy between a preset low frequency and preset high frequency to pass through a circuit unimpeded.

binaural interaction component That portion of an averaged evoked potential resulting from the brain's merging responses to signals presented simultaneously to both ears.

brainstem evoked potential Same as auditory brainstem response; designated by the initials BSEP.

central auditory nervous system Includes any neural structure wholly contained within the brain that can be activated by auditory signals.

central nervous system Entire brain and spinal cord.

cochlear microphonic Electric response from the cochlea that mirrors or reproduces the waveform of the eliciting acoustic signal.

cognitive potentials Term used interchangeably by some for event-related potentials.

common-mode noise Any noise in the measurement environment that appears as equal voltage and phase at both inputs of a differential amplifier.

common-mode rejection ratio Preamplifier's gain for common-mode signals or noise; value is always negative because the preamp's output of noise is less than its input.

composite AEP An average of two or more averaged evoked potentials obtained under identical signal and recording conditions.

condensation click Initial outward movement of the earphone diaphragm (i.e., toward the tympanic membrane) when electric pulse is delivered to the earphone.

contingent negative variation Large, low-frequency or direct current vertex-negative deflection after an alerting or warning signal that a second signal to which the subject must make a motor response is forthcoming.

derived response Response to specific frequency ranges determined by subtractions from an unmasked averaged evoked potential to a click the waveforms obtained with successively lower high-pass maskers.

deviant signal The infrequent signal in the oddball paradigm, that is, the signal whose probability of occurrence in a chain of signals is lower than the frequent or expected signal. It is also referred to as the unexpected, infrequent, rare, or oddball signal.

differential amplifier Instrument designed to accept two inputs and to produce an output proportional to their difference.

digital-to-analog conversion Process by which a computer converts the discrete digital values of an averaged evoked potential into continuously variable analog values.

digitize Take analog value of the EEG at each address or station in a preset analysis window and assign discrete positive or negative values to it.

early potentials Defined in this book as those replicable peaks of an averaged evoked potential occurring within the first 10 milliseconds after signal onset.

electrocardiogram Recording of the electric activity of the heart showing the form of heart beat as well as its rate.

electrocochleography Recording of cochlear microphonics, summating potentials, and action potentials from the ear.

electrodermogram Recording of electric resistance or of differences in electric potential between different portions of the skin.

electroencephalic activity General term for electric activity of the brain, usually recorded with extracranial electrodes.

electroencephalic response Change in electric activity of the brain evoked by auditory or other sensory signals.

electroencephalogram Recording made on the scalp of electric activity of the brain.

electroencephalograph Instrument for recording the electroencephalogram or EEG.

electrophysiologic audiometry Measurement of hearing in which the response index is a change in some electric property of the body in response to sound.

electrode Surface contact or interface between the patient's skin and the instrument; usually is a metal contact surface and a wire with a connecting pin at the other end.

emitted potential An event-related potential evoked by the absence of an expected signal in a sequence of regularly presented identical signals.

endogenous potentials Term used interchangeably by some for event-related potentials.

event-related potentials Components of averaged evoked potentials whose latencies and amplitudes depend upon the circumstances under which the eliciting or target signals are presented.

evoked potential audiometry Measurement of hearing in which the response index some change in the electroencephalogram (EEG).

exogenous potentials Term used interchangeably by some for signal-related potentials.

expected signal Signal in the oddball paradigm whose probability or occurrence in a chain of signals is higher than that of the oddball signal. It is also referred to as the frequent or the standard signal.

far-field Remote or distant from the structure(s) producing the measured potential, as opposed to recording directly from the neural generator in the ear or brain.

filter Instrument that allows desired frequencies to pass through a circuit while reducing or eliminating unwanted frequencies.

filter skirt Refers to the form and steepness of attenuation of frequencies beyond the high-pass or low-pass end of the filter.

frequency-following response Averaged evoked potential that reproduces the frequency of the eliciting tone-burst.

frequency response Output of an electric or acoustic system for a fixed input to the system over a broad range of frequencies.

frequent signal Same as expected or standard signal in the oddball paradigm.

gain Ratio of output of an amplifier to the input to the amplifier.

gated tone bursts Tone bursts whose rise-time, plateau, and fall-time are controlled by an electronic gate.

ground Common reference point for a pair of recording electrodes. Also can refer to an instrument-to-earth connection.

Heschl's gyrus Gyrus (or pair of gyri) on the superior surface of the temporal lobe that is the cortical terminal of the primary auditory projection system.

high-pass filter An instrument that reduces energy below a preset low frequencies but allows higher frequencies to pass through a circuit unimpeded.

horizontal montage Recording between the two earlobes or the two mastoids.

ignore condition During the oddball paradigm, the subject does not count or otherwise respond to the oddball (rare, unexpected, infrequent, deviant) signal.

infant In this book, a child between the ages of 11 days and 18 months.

infrequent signal Same as deviant, unexpected, rare, or oddball signal in the oddball paradigm.

input impedance Electric impedance across the input to a preamplifier; usually large in order not to drain current from the weak input source.

interpeak interval Time (usually in milliseconds) between designated peaks of an averaged evoked potential. Used interchangeably with interwave interval.

intersignal interval Time (usually in milliseconds) between successive acoustic or other signals.

interwave interval Time (usually in milliseconds) between designated peaks of an averaged evoked potential. Used interchangeably with interpeak interval.

intra-axial tumors Tumors contained entirely within the brainstem.

inverted Refers to the electrode (usually designated "reference") of a pair of recording electrodes whose electric polarity is reversed 180 degrees at the input to a differential amplifier.

K-complex Response noted in the electroencephalogram shortly after the onset of sound or other sensory stimuli; characterized by large, slow waves with smaller, faster activity riding on them.

latency Time between onset of a test signal and a particular peak or other portion of interest of an averaged evoked potential.

latency-intensity function Plot of latency of a peak (most often wave V of the early potentials) as a function of the strength or magnitude of the eliciting signal (usually a click).

late potentials Defined in this book as replicable peaks of an averaged evoked potential between 50 and 500 milliseconds.

lemniscal system Large-fiber sensory pathways in the central nervous system.

low-pass filter Instrument that reduces electric energy above a preset high frequency but allows lower frequencies to pass through a circuit unimpeded.

maximum length sequences Rapid signal presentation process, with an intersignal interval shorter than the analysis window, that still allows extraction of the time-amplitude configuration of the averaged evoked potential.

microvolt (μV) one-millionth of a volt.

middle latency responses Used interchangeably with middle potentials in this book.

middle potentials Defined in this book as replicable peaks of an averaged evoked potential between 10 and 50 milliseconds.

millisecond One-thousandth of a second.

mismatch negativity Event-related potential with a peak latency of about 175 milliseconds.

neonate Defined in this book as a child between birth and 10 days of age.

noncephalic lead An electrode attachment somewhere off the head.

noninverted Refers to the electrode (usually designated "active") of a pair of recording electrodes whose electric polarity is maintained at the input to a differential amplifier.

notch filter A narrow-band filter with steep skirts usually designed to cut out 60 Hz noise.

Nyquist frequency The highest frequency that can be reproduced accurately by an averaged response computer for given sampling rate or temporal resolution. For a specified high frequency to be reproduced, the temporal resolution of the computer must be fine enough to allow sampling of at least two points during one period of that frequency.

oddball paradigm A test protocol in which the frequent or expected signal in a chain of signals has a high probably of occurrence, and the deviant or oddball signal has a low probability of occurrence.

oddball signal Same as deviant, unexpected, infrequent, or rare signal in an oddball paradigm.

off-line analysis Analysis or processing of previously collected data.

on-line analysis Analysis or processing of data at the time that they are collected.

P300 Large, positive-going deflection at about 300 milliseconds in an averaged evoked potential elicited by the deviant or rare signal in an oddball paradigm.

peripheral auditory system All auditory-related structures from the pinna to the termination of the auditory (VIIIth) nerve in the cochlear nucleus of the brainstem.

phase lag Apparent delay of a peak caused by an analog filter.

phase lead Apparent earlier appearance of a peak caused by an analog filter.

phase shift Either an apparent delay or earlier appearance of a peak caused by an analog filter.

post-stimulus time histograms Plot of the frequency of discharge of a neuron as a function of time during which an eliciting signal is presented.

preamplifier Instrument into which electrodes are plugged that provides the initial boost or increase in the EEG from the patient.

primary auditory projection system Large-fiber pathway with interconnecting nuclei starting at the cochlear nucleus of the brainstem and terminating in Heschl's gyrus on the superior surface of the temporal lobe. Sometimes used interchangeably with the auditory lemniscal system.

primary auditory reception area Heschl's gyrus or the termination of the primary auditory projection system.

primary discharge pattern Post-stimulus time histogram that shows a burst of neural discharges at signal onset, sustained discharge rate throughout signal duration, and abrupt cessation of discharge at signal termination.

processing negativity Event-related potential with peak latency at about 75 milliseconds.

quantizing Part of the analog-to-digital process during which the magnitude of the analog signal is assigned a digital value.

rarefaction click Initial inward movement of the earphone diaphragm (i.e., away from the tympanic membrane) when electric pulse is delivered to the earphone.

rare signal Same as deviant, unexpected, infrequent, or oddball signal in an oddball paradigm.

recording epoch Selected time period, usually in milliseconds, after (or before) signal onset during which the EEG is digitized, quantified, and stored; used synonymously with "analysis window" in this book.

reticular formation Vaguely defined collection of gray matter that is found throughout the lower and upper brainstem.

shoulder An inflection in the large negative-going trace just beyond the most positive portion of wave V of the early potentials.

signal Has dual meaning in this book. Usually refers to the sound (or light or shock) delivered to the patient. In a different context, signal refers to the response portion of an averaged evoked potential in contrast to the noise portion.

signal artifact Electromagnetic radiation from the earphone during signal presentation that is picked up and registered by the recording electrodes.

signal magnitude General term for the size or largeness of the test signal; often expressed as signal intensity.

signal-related potentials Averaged evoked potentials whose peak latencies and amplitudes are dependent upon the frequency, magnitude, and other physical properties of the eliciting signals.

silent controls   Averaging of electroencephalic activity when no test signals are presented or when the test signals are inaudible.

site-of-lesion testing   Test procedures designed to determine where in the periphery or in the brain a patient's lesion is located.

smoothing   Post-stimulus process in which three or four adjacent points along an averaged evoked potential are averaged to reduce the high- frequency ripple that may be riding on the waveform.

somatosensory averaged evoked potentials   Averaged evoked potentials to electric shock or other signals applied to various areas of the skin.

somatosensory evoked potentials   Term used interchangeably with somatosensory averaged evoked potentials.

source loading   High-impedance load placed across the preamplifier input to reduce the drainage of the weak voltage from the source that is to be amplified.

standard signal   Same as the frequent or expected signal in the oddball paradigm.

stations   Equally spaced fixed points in time in the analysis window or recording epoch at which the EEG is digitized, quantified, and stored; used synonymously with "addresses" in this book.

stimulus   A sound or other signal strong enough to elicit a response from the ear or other end-organ; often used by others instead of "signal."

summating potential   A small cochlear potential, probably generated by the hair cells, that usually manifests itself as a direct current displacement of the cochlear microphonic.

summed evoked potentials   Sum or addition of segments of the EEG following a number of repetitions of the identical test signals.

sweep   Process by which the computer goes successively from address to address in a preset

analysis window, digitizing, quantifying, and storing the EEG.

temporal resolution   Smallest time interval that can be measured by the computer. The fineness or coarseness of the resolution will determine whether the latency of a particular peak in one averaged evoked potential can be considered earlier or later than a corresponding peak in another averaged evoked potential.

time-amplitude configuration   Usual display of an averaged evoked potential as positive and negative potentials over a fixed period of time.

time-locked   Implies that a particular peak or other component of an averaged evoked potential always occurs at a fixed time after the onset of the eliciting sound or other sensory signal.

tone pip   Brief, narrow-spectrum signal usually generated by electrically ringing a narrow-band filter and delivering the resultant electric pattern to the earphone.

transtympanic electrode   Electrode used during electrocochleography that penetrates the tympanic membrane and rests against the middle-ear promontory.

trigger   An electric signal that starts the computer to begin digitizing a preset time period of the EEG; the trigger usually starts at the same time that an electric signal is delivered to an earphone or other sensory signal device.

unexpected signal   Same as deviant, infrequent, rare, or oddball signal in an oddball paradigm.

visual averaged evoked potentials   Averaged evoked potentials to a reversing checkerboard or to a light flash.

visual evoked potentials   Term used interchangeably with visual averaged evoked potentials.

whole nerve action potential   Conglomerate response of the auditory (VIIIth) nerve recorded during electrocochleography or seen as waves I and II of the early potentials; usually referred to just as action potential.

Abbreviations

ABR: Auditory brainstem response.

AEP: Averaged evoked potential (usually preceded by an initial representing the applicable sensory modality: A for auditory, V for Visual, S for somatosensory. Because the emphasis of this book is auditory, the A for auditory is omitted most of the time.).

A-to-D: Analog-to-digital (also A/D).

AUTC: Area-under-the-curve.

BIC: Binaural interaction component.

BSEP: Brainstem evoked potential.

CANS: Central auditory nervous system.

CM: Cochlear microphonic.

CMRR: Common-mode rejection ratio.

CNS: Central nervous system.

CNV: Contingent negative variation.

D-to-A: Digital-to-analog (also D/A).

ECG: Electrocardiogram.

ECochG: Electrocochleography.

EEG: Electroencephalogram or electroencephalograph (the instrument used for recording the electroencephalogram).

EPA: Evoked potential audiometry.

EPs: Early potentials.

ERP: Event-related potential.

FFR: Frequency-following response.

HL: Hearing level.

HLn: Normal hearing level.

IPI: Interpeak interval.

ISI: Intersignal interval.

IWI: Interwave interval.

LPs: Late potentials.

μV: Microvolt.

MLR: Middle latency response.

MLS: Maximum length sequence.

MMN: Mismatch negativity.

MPs: Middle potentials.

ms: Millisecond.

n: Normal (when used in conjunction with hearing level).

nHL: Normal hearing level.

PAPS: Primary auditory projection system.

PAS: Peripheral auditory system.

PN: Processing negativity.

PST: Post-stimulus time histogram.

SAEP: Somatosensory averaged evoked potentials.

SEP: Somatosensory evoked potentials.

SP: Summating potential.

SRP: Signal (or stimulus)-related potential.

SSEP: Somatosensory evoked potentials.

VAEP: Visual averaged evoked potentials.

VEP: Visual evoked potentials.

WNAP: Whole nerve action potential.

Index